Study Guide for

Fundamentals of Nursing

Eleventh Edition

Study Guide for

Fundamentals of Nursing

Eleventh Edition

Geralyn Ochs, MSN, APRN, AGACNP-BC, ANP-BC, FAANP
Associate Professor of Nursing
Coordinator of the Adult Gerontological Acute Care Nurse Practitioner Program
St. Louis University School of Nursing
St. Louis, Missouri

ELSEVIER

Elsevier
3251 Riverport Lane
St. Louis, Missouri 63043

Study Guide for Fundamentals of Nursing,
ELEVENTH EDITION

ISBN: 978-0-323-81036-4

Previous editions copyrighted 2021, 2017, 2013, 2009, 2005, 2001, 1997, 1993, 1989, 1985.

Director, Traditional Education: Tamara Myers
Senior Content Development Manager: Lisa P. Newton
Senior Content Development Specialist: Tina A. Kaemmerer
Publishing Services Manager: Shereen Jameel
Project Manager: Nadhiya Sekar

Printed in India

Last digit is the print number: 9 8 7 6 5 4 3 2

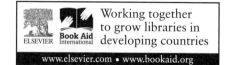

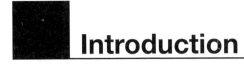

Introduction

The *Study Guide for Fundamentals of Nursing*, Eleventh Edition, has been developed to encourage independent learning for beginning nursing students. As a beginning nursing student, you may be wondering, "How will I possibly learn all of the material in this chapter?" The essential objective of this study guide is to assist you in this endeavor by helping you learn *what* you need to know and then testing what you have learned with hundreds of review questions.

This study guide follows the textbook layout chapter for chapter. For each chapter your instructor assigns, you will use the same chapter number in this study guide. Each chapter of this study guide has several sections to assist you to comprehend and recall.

The *Preliminary Reading* section is designed to teach prereading strategies. You will become familiar with the chapter by first reading the chapter title, key terms, objectives, key points (found at the end of each chapter), as well as all main headings. Also pay close attention to all illustrations, tables, and boxes. This can be done rather quickly and will give you an overall idea of the content of the chapter.

Next you will find the *Comprehensive Understanding* section. This will prove to be a very valuable tool not only as you first read the chapter but also as you review for exams. This section identifies both topics and main ideas for each chapter as an aid to concentration, comprehension, and retaining textbook information. By completing this section, you will learn to "pull out" key information in the chapter. As you write the answers in the study guide, you will be reinforcing that content. Once completed, this will serve as a review tool for exams.

The Case Study provides a short synopsis followed by one or more open-ended questions. This will give you an opportunity to apply the knowledge you have gained through working the previous sections.

The review questions in each chapter provide a valuable means of testing and reinforcing your knowledge of the material. All questions are multiple choice or multiple select. As a further means for independent learning, each answer requires a rationale (the reason *why* the option you selected is correct). After you have completed the review questions, you can check the answers in the back of the study guide.

Chapters 27 and 34-50 include exercises based on the care plans and concept maps found in the text. These exercises provide practice in synthesizing nursing process and critical thinking as you, the nurse, care for patients. Taking one aspect of the nursing process, you will be asked to imagine you are the nurse in the case study and write your answers to the questions. You will have to think about what knowledge, experiences, standards, and attitudes might be used in caring for the patient.

When you finish answering the review questions and exercises, take a few minutes for self-evaluation using the Answer Key. If you answered a question incorrectly, begin to analyze the thoughts that led you to the wrong answer:

1. Did you miss the key word or phrase?
2. Did you read into something that wasn't stated?
3. Did you not understand the subject matter?
4. Did you use an incorrect rationale for selecting your response?

Each incorrect response is an opportunity to learn. Go back to the text and reread any content that is still unclear. In the long run, it will be a time-saving activity.

The learning activities presented in this study guide will assist you in completing the semester with a firm understanding of nursing concepts and process that you can rely on for your entire professional career.

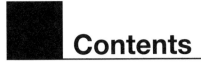

Contents

1 Nursing Today

PRELIMINARY READING

Chapter 1

COMPREHENSIVE UNDERSTANDING

Nursing as a Profession

1. According to Benner, an expert nurse goes through five levels of proficiency. Identify them.

    a. _____

    b. _____

    c. _____

    d. _____

    e. _____

2. What are the American Nursing Association (ANA, 2020) Standards of Nursing Practice?

    a. _____

    b. _____

    c. _____

    d. _____

    e. _____

    f. _____

3. Define *nursing* (according to the ANA, 2020).

    _____

    _____

4. Identify the ANA (2020) Standards of Professional Performance.

    a. _____

    b. _____

    c. _____

    d. _____

    e. _____

    f. _____

g. _____

h. _____

i. _____

j. _____

k. _____

l. _____

5. Describe ANA's Nursing Code of Ethics.

_____

_____

Professional Responsibilities and Roles

Match the following.

6. _____ Autonomy

7. _____ Caregiver

8. _____ Advocate

9. _____ Educator

10. _____ Communicator

11. _____ Manager

12. _____ Advanced Practice Registered Nurse (APRN)

13. _____ Clinical Nurse Specialist (CNS)

14. _____ Nurse Practitioner

15. _____ Certified Nurse-Midwife (CNM)

16. _____ Certified Registered Nurse Anesthetist (CRNA)

17. _____ Nurse educator

18. _____ Nursing administrator

19. _____ Nurse researcher

a. Conducts evidence-based practice and research to improve nursing care and to expand the scope of nursing practice
b. Independent nursing interventions that the nurse initiates without medical orders
c. Is essential for all nursing roles and activities
d. Helps the patient maintain and regain health, manage disease and symptoms, and attain a maximal level of function and independence
e. Manages patient care and the delivery of specific nursing services within a health care agency
f. Has personnel, policy, and budgetary responsibility for a specific nursing unit
g. Explains concepts and facts about health, describes the reason for activities, demonstrates, reinforces, and evaluates the patient's progress in learning
h. Works primarily in schools of nursing, staff development, departments of health care agencies, and patient education departments
i. Expert clinician in a specialized area of practice
j. Involves the independent care for women in normal pregnancy, labor and delivery, and care of newborns
k. Provides comprehensive health care to a group of patients in an inpatient, outpatient, ambulatory care, or community-based setting
l. Provides surgical anesthesia
m. Four roles: certified nurse-midwife, certified nurse practitioner, clinical nurse specialist, and certified registered nurse anesthetist
n. Protects patients' human and legal rights and provides assistance in asserting these rights

Historical Highlights

20. How did Florence Nightingale see the role of the nurse in the early 1800s?

_____

_____

Match the following.

21. _____ Clara Barton

22. _____ Lillian Wald and Mary Brewster

23. _____ Mary Adelaide Nutting

24. _____ Mary Mahoney

a. First professionally trained African-American nurse
b. Instrumental in moving nursing education into universities
c. Opened the Henry Street Settlement, focusing on the health needs of the poor
d. Founder of the American Red Cross

Contemporary Influences

25. What are the external forces that have affected nursing practice in the twentieth-first century?

a. _____

b. _____

c. _____

d. _____

e. _____

26. Explain *compassion fatigue*.

_____

_____

Trends in Nursing

27. Identify the competencies of the Quality and Safety Education for Nurses (QSEN) initiative.

a. _____

b. _____

c. _____

d. _____

e. _____

f. _____

28. Define the term *genomics*.

_____

_____

Professional Registered Nurse Education

Match the following.

29. _____ Associate degree

30. _____ Baccalaureate degree

31. _____ Master's degree

32. _____ Doctor of Philosophy

33. _____ Doctor of Nursing Practice

34. _____ In-service education

35. _____ Continuing education

a. A practice-focused doctorate

b. Emphasizes advanced knowledge in basic sciences and research-based clinical practice

c. Focuses on the basic sciences and theoretical and clinical courses related to the practice of nursing

d. A 4-year program that focuses on basic sciences theoretical and clinical courses and courses in social sciences, arts, and humanities

e. Rigorous research and theory development

f. Educational programs by various institutions and organizations

g. Instruction or training provided by health care agencies

Nursing Practice

36. What is the purpose of nurse practice act?

_____

_____

_____

37. The examination for Registered Nurse (RN) *licensure* provides:

_____

_____

_____

38. The value of *certification* is:

_____

_____

_____

Professional Nursing Organizations

39. The goals of any professional nursing organization are to:

_____

_____

_____

CASE STUDY

40. Tony, a student nurse, is preparing to participate in a team care conference for his patient. He listens to the registered dietitian and physical and occupational therapists detail the plan for the patient. Tony then describes the patient's concerns about walking to the group. Explain the QSEN competency here.

REVIEW QUESTIONS

Select the appropriate answer and cite the rationale for choosing that particular answer.

41. The factor that best advanced the practice of nursing in the twentieth-first century was:
    1. the growth of cities
    2. the teachings of Christianity
    3. better education of nurses
    4. improved conditions for women

    Answer: _____

    Rationale: _____

    _____

    _____

42. Graduate nurses must pass a licensure examination administered by the:
    1. State Boards of Nursing
    2. National League for Nursing
    3. Accredited School of Nursing
    4. American Nurses Association

    Answer: _____

    Rationale: _____

    _____

    _____

43. A group that lobbies at the state and federal levels for advancement of nurses' role, economic interests, and health care is the:
    1. State Boards of Nursing
    2. American Nurses Association
    3. American Hospital Association
    4. National Student Nurses Association

    Answer: _____

    Rationale: _____

    _____

    _____

2 The Health Care Delivery System

Chapter 2

COMPREHENSIVE UNDERSTANDING

1. Give examples of each of the levels of health care services available in the U.S. health care system.

   a. Primary care (health promotion): _____

   b. Preventive care: _____

   c. Secondary acute care: _____

   d. Tertiary care: _____

   e. Restorative care: _____

   f. Continuing care: _____

2. Levels of prevention describe the focus of health care-related activities, identify the three levels:

   a. _____

   b. _____

   c. _____

3. Explain what an integrated health care delivery system (IHCD) is _____

4. Identify the core mission of hospitals across the country: _____

5. Explain the focus of the following two acute care facilities:

   a. Intensive care units

   _____

   _____

   b. Mental health facilities

   _____

   _____

6. To improve care for patients residing in rural areas, rural hospitals are expected to:

   a. _____

   b. _____

   c. _____

   d. _____

   e. _____

7. Define what discharge planning is. _____

8. What is the focus of discharge planning? _____

9. Describe the following models of discharge planning that focus on the patient and their family caregiver:

   a. Care transitions program

   _____

   _____

   b. Transitional care model

   _____

   _____

   c. High-intensity care model (GRACE)

   _____

   _____

10. Identify the discharge instructions that are required by The Joint Commission (TJC):

   a. _____

   b. _____

   c. _____

   d. _____

   e. _____

11. List the tips on making a referral process.

   a. _____

   b. _____

   c. _____

   d. _____

12. The goal of *restorative care* is:

   _____

   _____

13. What is the focus of home health care?

   _____

   _____

14. _____ is a process aimed at enabling people with disabilities to reach and maintain their optimal physical, sensory, intellectual, psychological, and social functional levels.

Match the following.

15. _____ Extended care facility

16. _____ Continuing care

17. _____ Nursing center

18. _____ Assisted living

19. _____ Respite care

20. _____ Adult day care center

21. _____ Hospice

a. 24-hour intermediate and custodial care
b. Includes immediate care and skilled nursing facilities
c. Services are for people who are disabled, not functionally independent, or who suffer a terminal disease
d. Long-term care setting with an environment like home and greater resident autonomy
e. Provides short-term relief to the family members who care for the patient
f. Provides a variety of health and social services to specific patients populations who live in the community
g. Is a system of family-centered care that allows patients to live with comfort, independence, and dignity while easing the pains of a terminal illness

Issues in Health Care Delivery

Match the following health care payment models:

22. _____ Fee-for-service

23. _____ Pay-for-coordination

24. _____ Pay-for-performance (P4P)

25. _____ Episode-of-care payment

26. _____ Upside shared savings program

27. _____ Downside shared savings program

28. _____ Partial or full capitation

a. Includes both the gain share potential of an upside model, but also the downside risk of sharing the excess costs of health care delivery between provider and payer
b. Most traditional health care payment model; requires patients or payers to reimburse the provider for each service performed
c. Value-based reimbursement; providers are compensated only if they meet certain metrics for quality and efficiency
d. Provide incentives for providers treating specific patient populations; % of net savings go to providers
e. Coordinates care between the primary care provider and specialists
f. Payments are assigned a per-member per-month (PMPM) payment
g. Reimburses health care providers for specific episodes of care; a set amount of money will be paid

29. Identify the payment system that the Social Security Act established under Medicare A (hospital insurance):

_____

_____

30. Factors that have been identified to improve patient satisfaction are:

a. _____

b. _____

c. _____

d. _____

31. Identify the two main reasons for a nursing shortage.

a. _____

b. _____

32. Identify the Quality and Safety Education (QSEN) for Nurses competencies for registered nurses:

   a. _____

   b. _____

   c. _____

   d. _____

   e. _____

   f. _____

33. The Institute of Medicine (IOM) defines patient-centered care as:

   _____

   _____

34. Identify the eight principles of patient-centered care:

   a. _____

   b. _____

   c. _____

   d. _____

   e. _____

   f. _____

   g. _____

   h. _____

35. Health care organizations that apply for Magnet® status must demonstrate:

   a. _____

   b. _____

   c. _____

36. The revised Magnet® model has five components affected by global issues; please identify them.

   a. _____

   b. _____

   c. _____

   d. _____

   e. _____

37. Explain nurse-sensitive outcomes and give some examples.

   _____

   _____

   _____

38. Explain telemedicine.

_____

_____

39. Health care disparities are: _____

40. Identify the social determinants of health that are linked to health care disparities:

a. _____

b. _____

c. _____

d. _____

e. _____

f. _____

g. _____

h. _____

i. _____

j. _____

k. _____

l. _____

m. _____

n. _____

o. _____

CASE STUDY

41. A school nurse has been following a 9-year-old student who has behavioral problems in class. The student acts out and does not follow teacher instructions. The nurse plans to meet with the student's family and learn more about social determinants of health that might be affecting them. What specific factors would you consider in this assessment?

REVIEW QUESTIONS

Select the appropriate answer and cite the rationale for choosing that particular answer.

42. Health promotion programs are designed to help patients:
    1. Reduce the incidence of disease
    2. Maintain maximal function
    3. Reduce the need to use more expensive health care services
    4. All of the above

    Answer: _____

    Rationale: _____

    _____

    _____

43. Rehabilitation services begin:
    1. When the patient enters the health care system
    2. After the patient's physical condition stabilizes
    3. After the patient requests rehabilitation services
    4. When the patient is discharged from the hospital

    Answer: _____

    Rationale: _____

    _____

    _____

44. An example of an extended care facility is a:
    1. Home care agency
    2. Skilled nursing facility
    3. Suicide prevention center
    4. State-owned psychiatric hospital

    Answer: _____

    Rationale: _____

    _____

    _____

45. A patient and his or her family facing the end stages of a terminal illness might best be served by a:
    1. Hospice
    2. Rehabilitation center
    3. Extended care facility
    4. Crisis intervention center

    Answer: _____

    Rationale: _____

    _____

    _____

3 Community-Based Nursing Practice

Chapter 3

COMPREHENSIVE UNDERSTANDING

Community-Based Care

1. Community-based care focuses on: _____

2. Community-based health care focuses on: _____

3. Identify some of the challenges in community-based health care. _____

    _____

4. Improved delivery of health care involves three key components; identify them:

    a. _____

    _____

    b. _____

    _____

    c. _____

    _____

5. Identify five social determinants of health. _____

    _____

6. Define health disparities. _____

    _____

Community-Oriented Nursing

7. Briefly describe the differences between:

    a. Public health nursing focus: _____

    b. Community health nursing focus: _____

8. The community-oriented nurse's focus is on:

    a. _____

    b. _____

    c. _____

Community-Based Nursing

9. Community-based nursing care takes place in: _____

10. Vulnerable populations are those patients who:

    a. _____

    b. _____

    c. _____

Identify the risk factors for the following vulnerable groups.

11. Immigrant population: _____

12. Poverty and homelessness: _____

13. Abused patients: _____

14. Mental illness: _____

15. Older adults: _____

Competency in Community-Based Nursing

A nurse in a community-based practice must have a variety of skills and talents in assisting patients within the community. Briefly explain the competencies the nurse needs in the following roles.

16. Caregiver: _____

17. Case manager: _____

18. Change agent: _____

19. Patient advocate: _____

20. Collaborator: _____

21. Counselor: _____

22. Educator: _____

23. Epidemiologist: _____

Community Assessment

24. There are three components of a community that need to be assessed. Identify them and give an example of each.

    a. _____

    b. _____

    c. _____

25. While assessing an immigrant community, the nurse identifies that the children are under vaccinated. The nurse notes that there is a health clinic within a 3-mile radius. The nurse meets with the community leaders to develop a plan of improving the rate of vaccinations. What specific practices would the nurse provide?

REVIEW QUESTIONS

Select the appropriate answer and cite the rationale for choosing that particular answer.

26. Which of the following is an example of an intrinsic risk factor for homelessness?
    1. Severe anxiety disorders
    2. Psychotic mental disorders
    3. Living below the poverty line
    4. Progressive chronic alcoholism

    Answer: _____

    Rationale: _____

    _____

    _____

27. When the community health nurse refers patients to appropriate resources and monitors and coordinates the extent and adequacy of services to meet family health care needs, the nurse is functioning in the role of:
    1. Advocate
    2. Counselor
    3. Collaborator
    4. Case manager

    Answer: _____

    Rationale: _____

    _____

    _____

28. The first step in community assessment is determining the community's:
    1. Goals
    2. Set factors
    3. Boundaries
    4. Throughputs

    Answer: _____

    Rationale: _____

    _____

    _____

4 Theoretical Foundations of Nursing Practice

PRELIMINARY READING

Chapter 4

COMPREHENSIVE UNDERSTANDING

Theory

Match the following concepts that relate to theories.

1. _____ Nursing theory
2. _____ Theory
3. _____ Phenomenon
4. _____ Concepts
5. _____ Definitions
6. _____ Assumptions
7. _____ Grand theories
8. _____ Middle-range theories
9. _____ Descriptive theories
10. _____ Prescriptive theories

a. Label given to describe an idea about an event or group of situations
b. Address nursing interventions for a phenomenon, guide practice change, and predict consequences
c. More limited in scope, they address a specific phenomenon and reflect practice
d. Can be an abstract or concrete
e. A conceptualization of some aspect of nursing communicated for the purpose of describing, explaining, predicting, or prescribing nursing care
f. Concepts, explaining relationships, and predicting outcomes
g. Describe phenomena and identify circumstances in which the phenomena occur
h. Define a particular concept based on the theorist's perspective
i. "Taken for granted" statements
j. Theories that are abstract, broad in scope, and complex

Domains of Nursing

Match the following.

11. _____ Domain
12. _____ Paradigm
13. _____ Conceptual framework
14. _____ Nursing metaparadigm
15. _____ Person
16. _____ Environment
17. _____ Nursing

a. All possible conditions affecting the patient and the setting of health care delivery
b. The diagnosis and treatment of human responses to actual or potential health problems
c. Perspective or territory of a profession
d. Links science, philosophy, and theories accepted and applied by the discipline
e. Provides a way to organize major concepts and visualize the relationship
f. Is the recipient of nursing care
g. What nursing is, what it does, and what we do

Shared Theories

18. Shared theory explains: _____

19. Explain the following components of the nursing process as it pertains to systems.

   a. Input: _____

   b. Output: _____

c. Feedback: _____

d. Content: _____

Selected Nursing Theories

Match the following nursing theories and their focus

20. _____ Nightingale's   a. Five stages of skill acquisition of nurses

21. _____ Peplau's   b. Culturally specific nursing care

     c. Patient's self-care needs

22. _____ Henderson's   d. The patient's environment was the focus of nursing care

     e. Nurse-patient relationship

23. _____ Benner   f. Adaptation; help patient cope with changes

     g. Principles and practice of nursing; assist patient with 14 basic activities

24. _____ Orem's   h. Caring; transpersonal relationship

25. _____ Leininger's

26. _____ Roy's

27. _____ Watson's

Link Between Theory and Knowledge Development in Nursing

28. Research refines the knowledge base of nursing. Briefly explain each one.

     a. Theory generating: _____

     b. Theory testing: _____

CASE STUDY

29. You are taking care of Bob, who was recently transferred to the hospital with a diagnosis of pneumonia and weight loss.

     a. How might Florence Nightingale analyze this situation?

     b. How might Roy analyze this situation?

REVIEW QUESTIONS

Select the appropriate answer and cite the rationale for choosing that particular answer.

30. Which of the following models is based on the physiological, sociocultural, and dependence–independence adaptive modes?
   1. Roy's adaptation model
   2. Orem's model of self-care
   3. King's model of personal, interpersonal, and social systems
   4. Rogers' life process interactive person–environmental model

   Answer: _____

   Rationale: _____

   _____

   _____

31. Nursing metaparadigm includes which of the following linkages:
   1. Person
   2. Health
   3. Environment or situation
   4. All of the above

   Answer: _____

   Rationale: _____

   _____

   _____

5 Evidence-Based Practice

Chapter 5

COMPREHENSIVE UNDERSTANDING

The Need for Evidence-Based Practice

1. Define *evidence-based practice*. _____

    _____

2. Identify the steps of evidence-based practice.

    a. _____

    b. _____

    c. _____

    d. _____

    e. _____

    f. _____

    g. _____

3. Identify the five elements of a PICOT question.

    a. _____

    b. _____

    c. _____

    d. _____

    e. _____

4. Identify the sources where the evidence can be found.

    a. _____

    b. _____

    c. _____

    d. _____

5. A *peer-reviewed* article is one where: _____

6. A _____ is the highest level of experimental research.

7. To critique the evidence and determine its worth to practice, the nurse must consider what questions?

    a. _____

    b. _____

    c. _____

Critiquing the Evidence

Briefly explain the following elements of evidence-based articles.

8. Abstract: _____

9. Introduction: _____

10. Literature review: _____

11. A clinical article describes: _____

12. Identify and define the subsections that a research article contains in the manuscript narrative.

    a. _____

    b. _____

    c. _____

    d. _____

    e. _____

Nursing Research

13. Define *nursing research.* _____

14. Define *translation research.* _____

15. Define *outcomes research.* _____

16. Define *scientific method.* _____

17. List the five characteristics of scientific research.

    a. _____

    b. _____

    c. _____

    d. _____

    e. _____

18. Briefly describe the following quantitative methods.

    a. Experimental: _____

    b. Nonexperimental: _____

    c. Surveys: _____

    d. Evaluation: _____

19. Qualitative nursing research is: _____

Research Process

20. Identify the nursing process step that corresponds to each step in the research process.

    a. Identify the area of interest or clinical problem: _____

    b. Develop research question(s)/hypotheses: _____

    c. Determine how the study will be conducted: _____

    d. Conduct the study: _____

    e. Analyze results of the study: _____

21. Briefly explain informed consent in relation to conducting a study.

a. _____

b. _____

c. _____

d. _____

22. Explain confidentiality: _____

_____

CASE STUDY

23. The nurses on a medicine unit have seen an increase in the number of pressure injuries developing in their patients. The nurses decide to initiate a quality improvement project using the plan-do-study-act model. What would be a plan from the model?

REVIEW QUESTIONS

Select the appropriate answer and cite the rationale for choosing that particular answer.

24. Place the steps of the evidence-based practice (EBP) process in the appropriate order.
    1. Critically appraise the evidence you gather.
    2. Ask the clinical question in picot format.
    3. Evaluate the outcomes of the practice decision or change.
    4. Search for the most relevant and best evidence.
    5. Cultivate a spirit of inquiry.
    6. Integrate the evidence.
    7. Communicate the outcomes of the EBP change.
    8. Sustain the EPB change.

    Answer: _____

    Rationale: _____

    _____

    _____

25. Research studies can most easily be identified by:
    1. Examining the contents of the report
    2. Looking for the study only in research journals
    3. Reading the abstract and introduction of the report
    4. Looking for the word *research* in the title of the report

    Answer: _____

    Rationale: _____

    _____

    _____

26. A research report includes all of the following except:
    1. The researcher's interpretation of the study results
    2. A description of methods used to conduct the study
    3. A summary of other research studies with the same results
    4. A summary of literature used to identify the research problem

    Answer: _____

    Rationale: _____

    _____

    _____

6 Health and Wellness

PRELIMINARY READING

Chapter 6

COMPREHENSIVE UNDERSTANDING

Healthy People

1. Explain the framework of *Healthy People 2030*.

_____

Definition of Health

2. Define *health*.

_____

Models of Health and Illness

3. Identify some practices of each health behavior.

   a. Positive health behavior: _____

   b. Negative health behavior: _____

4. Describe the three components of the health belief model.

   a. _____

   b. _____

   c. _____

5. The health promotion model focuses on three areas. They are:

   a. _____

   b. _____

   c. _____

6. Define the main concepts of the holistic health model.

_____

_____

_____

Variables Influencing Health and Health Beliefs and Practices

7. Briefly describe the following internal variables.

   a. Developmental stage: _____

   b. Intellectual background: _____

   c. Perception of functioning: _____

   d. Emotional factors: _____

   e. Spiritual factors: _____

8. Briefly describe the following external variables.

   a. Family role and practices: _____

   b. Social determinants of health: _____

   c. Culture: _____

Health Promotion, Wellness, and Illness Prevention

9. Define *health promotion*.

   _____

   _____

10. Health education includes: _____

11. Define *illness prevention*.

    _____

    _____

12. Identify the differences between passive and active strategies for health promotion.

    _____

    _____

13. Define the following levels of preventive care.

    a. Primary: _____

    b. Secondary: _____

    c. Tertiary: _____

Risk Factors

14. Define *risk factor*.

    _____

    _____

15. Identify at least two risk factors for each of the following categories.

    a. Genetic and physiological factors: _____

    b. Age: _____

    c. Environment: _____

    d. Lifestyle: _____

Risk-Factor Identification and Changing Health Behaviors

16. Briefly explain the five stages of health behavior change.

    a. Precontemplation: _____

    b. Contemplation: _____

    c. Preparation: _____

    d. Action: _____

    e. Maintenance: _____

Illness

17. Define *illness*.

    _____

    _____

18. Explain the two general classifications of illness.

    a. Acute illness: _____

    b. Chronic illness: _____

19. Illness behavior involves: _____

20. Give examples of the following variables that influence illness.

    a. Internal variables: _____

    b. External variables: _____

Impact of Illness on the Patient and Family

21. The patient and family commonly experience the following. Briefly explain each one.

    a. Behavioral and emotional changes: _____

    b. Impact on body image: _____

    c. Impact on self-concept: _____

    d. Impact on family roles: _____

    e. Impact on family dynamics: _____

CASE STUDY

22. Mary, a student nurse is creating a plan of care for a patient with a new below-the-knee amputation. What factors does Mary need to consider for her patient?

Select the appropriate answer and cite the rationale for choosing that particular answer.

23. An interprofessional health care team is developing health education program for middle-school. Which health topics are consistent with the goals of *Health People 2020*? (Select all that apply.)
    1. Determining the best treatment for strep throat
    2. Explaining why it is important to get immunizations as scheduled
    3. Teaching about healthy snacks
    4. Describing why genetically modified foods are controversial
    5. Teaching different ways to fit exercise into the daily routine
    6. Explaining the problems related to lead exposure in the environment

    Answer: _____

    Rationale: _____

    _____

    _____

24. Internal variables influencing health beliefs and practices include:
    1. Developmental stage
    2. Intellectual background
    3. Emotional and spiritual factors
    4. All of the above

    Answer: _____

    Rationale: _____

    _____

    _____

25. Any variable increasing the vulnerability of an individual or a group to an illness or accident is a(an):
    1. Risk factor
    2. Illness behavior
    3. Lifestyle determinant
    4. Negative health behavior

    Answer: _____

    Rationale: _____

    _____

    _____

26. Marsha states, "My chubby size runs in our family. It's a glandular condition. Exercise and diet won't change things much." The nurse determines that this is an example of Marsha's:
    1. Health beliefs
    2. Active strategy
    3. Acute situation
    4. Positive health behavior

    Answer: _____

    Rationale: _____

    _____

    _____

7 Caring in Nursing Practice

Chapter 7

COMPREHENSIVE UNDERSTANDING

Theoretical Views on Caring

1. Define *caring*.

_____

_____

2. Explain Leininger's concept of care from a transcultural perspective.

_____

_____

3. Summarize Watson's transpersonal caring.

_____

_____

4. What does Watson mean by "transformative model"?

_____

_____

5. Swanson's theory of caring consists of five categories. Explain each.

   a. Knowing:

   _____

   _____

   b. Being with:

   _____

   _____

   c. Doing for:

   _____

   _____

   d. Enabling:

   _____

   _____

e. Maintaining belief:

_____

_____

6. List the common themes in nursing caring theories.

a. _____

b. _____

c. _____

d. _____

Ethics of Care

7. Identify the nurse's responsibilities in relation to the ethics of care.

_____

_____

Caring in Nursing Practice

8. Summarize the concept of presence.

_____

_____

9. The outcomes of nursing presence include:

a. _____

b. _____

c. _____

10. The use of touch is one comforting approach. Explain the differences between the three categories of touch.

a. Task-oriented:

_____

_____

b. Caring:

_____

_____

c. Protective:

_____

_____

11. Describe what listening involves.

_____

_____

_____

12. Two elements that facilitate knowing are:

   a. _____

   b. _____

13. List the 10 caring behaviors that are perceived by families.

   a. _____

   b. _____

   c. _____

   d. _____

   e. _____

   f. _____

   g. _____

   h. _____

   i. _____

   j. _____

The Challenge of Caring

14. Summarize the challenges facing nursing in today's health care system.

   _____

   _____

CASE STUDY

15. Sue is a nurse who is caring for an older man who is going to an assisted-living facility after discharge. Give an example of how Sue can listen to the patient that can display caring.

REVIEW QUESTIONS

Select the appropriate answer and cite the rationale for choosing that particular answer.

16. Touch is a caring intervention. Before implementing touch, what does the nurse need to know about touch? (Select all that apply.)
   1. Some cultures may have specific restrictions about non-skill-based touch.
   2. Touch is type of verbal communication.
   3. Touch forms a connection between nurse and patient.
   4. There is never a problem with using touch at any time.
   5. Touch reduces physical pain only.

   Answer: _____

   Rationale: _____

   _____

   _____

17. Leininger's care theory states that the patient's caring values and behaviors are derived largely from:
   1. gender
   2. culture
   3. experience
   4. religious beliefs

   Answer: _____

   Rationale: _____

   _____

   _____

18. The central common theme of the caring theories is:
    1. Maintenance of patient homeostasis
    2. Compensation for patient disabilities
    3. Pathophysiology and self-care abilities
    4. The nurse–patient relationship and psychosocial aspects of care

    Answer: _____

    Rationale: _____

    _____

    _____

19. For the nurse to effectively listen to the patient, he or she needs to:
    1. Lean back in the chair
    2. Sit with the legs crossed
    3. Maintain good eye contact
    4. Respond quickly with appropriate answers to the patient

    Answer: _____

    Rationale: _____

    _____

    _____

20. The nurse demonstrates caring by:
    1. Maintaining professionalism at all costs
    2. Doing all the necessary tasks for the patient
    3. Following all of the health care provider's orders accurately
    4. Helping family members become active participants in the care of the patient

    Answer: _____

    Rationale: _____

    _____

    _____

8 Caring for Patients With Chronic Disease

PRELIMINARY READING

Chapter 8

COMPREHENSIVE UNDERSTANDING

1. Chronic illness affects the _____, _____, and _____ aspects of a patient and family's life.

Prevalence and Costs of Chronic Disease

2. Chronic disease is _____.

3. Chronic illness is _____.

List the most common diseases by body systems:

4. Cardiac

   _____

   _____

5. Digestive

   _____

   _____

6. Endocrine

   _____

   _____

7. Pulmonary

   _____

   _____

8. Musculoskeletal

   _____

   _____

9. Neurologic/Psychiatric

   _____

   _____

10. Renal

    _____

    _____

Genetics and Chronic Illness

11. Define genetic mutation: _____

12. Give an example of the two types of autosomal disorders:

   a. Dominant

   _____

   _____

   b. Recessive

   _____

   _____

Interaction of Genetics, Environment, and Lifestyle

13. Explain multifactorial inheritance: _____

14. What factors should you consider when examining a family disease history:

   a. _____

   b. _____

   c. _____

15. Genetic counseling includes:

   a. _____

   b. _____

   c. _____

   d. _____

   e. _____

16. Identify some lifestyle and risk factors that are modifiable:

   a. _____

   b. _____

   c. _____

   d. _____

   e. _____

The Effect of Chronic Illness on Patients and Families

17. List the factors that affect adherence to chronic illness:

   a. _____

   b. _____

   c. _____

   d. _____

   e. _____

18. Explain the Five A's model that supports patients in self-managing their chronic disease:

   a. Assess: _____

   b. Advise: _____

   c. Agree: _____

   d. Assist: _____

   e. Arrange: _____

19. The physical effects and limitations of chronic illness vary depending on the _____ and _____.

20. The psychosocial needs of patient with chronic illness include _____, _____,

   _____, _____, _____, _____,

   and _____.

21. Patients who live with chronic illness often experience depression related to _____, _____,

   and _____.

22. Patients who experience depression often express _____, _____, _____,

   and _____.

23. Explain the reasons why social isolation can occur in chronic illness:

   a. _____

   b. _____

   c. _____

24. Give an example of the following personal strengths and strategies to cope with the psychosocial effects of chronic illness:

   a. Internal strengths

   _____

   _____

   b. External strengths

   _____

   _____

   c. Self-management strategies

   _____

   _____

25. The focus on caring for older adults with chronic illness is:

   a. _____

   b. _____

   c. _____

26. Identify the factors that put the caregiver at greatest risk for poor outcomes:

    a. _____

    b. _____

    c. _____

    d. _____

    e. _____

27. Briefly explain the chronic care model:

    _____

    _____

28. Identify the six essential elements of the chronic care model:

    a. _____

    b. _____

    c. _____

    d. _____

    e. _____

    f. _____

29. Give some examples of questions that you would ask when collecting a nursing history to assess the affect a chronic disease has on their lives:

    a. Symptoms

    _____

    _____

    b. Psychosocial problems

    _____

    _____

30. Identify the focus areas for chronic disease self-management:

    a. _____

    b. _____

    c. _____

31. Explain the purpose of the Chronic Disease Self-Management Resource Program (CDSMRP):

    _____

    _____

32. You are screening a woman at high risk for breast cancer for the BRCA genetic mutation; explain what a positive result will yield for the patient.

REVIEW QUESTIONS

33. All of the following are modifiable risk factors except:
    1. genetics
    2. smoking
    3. obesity
    4. alcohol intake

    Answer: _____

    Rationale: _____

    _____

    _____

34. The Five A's model includes the following, select all that apply:
    1. agree
    2. acknowledge
    3. advise
    4. arrange
    5. assist

    Answer: _____

    Rationale: _____

    _____

    _____

35. As a nurse, you are caring for an elderly woman who is caring for her husband who has dementia. The woman states, "I just cannot stand watching him suffer any more. It makes me so angry that he has dementia. Why did it have to happen to us? He makes me so upset sometimes, I cannot remember any of the good times we used to have together." Which statement is the most appropriate response by the nurse?
    1. "Why don't you love your husband anymore?"
    2. "It sounds like you need a break. Can't your children help you?"
    3. "I understand your frustration. Is there something you would like to talk about now?"
    4. "I will ask the social worker to come see you to arrange for someone to come help you at home."

    Answer: _____

    Rationale: _____

    _____

    _____

9 | Cultural Competence

PRELIMINARY READING

Chapter 9

COMPREHENSIVE UNDERSTANDING

Health Disparities

1. Define *health disparity*.

   _____

   _____

2. Social determinants of health are:

   _____

   _____

3. Health care disparities are:

   _____

   _____

Culture

Match the following.

4. _____ Culture

5. _____ Intersectionality

6. _____ Oppression

7. _____ Marginalized groups

8. _____ Culturally congruent care

9. _____ Cultural competence

10. _____ Emic worldview

11. _____ Etic worldview

12. _____ Stereotype

13. _____ Social determinants

a. A formal and informal system of advantages and disadvantages tied to a membership in social groups

b. Transcultural care

c. Learned and shared beliefs, values, norms, and traditions of a particular group

d. Conditions in which people are born, grow, live, work, and age

e. Health care must be culturally sensitive and appropriate to the needs of the patient

f. Research and policy model to study the complexities of people's lives and experiences

g. Outsider perspective

h. Have poorer health outcomes because of complex interactions due to behaviors, environment, and clinical care received

i. Insider perspective

j. Assumed belief regarding a particular group

Race, Ethnic, and Cultural Diversity

Define the following.

14. Racial identity _____

15. Ethnic and cultural identity _____

16. Acculturation _____

17. Assimilation _____

33

Core Measures

18. Define *Core measures* and their purpose: _____

A Model of Cultural Competence

19. Briefly explain the five interrelated constructs of cultural competency:

    a. Cultural awareness

    _____

    _____

    b. Cultural knowledge

    _____

    _____

    c. Cultural skill

    _____

    _____

    d. Cultural encounter _____

    _____

    _____

    e. Cultural desire

    _____

    _____

Cultural Awareness and Knowledge

20. Identify the *areas* to focus on in conducting a comprehensive cultural assessment:

    a. _____

    b. _____

    c. _____

    d. _____

    e. _____

    f. _____

21. List the domains of transcultural assessment model:

    a. _____

    b. _____

    c. _____

    d. _____

    e. _____

    f. _____

    g. _____

h. _____

i. _____

j. _____

k. _____

l. _____

22. Linguistic *competence* is: _____

23. State the *recommendations* that all organizations are to follow to provide culturally and linguistically appropriate services:

a. _____

b. _____

c. _____

d. _____

24. Define health *literacy*: _____

25. Explain the teach-back method: _____

_____

26. Explain the *following* mnemonic *LEARN* model that assists the nurse to reflect upon in each patient encounter:

a. L _____

b. E _____

c. A _____

d. R _____

e. N _____

CASE STUDY

27. A 35-year-old woman has Medicaid coverage for herself and two young children. She missed an appointment at the local health clinic to get an annual mammogram because she had no transportation. She gets the annual screening because her mother had breast cancer. Identify some social determinants of this woman's health?

Select the appropriate answer and cite the rationale for choosing that particular answer.

28. When providing care to patients with varied cultural backgrounds, it is imperative for the nurse to *recognize* that:
    1. Cultural considerations must be put aside if basic needs are in jeopardy.
    2. Generalizations about the behavior of a particular group may be inaccurate.
    3. Current health standards should determine the acceptability of cultural practices.
    4. Similar reactions to stress will occur when individuals have the same cultural background.

    Answer: _____

    Rationale: _____

    _____

    _____

29. To be *effective* in meeting various ethnic needs, the nurse should:
    1. Treat all patients alike
    2. Be aware of patients' cultural differences
    3. Act as if he or she is comfortable with the patient's behavior
    4. Avoid asking questions about the patient's cultural background

    Answer: _____

    Rationale: _____

    _____

    _____

30. The *most* important factor in providing nursing care to patients in a specific ethnic group is:
    1. Communication
    2. Time orientation
    3. Biological variation
    4. Environmental control

    Answer: _____

    Rationale: _____

    _____

    _____

31. Which of the following is an example of a health disparity? (Select all that apply.)
    1. A patient who has a homosexual sexual preference
    2. A patient unable to access primary care services
    3. Patients living with chronic disease
    4. A family who relies on public transportation
    5. A patient who has had a history of smoking for 10 years

    Answer: _____

    Rationale: _____

    _____

    _____

10 Family Dynamics

Chapter 10

COMPREHENSIVE UNDERSTANDING

The Family

1. Define the three important attributes that characterize contemporary families.

    a. Family durability: _____

    b. Family resiliency: _____

    c. Family diversity: _____

2. A family is defined as:

    _____

    _____

Family Forms and Current Trends

3. Summarize the various family forms.

    a. Nuclear family: _____

    b. Extended family: _____

    c. Single-parent family: _____

    d. Blended family: _____

    e. Alternative family: _____

4. Explain the following threats and concerns facing the family.

    a. Family caregivers: _____

    b. Poverty: _____

    _____

    c. Homelessness: _____

    d. Domestic violence: _____

5. Define the following:

    a. Structure: _____

    _____

    b. Function: _____

    _____

6. Structure may enhance or detract from the family's ability to respond to stressors. Briefly explain each of the following.

    a. Rigid structure: _____

    b. Open or flexible structure: _____

Identify the three levels and focuses proposed for family nursing practice. Briefly explain each.

7. Family as context: _____

8. Family as patient: _____

9. Family as system: _____

10. Explain the following attributes of healthy families:

    a. Hardiness:

    _____

    _____

    b. Resiliency:

    _____

    _____

11. Identify how the following affect heath:

    a. Genetics: _____

    b. Chronic illness and/or trauma: _____

    c. End-of-life care: _____

Family–Centered Care and the Nursing Process

12. Three factors underlie the family approach to the nursing process. Name them.

    a. _____

    b. _____

    c. _____

13. Identify and define the areas to include in a family assessment.

    a. _____

    b. _____

    c. _____

14. A comprehensive, culturally sensitive family assessment is critical in order to:

    a. _____

    b. _____

    c. _____

    d. _____

15. Give some examples of nursing diagnoses applicable to family care:

a. _____

b. _____

c. _____

d. _____

e. _____

f. _____

g. _____

16. When planning family-centered care, the goals and outcomes are: _____

_____

Implementing Family-Centered Care

17. When implementing family-centered care, the following need to be addressed. Briefly explain.

a. Health promotion: _____

b. Acute care: _____

c. Discharge planning: _____

d. Communication: _____

e. Restorative and continuing care: _____

CASE STUDY

18. John is a 55-year-old male who was severely injured in a motor vehicle accident 2 weeks ago. He is now stable and is prepared for rehabilitation to assist him to return home. What are some teaching strategies to give to his family to avoid caregiver role strain?

Select the appropriate answer and cite the rationale for choosing that particular answer.

19. A married couple has three children. The youngest child has graduated from college and is moving to a different city to take a job. The other two children left the home several years ago. What developmental tasks does the nurse expect this family to experience at this point in time? (Select all that apply.)
    1. Take on parenting roles
    2. Making room for the wisdom of older adults
    3. Refocusing on marital issues
    4. Determining new focus on recreational activities
    5. Developing intimate relations with others

    Answer: _____

    Rationale: _____

    _____

    _____

20. Family structure can best be described as:
    1. A complex set of relationships
    2. A basic pattern of predictable stages
    3. The pattern of relationships and ongoing membership
    4. Flexible patterns that contribute to adequate functioning

    Answer: _____

    Rationale: _____

    _____

    _____

21. When planning care for a patient and using the concept of family as patient, the nurse:
    1. Includes only the patient and his or her significant other
    2. Considers the developmental stage of the patient and not the family
    3. Understands that the patient's family will always be a help to the patient's health goals
    4. Realizes that cultural background is an important variable when assessing the family

    Answer: _____

    Rationale: _____

    _____

    _____

22. Interventions used by the nurse when providing care to a rigidly structured family include:
    1. Attempting to change the family structure
    2. Providing solutions for problems as they arise
    3. Exploring with the family the benefits of moving toward more flexible modes of action
    4. Administering nursing care in a manner that provides minimal opportunity for change

    Answer: _____

    Rationale: _____

    _____

    _____

11 Developmental Theories

PRELIMINARY READING

Chapter 11

COMPREHENSIVE UNDERSTANDING

Developmental Theories

1. Briefly summarize Gesell's theory of development.

   _____

   _____

2. Briefly summarize theories of psychoanalytical/psychosocial theory.

   _____

   _____

3. Explain the five stages of Freud's psychoanalytic model of personal development.

   a. Stage 1: Oral: _____

   b. Stage 2: Anal: _____

   c. Stage 3: Phallic: _____

   d. Stage 4: Latency: _____

   e. Stage 5: Genital: _____

Match the following stages of Erickson (psychosocial development) with the appropriate years.

4. _____ Trust vs. mistrust		a. 3–6 years
5. _____ Autonomy vs. shame		b. Birth to 1 year
6. _____ Initiative vs. guilt		c. Puberty
7. _____ Industry vs. inferiority		d. 1–3 years
8. _____ Identity vs. role confusion		e. 6–11 years
9. _____ Intimacy vs. isolation		f. Middle-age
10. _____ Generativity vs. self-absorption		g. Young adult
11. _____ Integrity vs. despair		h. Old age

12. Define *temperament*.

   _____

   _____

13. Identify the three basic classes of temperament and briefly explain each.

a. _____

b. _____

c. _____

14. Contemporary life-span approach considers:

_____

_____

15. Identify the four periods of Piaget's theory of cognitive development.

a. _____

b. _____

c. _____

d. _____

Kohlberg identified six stages of moral development under three levels. Briefly describe each.

16. Level I: Preconventional level: _____

_____

a. Stage 1: _____

_____

b. Stage 2: _____

_____

17. Level II: Conventional level: _____

_____

a. Stage 3: _____

_____

b. Stage 4: _____

_____

18. Level III: Postconventional level: _____

_____

a. Stage 5: _____

_____

b. Stage 6: _____

_____

19. Connor is a shy 9-year-old boy who presents to the clinic for a physical exam prior to summer camp. Initially he seems uncomfortable with the experience of the exam. You ask Connor if he wants his parents in the room for the exam. The mother responds before Connor can answer and states, "of course I'll come in with you."

  a. According to Erickson, at what stage of development is Connor?

  b. How do you think Connor might respond to his mother's comment?

  c. According to temperamental theory and based on your observations, what temperament style is Connor most likely displaying?

REVIEW QUESTIONS

Select the appropriate answer and cite the rationale for choosing that particular answer.

20. According to Piaget, the school-age child is in the third stage of cognitive development, which is characterized by:
   1. Concrete operations
   2. Conventional thought
   3. Postconventional thought
   4. Identity vs. role diffusion

   Answer: _____

   Rationale: _____

   _____

   _____

21. According to Erikson, the developmental task of adolescence is:
   1. Industry vs. inferiority
   2. Identity vs. role confusion
   3. Autonomy vs. shame and doubt
   4. Role acceptance vs. role confusion

   Answer: _____

   Rationale: _____

   _____

   _____

22. According to Erikson's developmental theory, the primary developmental task of the middle years is to:
   1. Achieve intimacy
   2. Achieve generativity
   3. Establish a set of personal values
   4. Establish a sense of personal identity

   Answer: _____

   Rationale: _____

   _____

   _____

23. According to Kohlberg, children develop moral reasoning as they mature. Which of the following is most characteristic of a preschooler's stage of moral development?
   1. The rules of correct behavior are obeyed.
   2. Behavior that pleases others is considered good.
   3. Showing respect for authority is important behavior.
   4. Actions are determined as good or bad in terms of their consequences.

   Answer: _____

   Rationale: _____

   _____

   _____

12 Conception Through Adolescence

PRELIMINARY READING

Chapter 12

COMPREHENSIVE UNDERSTANDING

Intrauterine Life

1. Identify the three stages of a full-term pregnancy, and state when each occurs.

   a. _____

   b. _____

   c. _____

2. Identify some of the common concerns that are verbalized by the expectant mother that are attributable to fetal growth and hormonal changes.

   _____

   _____

Transition From Intrauterine to Extrauterine Life

3. The assessment tool used to assess newborns is the Apgar score. Identify the components.

   a _____

   b _____

   c. _____

   d. _____

   e. _____

4. Direct nursing care at birth includes _____, _____, and _____.

5. Give some examples of how to encourage parent–child attachment immediately after birth.

   _____

   _____

Newborn

Match the following terms that address the newborn.

6. _____ Neonatal period

7. _____ Molding

8. _____ Anterior fontanel

9. _____ Early cognitive development

10. _____ Infant positioning

11. _____ Posterior fontanel

12. _____ Normal behavior

13. _____ Health promotion of the infant

a. Screenings, car seats, and cribs
b. Closes at the end of the second to third month
c. Overlapping of the soft skull bones
d. First month of life
e. Innate behavior, reflexes, and sensory functions
f. Sleep on their back
g. Sucking, crying, sleeping, and activity
h. Closes at 12–18 months

Infant

14. Infancy is the period from _____ to _____.

15. Summarize the changes in size, weight, and height that occur in the first 12 months.

_____

_____

16. Describe the cognitive changes that occur in infants.

_____

_____

17. Identify the language development in infants and how to help parents further develop infants' language.

_____

_____

18. Explain the following psychosocial changes that occur.

a. Separation and individuation: _____

b. Play: _____

19. Explain the following in relation to health risks of the infant.

a. Injury prevention: _____

b. Child maltreatment: _____

20. Give an example of health promotion activities for the following.

a. Nutrition: _____

b. Supplementation: _____

c. Immunizations: _____

d. Sleep: _____

Chapter **12 Conception Through Adolescence**

Toddler

21. Toddlerhood ranges from _____ to _____.

22. Summarize the fine motor capabilities that occur during this stage.

    _____

    _____

23. Summarize the cognitive changes that occur during this stage.

    _____

    _____

24. Describe language ability at this stage.

    _____

    _____

25. Describe the psychosocial changes of a toddler.

    _____

    _____

26. Describe the play of a toddler.

    _____

    _____

27. Identify the health risks of a toddler.

    _____

    _____

28. Identify the health promotion activities for this age-group related to the following.

    a. Nutrition: _____

    b. Toilet training: _____

Preschoolers

29. The preschool period ranges from _____ to _____.

30. Summarize the height and weight changes that occur in preschoolers.

    _____

    _____

31. Describe the more complex thinking processes a preschooler develops.

    _____

    _____

32. Explain the following.

    a. Psychosocial: _____

    b. Language: _____

    c. Focus of fear: _____

33. Describe the concept of play for the preschooler.

_____

_____

34. Explain health promotion activities related to the following for this group.

    a. Nutrition: _____

    b. Sleep: _____

    c. Vision: _____

School-Age Children

35. The school-age years range from _____ to _____.

36. Puberty begins at _____.

37. Summarize the physical changes that occur in school-age children.

_____

_____

38. Define the cognitive skills that develop in school-age children.

_____

_____

39. Summarize psychosocial development in relation to the following.

    a. Psychosocial changes: _____

    b. Peer relationships: _____

    c. Sexual identity: _____

    d. Stress: _____

40. Identify the health risks for school-age children.

_____

_____

41. Give an example of a health promotion intervention that is appropriate for school-age children.

   a. Perceptions: _____

   b. Health education: _____

   c. Health maintenance:_____

   d. Safety: _____

   e. Nutrition: _____

Adolescents

42. The adolescent period ranges from _____ to _____.

43. List the four major physical changes that occur.

   a. _____

   b. _____

   c. _____

   d. _____

44. Briefly explain the cognitive abilities of this group.

   _____

   _____

45. Identify some strategies for communicating with adolescents.

   a. _____

   b. _____

   c. _____

   d. _____

   e. _____

46. Explain the following components of personal total identity.

   a. Sexual identity: _____

   b. Peer group identity: _____

   c. Family identity: _____

   d. Health identity: _____

47. Identify the leading causes of death for adolescents.

   a. _____

   b. _____

   c. _____

48. List the six warning signs of suicide for adolescents.

a. _____

b. _____

c. _____

d. _____

e. _____

f. _____

49. Define the two eating disorders that follow.

a. Anorexia nervosa: _____

b. Bulimia nervosa: _____

50. Identify health promotion interventions for adolescents in regard to the following.

a. Substance abuse: _____

b. Sexually transmitted infections: _____

c. Pregnancy: _____

51. Identify the concerns of minority adolescents.

_____

_____

52. Explain how a nurse could help a teen disclose his or her sexual orientation.

_____

_____

CASE STUDY

53. Jordynn, a 13-year-old female, presents to the clinic with her mother for an annual physical exam for school. Her weight is > 80% and her height is within 50%.

a. What stage of development is Jordynn?

b. What are some nursing actions most appropriate to this age group?

c. Would you encourage a low-fat diet to prevent fat disposition?

Select the appropriate answer and cite the rationale for choosing that particular answer.

54. The mother of a 2-year-old expresses concern that her son's appetite has diminished and that he seems to prefer milk to other solid foods. Which response by the nurse reflects knowledge of principles of communication and nutrition?
    1. "Have you considered feeding him when he doesn't seem interested in feeding himself?"
    2. "Oh, I wouldn't be too worried; children tend to eat when they're hungry. I just wouldn't give him dessert unless he eats his meal."
    3. "That is not uncommon in toddlers. You might consider increasing his milk to two quarts per day to be sure he gets enough nutrients."
    4. "A toddler's rate of growth normally slows down. It's common to see a toddler's appetite diminish in response to decreased calorie needs."

    Answer: _____

    Rationale: _____

    _____

    _____

55. To stimulate cognitive and psychosocial development of the toddler, it is important for parents to:
    1. Set firm and consistent limits
    2. Foster sharing of toys with playmates and siblings
    3. Provide clarification about what is right and wrong
    4. Limit confusion by restricting exploration of the environment

    Answer: _____

    Rationale: _____

    _____

    _____

56. Which of the following is true of the developmental behaviors of school-age children?
    1. Fears center on the loss of self-control.
    2. Positive feedback from parents and teachers is crucial to development.
    3. Formal and informal peer group membership is the key in forming self-esteem.
    4. A full range of defense mechanisms is used, including rationalization and intellectualization.

    Answer: _____

    Rationale: _____

    _____

    _____

13 Young and Middle Adults

Chapter 13

COMPREHENSIVE UNDERSTANDING

Young Adults

1. Describe the period of life called *emerging adulthood*.

   _____

   _____

2. Summarize the physical changes that occur in young adults.

   _____

   _____

3. Briefly explain the cognitive development of the period.

   _____

   _____

4. Explain the psychosocial patterns of the following age groups.

   a. 23–28 years: _____

   _____

   b. 29–34 years: _____

   _____

   c. 35–43 years: _____

   _____

5. Briefly explain the psychosocial development of a young adult in relation to the following.

   a. Lifestyle: _____

   _____

   b. Career: _____

   _____

   c. Sexuality: _____

   _____

   d. Childbearing cycle: _____

   _____

6. Describe the following types of families.

   a. Singlehood: _____

   _____

   b. Parenthood: _____

   _____

   c. Alternative family structures and parenting: _____

   _____

Briefly explain the risk factors for young adults in regard to the following.

7. Family history: _____

   _____

8. Personal hygiene habits: _____

   _____

9. Violent death and injury: _____

   _____

10. Substance abuse: _____

    _____

11. Human trafficking: _____

    _____

12. Unplanned pregnancies: _____

    _____

13. Sexually transmitted infections: _____

    _____

14. Environmental and occupational risks: _____

    _____

Explain how you would assess the psychosocial health concerns of the young adult related to:

15. Job stress: _____

    _____

16. Family stress: _____

    _____

17. Infertility: _____

    _____

18. Obesity: _____

    _____

19. Exercise: _____

    _____

Explain the physiological changes that occur to pregnant women and childbearing families.

20. Prenatal care: _____

_____

21. Physiological changes during pregnancy: _____

_____

    a. First trimester: _____

_____

    b. Second trimester: _____

_____

    c. Third trimester: _____

_____

Middle Adults

22. Middle adulthood is the period from _____ to _____.

23. Identify the major physiological changes that occur between 40 and 65 years of age.

_____

_____

24. Define the following.

    a. Perimenopause: _____

_____

    b. Menopause: _____

_____

    c. Climacteric: _____

_____

Summarize the psychosocial development of middle adults in the following areas.

25. "Sandwich generation": _____

_____

26. Career transition: _____

_____

27. Sexuality: _____

_____

28. Singlehood: _____

_____

29. Marital changes: _____

_____

30. Family transitions: _____

_____

The following are health concerns for middle adults. Identify strategies for each one.

31. Stress: _____

_____

32. Obesity: _____

_____

33. Summarize two psychosocial concerns of middle adults.

    a. Anxiety: _____

    _____

    b. Depression: _____

    _____

CASE STUDY

34. Bill, a 25-year-old unemployed carpenter, comes to your health center for immunizations so that he can work in a restaurant. During the encounter he states that he has not seen a health care provider since he was in high school. Before you administer his immunizations, you do a thorough history and physical exam. During the history Bill tells you he likes to drink beers with his friends and date lots of women.

    a. What questions would you ask Bill about his usual health promotion activities?

    b. How would you ask Bill about his risk for STDs?

    c. What health screening activities would you suggest to Bill?

Select the appropriate answer and cite the rationale for choosing that particular answer.

35. The greatest cause of illness and death in the young adult population is:
    1. Violence
    2. Substance abuse
    3. Cardiovascular disease
    4. Sexually transmitted disease

    Answer: _____

    Rationale: _____

    _____

    _____

36. Which physiological change would be a normal assessment finding in a middle adult?
    1. Increased breast size
    2. Reduced auditory acuity
    3. Thickening of the waistline
    4. Increased anteroposterior diameter of the thorax

    Answer: _____

    Rationale: _____

    _____

    _____

37. In planning patient education for Mrs. Smith, a 45-year-old woman who had an ovarian cyst removed, which of the following facts is true about the sexuality of middle-aged adults?
    1. Menstruation ceases after menopause.
    2. Estrogen is produced after menopause.
    3. With removal of the ovarian cyst, pregnancy cannot occur.
    4. After reaching climacteric, a man is unable to father a child.

    Answer: _____

    Rationale: _____

    _____

    _____

14 Older-Adults

PRELIMINARY READING

Chapter 14

COMPREHENSIVE UNDERSTANDING

Myths and Stereotypes

1. Older-adults are persons age _____ and over.

2. Identify three myths or stereotypes regarding older-adults.

   a. _____

   b. _____

   c. _____

3. *Agism* is: _____

   _____

Developmental Tasks for Older-Adults

4. List the seven developmental tasks of older-adults.

   a. _____

   b. _____

   c. _____

   d. _____

   e. _____

   f. _____

   g. _____

Community-Based and Institutional Health Care Services

5. A quality nursing home has the following features:

   a. _____

   b. _____

   c. _____

   d. _____

   e. _____

   f. _____

   g. _____

   h. _____

   i. _____

Assessing the Needs of Older-Adults

6. Nurses need to consider three key points to ensure an age-specific approach.

   a. _____

   b. _____

   c. _____

7. Identify the early indicators of an acute illness.

   a. _____

   b. _____

   c. _____

   d. _____

   e. _____

Match the following common physiological changes to the system.

8. _____ Integumentary

9. _____ Respiratory

10. _____ Cardiovascular

11. _____ Gastrointestinal

12. _____ Musculoskeletal

13. _____ Neurological

14. _____ Sensory

15. _____ Genitourinary

16. _____ Reproductive

17. _____ Endocrine

a. Decreased estrogen production, atrophy of vagina, uterus, and breasts
b. Decrease in saliva, gastric secretions, and pancreatic enzymes
c. Decreased ability to respond to stress
d. Pigmentation changes, glandular atrophy, thinning hair
e. 50% decrease in renal blood flow, decreased bladder capacity
f. Decreased cough reflex and vital capacity, increased airway resistance
g. Lower cardiac output, decreased baroreceptor sensitivity
h. Presbyopia, presbycusis, decreased proprioception
i. Decalcification of bones, degenerative changes, dehydration of intervertebral disks
j. Degeneration of nerve cells, decrease in neurotransmitters

18. Functional status in older-adults refers to: _____

    _____

19. Explain the three common conditions that affect cognition.

    a. Delirium: _____

    _____

    b. Dementia: _____

    _____

    c. Depression: _____

    _____

20. Identify the psychosocial changes that occur in older-adults.

    a. Retirement: _____

    _____

    b. Social isolation: _____

    _____

c. Sexuality: _____

_____

d. Housing and environment: _____

_____

e. Death: _____

_____

Addressing the Health Concerns of Older-Adults

21. *Healthy People 2020* for older-adults focuses on:

a. _____

b. _____

c. _____

d. _____

22. List general preventive measures to recommend to older-adults.

a. _____

b. _____

c. _____

d. _____

e. _____

f. _____

g. _____

h. _____

i. _____

Match the following health concerns.

23. _____ Heart disease

24. _____ Cancer

25. _____ Stroke

26. _____ Smoking

27. _____ Alcohol abuse

28. _____ Nutrition

29. _____ Dental problems

30. _____ Exercise

31. _____ Polypharmacy

32. _____ Falls

33. _____ Sensory impairments

34. _____ Pain

35. _____ Medication use

a. Concurrent use of many medications
b. Changes in vision, hearing, taste, and smell
c. Leading cause of death
d. Consequences can include depression, loss of appetite, sleep difficulties
e. Third leading cause of death
f. Risk factors: impaired vision, arthritis, incontinence, medication reactions
g. Risk factor in the four most common causes of death
h. Second most common cause of death
i. Situational factors and clinical conditions affect older adults' needs
j. Adverse effects include confusion, impaired balance, dizziness, and nausea
k. Caused by depression, loneliness, and lack of social support
l. Caries, gingivitis, and ill-fitting dentures
m. Maintains and strengthens functional ability and promotes well-being

58

Match the following interventions used to maintain the psychosocial health of older-adults.

36. _____ Therapeutic communication

37. _____ Touch

38. _____ Reality orientation

39. _____ Validation therapy

40. _____ Reminiscence

41. _____ Body image

a. Assisting with grooming and hygiene
b. An alternative approach to communication with a confused adult
c. Nurse expresses attitudes of concern, kindness, and compassion
d. Technique to make older-adults aware of time, place, and person
e. Can significantly lower agitation levels in older-adults with dementia
f. Recalling the past

42. *Elder mistreatment* is defined as: _____

_____

43. Identify types of elder abuse:

_____

_____

Describe the following therapeutic communication tools.

44. Touch: _____

_____

45. Reality orientation: _____

_____

46. Validation therapy: _____

_____

47. Reminiscence: _____

_____

Older-Adults and the Acute Care Setting
Explain why older adults are at risk for each of the following.

48. Delirium: _____

_____

49. Dehydration and malnutrition: _____

_____

50. Health-associated infections (HAIs): _____

_____

51. Transient urinary incontinence: _____

_____

52. Skin breakdown: _____

_____

53. Falls: _____

_____

Older-Adults and Restorative Care

54. Summarize the two types of ongoing care for older-adults.

a. _____

b. _____

CASE STUDY

55. As a nurse in a long-term care facility, you are caring several elders with noticeable hearing losses.

a. What would be the best way to communicate with these patients?

b. What if they also had a memory deficit, how would you complete your assessment?

REVIEW QUESTIONS

Select the appropriate answer and cite the rationale for choosing that particular answer.

56. Which statement describing delirium is correct?
    1. Symptoms of delirium are irreversible.
    2. The onset of delirium is slow and insidious.
    3. Symptoms of delirium are stable and unchanging.
    4. Causes include electrolyte imbalances and cerebral anoxia.

    Answer: _____

    Rationale: _____

    _____

    _____

57. Ms. Dale states that she does not need the TV turned on because she cannot see very well. Normal visual changes in older-adults include all of the following except:
    1. Double vision
    2. Sensitivity to glare
    3. Decreased visual acuity
    4. Decreased accommodation to darkness

    Answer: _____

    Rationale: _____

    _____

    _____

58. Mr. DeLone states that he is worried about his parents' plans to retire. All of the following would be appropriate responses regarding retirement of older-adults except:
    1. Retirement may affect an individual's physical and psychological functioning.
    2. Positive adjustment is often related to how much a person planned for the retirement.
    3. Reactions to retirement are influenced by the importance that has been attached to the work role.
    4. Retirement for most persons represents a sudden shock that is irreversibly damaging to self-image and self-esteem.

    Answer: _____

    Rationale: _____

    _____

    _____

15 Critical Thinking and Clinical Judgment

PRELIMINARY READING

Chapter 15

COMPREHENSIVE UNDERSTANDING

Clinical Judgment in Nursing Practice

1. A clinical judgment is: _____

   _____

2. Define *evidence-based knowledge*.

   _____

   _____

3. Critical thinking is a way of thinking about clinical situations by asking questions such as:

   a. _____

   b. _____

   c. _____

   d. _____

   e. _____

   f. _____

   g. _____

   h. _____

Levels of Critical Thinking in Nursing

4. Identify the six cognitive skills that enable nurses to apply the process in clinical decision making:

   a. _____

   b. _____

   c. _____

   d. _____

   e. _____

   f. _____

Critical Thinking Competencies

Match the following cognitive processes to critical thinking competencies.

5. _____ Scientific method

6. _____ Problem solving

7. _____ Decision making

8. _____ Diagnostic reasoning

9. _____ Inference

10. _____ Clinical decision making

11. _____ Nursing process

a. Focuses on problem resolution
b. Process of drawing conclusions from related pieces of evidence
c. Systematic, ordered approach to gathering data and solving problems
d. Obtain information and then use the information plus what you already know to find a solution
e. Five-step clinical decision-making approach
f. Careful reasoning so the best options are chosen for the best outcomes
g. Determining a patient's health status after you have assigned meaning to the behaviors and symptoms presented

12. Explain the two types of interpretation of facts and observations:

 a. Inductive reasoning: _____

 _____

 b. Deductive reasoning: _____

 _____

Components of Critical Thinking in the Clinical Judgment Model

13. The clinical thinking model includes six components of critical thinking in nursing judgment; identify them and give an example:

 a. _____

 b. _____

 c. _____

 d. _____

 e. _____

 f. _____

Match the following critical thinking attitudes with the appropriate application to practice.

14. _____ Confidence

15. _____ Thinking independently

16. _____ Fairness

17. _____ Responsibility

18. _____ Risk taking

19. _____ Discipline

20. _____ Perseverance

21. _____ Creativity

22. _____ Curiosity

23. _____ Integrity

24. _____ Humility

a. Refer to policy and procedure manual to review steps of a skill
b. Explore and learn more about a patient to make appropriate clinical judgments
c. Speak with conviction and always be prepared to perform care safely
d. Be cautious of an easy answer; look for a pattern and find a solution
e. Be willing to recommend alternative approaches to nursing care
f. Look for different approaches if interventions are not working
g. Read the nursing literature
h. Take time to be thorough and manage your time effectively
i. Do not compromise nursing standards or honesty in delivering nursing care
j. Listen to both sides in any discussion
k. Recognize when you need more information to make a decision

Evaluation of Clinical judgments

25. List the steps of a model for using reflection in your practice:

R. _____

E. _____

F. _____

L. _____

E. _____

C. _____

T. _____

26. List some examples of questions that you would use in your journal for self-evaluation:

a. _____

b. _____

c. _____

d. _____

e. _____

27. List ways the nurse can evaluate his or her clinical judgments:

a. _____

b. _____

c. _____

CASE STUDY

28. You are removing your patient's food tray and notice that the food is still on the tray. When you assess the patient, he states he feels hungry but does not eat his food when it is served.

a. Using critical thinking skills, the nurse would perform what?

b. What specific questions could I ask this patient to better understand the issue?

Select the appropriate answer and cite the rationale for choosing that particular answer.

29. Clinical decision making requires the nurse to:
    1. Improve a patient's health
    2. Standardize care for the patient
    3. Follow the health care provider's orders for patient care
    4. Establish and weigh criteria in deciding the best choice of therapy for a patient

    Answer: _____

    Rationale: _____

    _____

    _____

30. Which of the following is not one of the five steps of the nursing process?
    1. Planning
    2. Evaluation
    3. Assessment
    4. Hypothesis testing

    Answer: _____

    Rationale: _____

    _____

    _____

16 Nursing Assessment

PRELIMINARY READING

Chapter 16

COMPREHENSIVE UNDERSTANDING

Critical Thinking in Assessment

1. Identify the two steps of a nursing assessment.

   a. _____

   b. _____

2. List some types of nursing assessments.

   _____

   _____

3. List Gordon's 11 functional health patterns.

   a. _____

   b. _____

   c. _____

   d. _____

   e. _____

   f. _____

   g. _____

   h. _____

   i. _____

   j. _____

   k. _____

4. Discuss the two primary types of data.

   a. Subjective data: _____

   _____

   b. Objective data: _____

   _____

5. Identify the variety of sources where data can be obtained.

a. _____

b. _____

c. _____

d. _____

e. _____

The Patient-Centered Interview

6. A patient-centered interview is:

_____

7. List the effective communication skills to use with patients during assessment interviews:

a. _____

b. _____

c. _____

d. _____

8. List the three phases of all patient-centered interviews.

a. _____

b. _____

c. _____

9. During an interview, the following are used. Briefly explain.

a. Observation: _____

_____

b. Open-ended questions: _____

_____

c. Leading questions: _____

_____

d. Back channeling: _____

_____

e. Probing: _____

_____

f. Direct closed-ended questions: _____

_____

Nursing Health History

Match the following basic components of the health history.

10. _____ Biographical information

11. _____ Reasons for seeking health care

12. _____ Patient expectations

13. _____ Present illness/health concerns

14. _____ Health history

15. _____ Family history

16. _____ Environmental history

17. _____ Psychosocial history

18. _____ Spiritual health

19. _____ Review of systems (ROS)

a. Represents the totality of one's being
b. Reveals the patient's support systems and coping mechanisms
c. To determine whether the patient is at risk for illnesses of a genetic or a familial nature
d. Systematic approach for collecting the patient's self-reported data on all body systems
e. Patient's understanding of why he or she is seeking health care
f. Factual demographic data about the patient
g. Chief concerns or problems
h. Essential and relevant data about the nature and onset of symptoms
i. Health care experiences and current health habits and lifestyle patterns
j. Patient's home and work, focusing on determining the patient's safety

20. Diagnostic and laboratory data provide: _____

_____

21. Define the term *data validation*: _____

_____

22. A concept map is: _____

_____

CASE STUDY

23. Mrs. Smith, an 80-year-old, is in the hospital for hip replacement.

   a. Any specific considerations for this patient?

   b. What are the key components of the nursing history that you would obtain?

   c. What sources could you use?

Select the appropriate answer and cite the rationale for choosing that particular answer.

24. The interview technique that is most effective in strengthening the nurse–patient relationship by demonstrating the nurse's willingness to hear the patient's thoughts is:
    1. Direct question
    2. Problem solving
    3. Problem seeking
    4. Open-ended question

    Answer: _____

    Rationale: _____

    _____

    _____

25. While obtaining a health history, the nurse asks Mr. Jones if he has noted any change in his activity tolerance. This is an example of which interview technique?
    1. Direct question
    2. Problem solving
    3. Problem seeking
    4. Open-ended question

    Answer: _____

    Rationale: _____

    _____

    _____

26. Mr. Davis tells the nurse that he has been experiencing more frequent episodes of indigestion. The nurse asks if the indigestion is associated with meals or a reclining position and asks what relieves the indigestion. This is an example of which interview technique?
    1. Direct question
    2. Problem solving
    3. Problem seeking
    4. Open-ended question

    Answer: _____

    Rationale: _____

    _____

    _____

27. The information obtained in a review of systems (ROS) is:
    1. Objective
    2. Subjective
    3. Based on the nurse's perspective
    4. Based on physical examination findings

    Answer: _____

    Rationale: _____

    _____

    _____

Analysis and Nursing Diagnosis

Chapter 17

COMPREHENSIVE UNDERSTANDING

Match the following terms that relate to diagnostic conclusions.

1. _____ Medical diagnosis

2. _____ Collaborative problem

3. _____ Defining characteristics

4. _____ Nursing diagnosis

5. _____ Health promotion nursing diagnosis

6. _____ Problem-focused nursing diagnosis

a. Desire to increase well-being and actualize human health potential

b. The clinical criteria or assessment findings that support an actual nursing diagnosis

c. Identification of a disease condition based on a specific evaluation of the history and physical exam

d. Is a problem that requires both medicine and nursing interventions to treat

e. Patient's responses or vulnerability to health conditions or live events that a nurse is licensed to treat

f. Clinical judgment concerning an undesirable human response to a health condition or life processes

Critical Thinking in Analysis and Nursing Diagnosis

Define the following components of the diagnostic reasoning process.

7. Data cluster: _____

_____

8. Data interpretation: _____

_____

Explain the following components of the formulation of a nursing diagnosis.

9. Diagnostic label or diagnosis: _____

_____

10. Related factor: _____

_____

11. Related factors are categorized into four groups, identify them:

a._____

b._____

c._____

d._____

12. The following are necessary for an accurate diagnostic statement, explain briefly:

    a. diagnostic validity

    b. prioritization

Sources of Diagnostic Errors

Identify the sources of error in the steps of the nursing process related to:

13. Errors in data collection: _____

14. Errors in data clustering: _____

    _____

15. Errors in interpretation and analysis of data: _____

    _____

16. Errors in the diagnostic statement: _____

    _____

17. State the guidelines to use to reduce errors when formulating the diagnostic statement.

    a. _____

    b. _____

    c. _____

    d. _____

    e. _____

    f. _____

    g. _____

    h. _____

    i. _____

    j. _____

    k. _____

    l. _____

18. Explain the process of documenting a patient's nursing diagnoses.

    _____

    _____

19. A collaborative (multidisciplinary) problem is indicated instead of a nursing or medical diagnoses.

    a. List two types of collaborative problems.

REVIEW QUESTIONS

Select the appropriate answer and cite the rationale for choosing that particular answer.

20. A nursing diagnosis:
    1. Identifies nursing problems
    2. Is not changed during the course of a patient's hospitalization
    3. Is derived from the physician's history and physical examination
    4. Is a statement of a patient response to a health problem that requires nursing intervention

    Answer: _____

    Rationale: _____

    _____

    _____

21. The first part of the nursing diagnosis statement:
    1. May be stated as a medical diagnosis
    2. Identifies the cause of the patient problem
    3. Identifies appropriate nursing interventions
    4. Identifies an actual or potential health problem

    Answer: _____

    Rationale: _____

    _____

    _____

22. The second part of the nursing diagnosis statement:
    1. Is usually stated as a medical diagnosis
    2. Identifies the expected outcomes of nursing care
    3. Identifies the probable cause of the patient problem
    4. Is connected to the first part of the statement with the phrase "related to"

    Answer: _____

    Rationale: _____

    _____

    _____

23. Which of the following is the correctly stated nursing diagnosis?
    1. Needs to be fed related to broken right arm
    2. Impaired skin integrity related to fecal incontinence
    3. Abnormal breath sounds caused by weak cough reflex
    4. Impaired physical mobility related to rheumatoid arthritis

    Answer: _____

    Rationale: _____

    _____

    _____

18 Planning Nursing Care

PRELIMINARY READING

PRELIMINARY READING

Chapter 18

COMPREHENSIVE UNDERSTANDING

Establishing Priorities

1. Planning involves _____

   _____

2. Nurses establish priorities in relation to importance and time. Briefly explain the following.

   a. High priority: _____

   b. Intermediate priority: _____

   c. Low priority: _____

3. Identify some factors within the health care environment that affect the ability to set priorities.

   a. _____

   b. _____

   c. _____

   d. _____

Critical Judgment in Setting Outcomes

Identify whether the outcomes are patient centered or nurse sensitive.

4. pressure injury reduces in diameter by discharge

5. pressure injury prevalence

6. patient satisfaction

7. patient will achieve improved flexion in elbow

8. urinary catheter-associated blood stream infection rate for patients in the ICU

9. patient reports pain at a level of 3 or below by discharge

    a. Patient-centered outcome

    b. Nurse-sensitive outcome

10. The SMART approach for writing goals and outcome statement stands for: _____

   _____

Briefly explain the guidelines to follow when writing goals and expected outcomes.

11. Specific: _____

   _____

12. Measurable: _____

_____

13. Attainable: _____

_____

14. Realistic: _____

_____

15. Timed: _____

Planning Nursing Interventions

There are three categories of interventions, and category selection is based on the patient's needs. Define each.

16. Independent nursing interventions: _____

_____

17. Dependent nursing interventions: _____

_____

18. Interdependent interventions: _____

_____

19. Identify the six factors the nurse uses to select nursing interventions for a specific patient.

a. _____

b. _____

c. _____

d. _____

e. _____

f. _____

Systems for Planning Nursing Care

20. Define the purposes of the *nursing care plan.*

_____

_____

Briefly explain the following types of care plans.

21. Briefly explain what a interprofessional care plan is: _____

_____

22. Explain the process of "nursing handoffs" as a practice of communication information at the end of the shift.

_____

_____

Consulting With Health Care Professionals

23. Consultation is a process in which: _____

_____

24. List the six steps of the nurse's role when seeking consultation.

a. _____

b. _____

c. _____

d. _____

e. _____

f. _____

CASE STUDY

25. A nurse completes a respiratory assessment on a patient who had abdominal surgery 1 day ago. During the assessment, the nurse auscultates crackles in both lower lobes, and the patient coughs, producing light yellow sputum. The patient's temperature is 37° C, pulse is 110 beats/min, respiratory rate is 28 breaths/min, and blood pressure is 118/82 mm Hg. Pulse oximetry was 99% and is now 93%. The nurse identifies a nursing diagnosis of impaired gas exchange.

a. What type of priority is this?

b. What is a goal for this patient?

REVIEW QUESTIONS

Select the appropriate answer and cite the rationale for choosing that particular answer.

26. The following statement appears on the nursing care plan for an immunosuppressed patient: "The patient will remain free from infection throughout hospitalization." This statement is an example of a (an):
1. Long-term goal
2. Short-term goal
3. Nursing diagnosis
4. Expected outcome

Answer: _____

Rationale: _____

_____

_____

27. The following statements appear on a nursing care plan for a patient after a mastectomy: "Incision site approximated; absence of drainage or prolonged erythema at incision site; and patient remains afebrile." These statements are examples of:
1. Long-term goals
2. Short-term goals
3. Nursing diagnosis
4. Expected outcomes

Answer: _____

Rationale: _____

_____

_____

28. The planning step of the nursing process includes which of the following activities?
1. Assessing and diagnosing
2. Evaluating goal achievement
3. Setting goals and selecting interventions
4. Performing nursing actions and documenting them

Answer: _____

Rationale: _____

_____

_____

19 Implementing Nursing Care

PRELIMINARY READING

Chapter 19

COMPREHENSIVE UNDERSTANDING

1. Define the fourth step of the nursing process.

   _____

   _____

2. Define the following terms related to a nursing intervention.

   a. Direct care: _____

   b. Indirect care: _____

3. List the domains of nursing practice when intervening with patients.

   a. _____

   b. _____

   c. _____

   d. _____

   e. _____

   f. _____

   g. _____

Standard Nursing Interventions

Define the following terms.

4. Clinical practice guideline: _____

   _____

5. Standing order: _____

   _____

6. Nursing Interventions Classification (NIC): _____

   _____

Critical Thinking in Implementation

7. Briefly explain the activities for making decisions during implementation.

   a. _____

   b. _____

   c. _____

   d. _____

75

Implementation Process

Briefly explain the five preparatory activities for implementation of safe and effective nursing care.

8. Reassess the patient: _____

_____

9. Review and revise the existing nursing care plan: _____

_____

10. Organize resources and care delivery: _____

_____

11. Anticipate and prevent complications: _____

_____

12. Implement nursing interventions: _____

_____

Direct Care

13. Define activities of daily living (ADLs).

_____

_____

14. Instrumental activities of daily living (IADLs) include: _____

_____

_____

15. Physical care techniques include: _____

_____

_____

16. Lifesaving measures are: _____

_____

_____

17. Counseling is: _____

_____

_____

18. Teaching involves: _____

_____

_____

19. An adverse reaction is: _____

_____

_____

20. Preventive nursing interventions are: _____

_____

_____

21. Indirect care measures: _____

_____

_____

Achieving Patient Outcomes

22. Patient adherence is: _____

_____

_____

CASE STUDY

23. You are beginning your day shift, and one of you have been assigned to care for an 84-year-old patient who recently was admitted with symptoms of a lung infection. You are reviewing and revising the nursing care plan. Identify the steps that you would take.

REVIEW QUESTIONS

Select the appropriate answer and cite the rationale for choosing that particular answer.

24. Which of the following is not true of standing orders?
    1. Standing orders are commonly found in critical care and community health settings.
    2. Standing orders are approved and signed by the health care provider in charge of care before implementation.
    3. With standing orders, nurses have the legal protection to intervene appropriately in the patient's best interest.
    4. With standing orders, the nurse relies on the health care provider's judgment to determine if the intervention is appropriate.

    Answer: _____

    Rationale: _____

    _____

    _____

25. The nursing care plan calls for the patient, a 300-lb woman, to be turned every 2 hours. The patient is unable to assist with turning. The nurse knows that she may hurt her back if she attempts to turn the patient by herself. The nurse should:
    1. Turn the patient by herself
    2. Ask another nurse to help her turn the patient
    3. Rewrite the care plan to eliminate the need for turning
    4. Ignore the intervention related to turning in the care plan

    Answer: _____

    Rationale: _____

    _____

    _____

77

26. Mrs. Kay comes to the family clinic for birth control. The nurse obtains a health history and performs a pelvic examination and Pap test. The nurse is functioning according to:
    1. Protocol
    2. Standing order
    3. Nursing care plan
    4. Intervention strategy

    Answer: _____

    Rationale: _____

    _____

    _____

27. Mary Jones is a newly diagnosed patient with diabetes. The nurse shows Mary how to administer an injection. This intervention activity is:
    1. Teaching
    2. Managing
    3. Counseling

    Answer: _____

    Rationale: _____

    _____

    _____

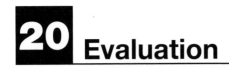

Evaluation

PRELIMINARY READING

Chapter 20

COMPREHENSIVE UNDERSTANDING

Critical Judgment and Critical Thinking in Evaluation

1. Evaluation is the fifth step of the nursing process that determines:

   _____

   _____

2. Identify the four actions that show a nurse is competent to perform an evaluation.

   a. _____

   b. _____

   c. _____

   d. _____

Experience

3. Identify the three key themes for recognizing patient deterioration:

   a. _____

   b. _____

   c. _____

Standards and Attitudes for Evaluation

4. Identify the competencies for evaluation:

   a. _____

   b. _____

   c. _____

   d. _____

5. Briefly explain criterion-based standards that are used in the evaluation process:

   _____

Evaluation Process

6. Evaluation is an ongoing process that includes a _____ or _____ with an established standard.

7. Evaluative measures are _____.

8. The benefits of the use of the Nursing Outcomes Classification (NOC) include:

    a. _____

    b. _____

    c. _____

9. List the steps to objectively evaluate the level of your patients success in achieving outcomes of care:

    a. _____

    b. _____

    c. _____

    d. _____

    e. _____

10. Reflection-in-action involves: _____

    _____

Briefly explain the following parts of the evaluative process.

11. Care plan revision: _____

    _____

    _____

12. Discontinuing a care plan: _____

    _____

13. Redefining the diagnosis: _____

14. Revising expected outcomes: _____

15. Revising interventions: _____

Document Outcomes

16. Identify the responsibilities of documenting and reporting.

    _____

    _____

Evaluation of Health care

17. Nurse-sensitive quality outcomes are significant health care problems because they _____,

    _____, and _____.

18. List the nurse-sensitive outcomes identified by National Data Base of Nursing Quality Indicators (NDNQI):

    a. _____

    b. _____

    c. _____

    d. _____

    e. _____

f. _____

g _____

h _____

i. _____

j. _____

CASE STUDY

19. A patient has a pressure injury resulting from urinary incontinence and sustained pressure over the coccyx. The nursing care plan includes a goal of "pressure injury heals in 3 weeks." Identify some appropriate evaluative measures for this goal.

REVIEW QUESTIONS

Select the appropriate answer and cite the rationale for choosing that particular answer.

20. Measuring the patient's response to nursing interventions and his or her progress toward achieving goals occurs during which phase of the nursing process?
    1. Planning
    2. Evaluation
    3. Assessment
    4. Nursing diagnosis

    Answer: _____

    Rationale: _____

    _____

    _____

21. The criteria used to determine the effectiveness of a nursing action are based on the:
    1. Nursing diagnosis
    2. Expected outcomes
    3. Patient's satisfaction
    4. Nursing interventions

    Answer: _____

    Rationale: _____

    _____

    _____

22. When a patient-centered goal has not been met in the projected time frame, the most appropriate action by the nurse would be to:
    1. Rewrite the plan using different interventions
    2. Continue with the same plan until the goal is met
    3. Repeat the entire sequence of the nursing process to discover needed changes
    4. Conclude that the goal was inappropriate or unrealistic and eliminate it from the plan

    Answer: _____

    Rationale: _____

    _____

    _____

23. Which of the following statements correctly describes the evaluation process? (Select all that apply.)
    1. Evaluation is an ongoing process.
    2. Evaluation usually reveals obvious changes in a patient.
    3. Evaluation involves making clinical decisions.
    4. Evaluation requires the use of assessment skills
    5. Evaluation is performed only when the patient's condition changes.

    Answer: _____

    Rationale: _____

    _____

    _____

21 Managing Patient Care

PRELIMINARY READING

Chapter 21

COMPREHENSIVE UNDERSTANDING

Building a Nursing Team

1. Effective team development requires _____, _____, _____, and _____.

2. When a nurse manager uses transformational leadership, they:

   a. _____

   b. _____

   c. _____

3. Identify the 12 characteristics of an effective nurse leader.

   a. _____

   b. _____

   c. _____

   d. _____

   e. _____

   f. _____

   g. _____

   h. _____

   i. _____

   j. _____

   k. _____

   l. _____

Match the following terms.

4. _____ Magnet recognition

5. _____ Team nursing

6. _____ Primary care

7. _____ Case management

8. _____ Shared governance

9. _____ Responsibility

10. _____ Autonomy

11. _____ Authority

12. _____ Accountability

13. _____ Interprofessional collaboration

a. Bringing representatives of various disciplines together to work with patients to improve quality of care
b. One RN assumes the responsibility for a caseload of patients throughout their hospitalization
c. Is the typical decentralized structure where managers and staff become more actively involved in decision making
d. The hospital has clinical promotion systems and research and evidence-based practice programs; nurses have professional autonomy over their practice
e. Care is provided by a group of people led by an RN
f. Duties and activities that an individual is employed to perform
g. Responsibility for the outcomes of the actions
h. Freedom of choice and responsibility for choices
i. Legal ability to perform a task
j. Approach that coordinates and links health care services to patients, streamlining costs and maintaining quality

14. List the responsibilities of nursing managers.

a. _____

b. _____

c. _____

d. _____

e. _____

f. _____

g. _____

h. _____

i. _____

j. _____

k. _____

l. _____

m. _____

n. _____

15. Identify the five approaches the nurse manager uses to support staff involvement.

a. _____

b. _____

c. _____

d. _____

e. _____

Leadership Skills for Nursing Students

Summarize each of the following skills.

16. Clinical judgement: _____
_____

17. Priority setting: _____
_____

18. Organizational skills: _____
_____

19. Use of resources: _____
_____

20. Time management: _____
_____

21. Evaluation: _____
_____

22. Team communication: _____
_____

23. List the principles of time management.

   a. _____
   b. _____
   c. _____
   d. _____
   e. _____

24. Identify the five rights of delegation.

   a. _____
   b. _____
   c. _____
   d. _____
   e. _____

25. Summarize the requirements for appropriate delegation.

   a. _____
   b. _____
   c. _____
   d. _____
   e. _____

26. As an RN caring for a patient who had bronchitis, what tasks can you delegate to a nursing assistant?

REVIEW QUESTIONS

Select the appropriate answer and cite the rationale for choosing that particular answer.

27. A student nurse practicing primary leadership skills would demonstrate all of the following except:
    1. Being sensitive to the group's feelings
    2. Recognizing others for their contributions
    3. Developing listening skills and being aware of personal motivation
    4. Assuming primary responsibility for planning, implementation, follow-up, and evaluation

    Answer: _____

    Rationale: _____

    _____

    _____

22 Ethics and Values

PRELIMINARY READING

Chapter 22

COMPREHENSIVE UNDERSTANDING

Basic Terms in Health Ethics

Match the following terms in health ethics.

1. _____ Autonomy

2. _____ Beneficence

3. _____ Nonmaleficence

4. _____ Justice

5. _____ Fidelity

a. The agreement to keep promises and the unwillingness to abandon patients
b. The best interests of the patient remain more important than self-interest
c. Fairness
d. Commitment to include patients in decisions about care
e. Avoidance of harm or hurt

Professional Nursing Code of Ethics

6. Identify and define the four basic principles of the code of ethics.

a. _____

b. _____

c. _____

d. _____

Values

Define the following terms.

7. Value: _____

_____

8. Values clarification: _____

_____

Approaches to Ethics

Briefly explain the following philosophical constructs in relation to ethical systems.

9. Deontology: _____

_____

10. Utilitarianism: _____

_____

11. Feminist ethics: _____

_____

86

12. Ethic of care: _____

_____

13. Casuistry: _____

_____

Nursing Point of View

14. List the key steps in the resolution of an ethical dilemma.

   a. _____

   b. _____

   c. _____

   d. _____

   e. _____

   f. _____

   g. _____

15. Identify the three major functions of the ethics committee.

   a. _____

   b. _____

   c. _____

Issues in Health Care Ethics

Briefly describe the current sources of ethical concerns.

16. Social media: _____

_____

17. Quality of life: _____

_____

18. Disabilities: _____

_____

19. End-of-life care: _____

_____

CASE STUDY

20. A nurse is caring for a 36-year-old with a brain tumor who is dying. The patient has undergone surgery and chemotherapy, but nothing has worked so far to stop the growth of the tumor. The physician offered the patient one further treatment plan that could prolong life for a few weeks, but the treatment has painful side effects. The patient tells his nurse that he is at peace with the prognosis and wants to stop all further treatment. The nurse is troubled by the patient's response. She feels confident that the side effects could be managed, and, for her, refusing treatment violates a belief in the sanctity of life. Identify the ethical principles at stake in this situation.

   a. _____

   b. _____

   c. _____

Select the appropriate answer and cite the rationale for choosing that particular answer.

21. A health care issue often becomes an ethical dilemma because:
    1. Decisions must be made based on value systems.
    2. The choices involved do not appear to be clearly right or wrong.
    3. Decisions must be made quickly, often under stressful conditions.
    4. A patient's legal rights coexist with a health professional's obligations.

    Answer: _____

    Rationale: _____

    _____

    _____

22. Which statement about an institutional ethics committee is correct?
    1. The ethics committee would be the first option in addressing an ethical dilemma.
    2. The ethics committee replaces decision making by the patient and health care providers.
    3. The ethics committee relieves health care professionals from dealing with ethical issues.
    4. The ethics committee provides education, policy recommendations, and case consultation.

    Answer: _____

    Rationale: _____

    _____

    _____

23. The nurse is working with the parents of a seriously ill newborn. Surgery has been proposed for the infant, but the chances of success are unclear. In helping the parents resolve this ethical conflict, the nurse knows that the first step is:
    1. Exploring reasonable courses of action
    2. Identifying people who can solve the difficulty
    3. Clarifying values related to the cause of the dilemma
    4. Collecting all available information about the situation

    Answer: _____

    Rationale: _____

    _____

    _____

24. The ANA *Code of Ethics for Nurses* articulates that the nurse "promotes, advocates for, and strives to protect the health, safety, and right of the patient." This promise to protect includes a promise to protect patient privacy. On the basis of this principle, if you participate in a public online social network such as Facebook, could you post images of a patient's x-ray film if you obscured or deleted all patient identifiers?
    1. Yes. Patient privacy would not be violated because patient identifiers were removed.
    2. Yes. Respect for autonomy implies that you have the autonomy to decide what constitutes privacy.
    3. No. A viewer might identify the patient based on other comments that you make online about the patient's condition and your place of work.
    4. No. The principle of justice requires you to allocate resources fairly.

    Answer: _____

    Rationale: _____

    _____

    _____

Legal Implications in Nursing Practice

PRELIMINARY READING

Chapter 23

COMPREHENSIVE UNDERSTANDING

Legal limits of Nursing

Match the following sources of law:

1. _____ Nurse Practice Acts

2. _____ Constitutional law

3. _____ Common law

4. _____ Criminal laws

5. _____ Statutory law

6. _____ Administrative law

7. _____ Civil laws

8. _____ Case Law

a. Decisions made in legal cases that were resolved in courts
b. Prevent harm to society and provide punishment for crimes
c. Derived from statues passed by the U.S. Congress and state legislatures
d. Protect the rights of individual persons within our society and encourage fair and equitable treatment
e. Describe and define the legal boundaries of nursing practice within each state
f. Judicial decisions made in courts when individual legal cases are decided
g. Reflects decisions made by administrative bodies
h. Is derived from federal and state constitutions

Scope and Standards of Nursing

9. Define the following:

a. Scope of nursing practice

_____

_____

b. Standards of nursing care

_____

_____

10. Standards of Nursing care are derived from:

a. _____

b. _____

c. _____

d. _____

e. _____

Federal Statutes Impacting Nursing Practice

Briefly explain the following.

11. Accountable Care Act (ACA): _____

_____

12. The ACA intends to reduce overall medical cost by:

a. _____

b. _____

c. _____

13. Americans With Disabilities Act (ADA): _____

_____

14. Health Information Technology for Economic and Clinical Health Act (HITECH act): _____

_____

15. Mental Health Parity and Addiction Equity Act (MHPAEA): _____

_____

16. Patient Self-Determination Act (PSDA): _____

_____

17. Uniform Anatomical Gift Act (UAGA): _____

_____

18. Health Information Technology Act (HITECH): _____

_____

19. Describe the focus of Omnibus Budget Reconciliation Act (OBRA): _____

_____

20. The Joint Commission's specific guidelines for the use of restraints are:

a. _____

b. _____

c. _____

State Statutes Impacting Nursing Practice

Explain the following issues that affect nursing practice on a state level.

21. Licensure: _____

_____

Explain the following statutory guidelines for legal consent.

22. Adults:

a. _____

b. _____

c. _____

d. _____

e. _____

23. Minors:

    a. _____

    b. _____

    c. _____

24. Unemancipated minors:

    a. _____

    b. _____

    c. _____

    d. _____

    e. _____

25. List the key elements of informed consent.

    a. _____

    b. _____

    c. _____

    d. _____

    e. _____

    f. _____

26. Good Samaritan laws: _____

_____

27. Public health laws: _____

_____

28. Uniform Determination of Death Act: _____

_____

Legal Implications and Reducing your Legal Risks

Match the following terms.

29. _____ Torts

30. _____ Unintentional torts

31. _____ Battery

32. _____ False imprisonment

33. _____ Invasion of privacy

34. _____ Slander

35. _____ Libel

36. _____ Negligence

37. _____ Malpractice

38. _____ Defamation of character

a. Publication of false statements that result in damage to a person's reputation
b. Referred to as professional negligence; below the standard of care
c. When one person speaks falsely about another person
d. Civil wrongful acts or omissions made against a person or property
e. Any intentional touching without consent
f. Written defamation of character
g. Arise when a person is harmed, and the person inflicting the harm knew, and the actions were less than the standard of practice
h. Unjustified restraining of a person without legal warrant
i. The release of a patient's medical information to an unauthorized person
j. Conduct that falls below the standard of care

Chapter **23 Legal Implications in Nursing Practice**

39. List the criteria that are necessary to establish nursing malpractice.

    a. _____

    b. _____

    c. _____

    d. _____

40. Briefly explain the following issues.

    a. Termination of pregnancy: _____

    b. Death with dignity: _____

Nursing Workforce guidelines

41. Briefly explain the following.

    a. Nursing student's liability:

    _____

    b. Staffing and nurse-to-patient ratio:

    _____

42. Prior to establishing a relationship, a nurse may refuse an assignment and it is not considered abandonment when:

    a. _____

    b. _____

    c. _____

    d. _____

    e. _____

    f. _____

Reducing legal risks

43. Identify the components of risk management. _____

    _____

44. Identify the purpose of the occurrence (incident) report.

    _____

    _____

CASE STUDY

45. You are a new graduate nurse working on a medical/surgical unit. One morning, you are floated to the labor and delivery unit for the day because it is very short staffed. You tell your charge nurse that you are uncomfortable working on a unit so different from your own. The charge nurse tells you that the labor and delivery charge nurse will make sure you have easy patients and will help you with anything you need. What should you do?

REVIEW QUESTIONS

Select the appropriate answer and cite the rationale for choosing that particular answer.

46. The scope of nursing practice is legally defined by:
    1. State nurse practice acts
    2. Professional nursing organizations
    3. Hospital policy and procedure manuals
    4. Health care providers in the employing institutions

    Answer: _____

    Rationale: _____

    _____

    _____

47. A student nurse who is employed as a nursing assistant may perform any functions that:
    1. Have been learned in school
    2. Are expected of a nurse at that level
    3. Are identified in the position's job description
    4. Require technical rather than professional skill

    Answer: _____

    Rationale: _____

    _____

    _____

48. A confused patient who fell out of bed because side rails were not used is an example of which type of liability?
    1. Felony
    2. Battery
    3. Assault
    4. Negligence

    Answer: _____

    Rationale: _____

    _____

    _____

49. The nurse puts restraints on a patient without the patient's permission and without a physician's order. The nurse may be guilty of:
    1. Battery
    2. Assault
    3. Neglect
    4. Invasion of privacy

    Answer: _____

    Rationale: _____

    _____

    _____

50. In a situation in which there is insufficient staff to implement competent care, a nurse should:
    1. Organize a strike
    2. Refuse the assignment
    3. Inform the patients of the situation
    4. Accept the assignment but make a protest in writing to the administration

    Answer: _____

    Rationale: _____

    _____

    _____

24 Communication

PRELIMINARY READING

Chapter 24

COMPREHENSIVE UNDERSTANDING

Communication and Nursing Practice

1. Communication is: _____

_____

2. For the nurse to be able to relate to others, he or she must have the ability to:

    a. _____

    b. _____

    c. _____

3. Critical thinking and clinical judgment help nurses over come _____ or _____ that interfere with accurately perceiving and interpreting messages from others.

Match the following levels of communication.

4. _____ Intrapersonal

5. _____ Interpersonal

6. _____ Small group

7. _____ Public

8. _____ Electronic

a. Interaction with an audience
b. The use of technology to create ongoing relationships
c. Develops self-awareness and a positive self-esteem
d. One-to-one interaction between a nurse and another person
e. Interaction that occurs with a small number of persons

Elements of the Communication Process

Match the following terms that address communication.

9. _____ Referent

10. _____ Sender

11. _____ Receiver

12. _____ Message

13. _____ Channels

14. _____ Feedback

15. _____ Interpersonal variables

16. _____ Environment

17. _____ Verbal communication

18. _____ Connotative meaning

19. _____ Intonation

20. _____ Timing

21. _____ Pacing

22. _____ Clarity and brevity

a. Factors within both the sender and the receiver that influence communication

b. Code that conveys specific meaning through the combination of spoken words

c. Person who encodes and delivers the message

d. Simple, brief, and direct

e. Thinking before speaking and developing an awareness of the rhythm of your speech

f. Person who decodes the message

g. Motivates one person to communicate with another

h. Setting for the sender–receiver interaction

i. Interpretation of a word's meaning influenced by the thoughts and feelings that people have about the word

j. Content of the communication

k. Tone of voice

l. Means of conveying and receiving messages through the senses

m. Indicates whether the receiver understood the meaning of the sender's message

n. When a patient expresses an interest in communicating

23. State three aspects of nonverbal communication.

a. _____

b. _____

c. _____

24. Identify the four zones of personal space.

a. _____

b. _____

c. _____

d. _____

Professional Nursing Relationships

25. List the four goal-directed phases that characterize the nurse–patient relationship.

a. _____

b. _____

c. _____

d. _____

26. Motivational interviewing (MI) is a: _____

_____

Explain the focus of the following relationships.

27. Nurse–family: _____

_____

28. Nurse–health care team: _____

    _____

29. Give some examples of lateral violence or workplace bullying. _____

    _____

30. Identify some techniques the nurse can use when experiencing lateral violence.

    a. _____

    b. _____

    c. _____

    d. _____

    e. _____

    f. _____

    g. _____

Elements of Professional Communication

31. List the elements of professional communication.

    a. _____

    b. _____

    c. _____

    d. _____

    e. _____

32. Define the following terms.

    a. Autonomy: _____

    _____

    b. Assertiveness: _____

    _____

Nursing Process

Assessment

33. Explain the following factors that affect communication.

    a. Psychophysiological context: _____

    _____

    b. Relational context: _____

    _____

    c. Situational context: _____

    _____

    d. Environmental context: _____

    _____

    e. Cultural context: _____

    _____

96

34. Give some examples of how to communicate with the older adults who have a hearing loss.

a. _____

b. _____

c. _____

d. _____

e. _____

f. _____

g. _____

h. _____

i. _____

35. Gender influences communication. Explain how communication differs in regard to gender.

a. Male: _____

_____

b. Female: _____

_____

Analysis and Nursing Diagnosis

36. The primary diagnosis used to describe the patient with limited or no ability to communicate is: _____

_____

37. Identify the defining characteristics of the diagnosis above.

_____

_____

38. Identify the related factors that contribute to the above diagnosis.

_____

_____

Planning and Outcomes Identification

39. List the goals and outcomes for the patient with the above diagnosis.

a. _____

b. _____

c. _____

d. _____

Implementation

Match the following therapeutic communication techniques.

40. _____ Active listening

41. _____ Sharing observations

42. _____ Sharing empathy

43. _____ Sharing hope

44. _____ Sharing humor

45. _____ Sharing feelings

46. _____ Using touch

47. _____ Using silence

48. _____ Providing information

49. _____ Clarifying

50. _____ Focusing

51. _____ Paraphrasing

52. _____ Asking relevant questions

53. _____ Summarizing

54. _____ Self-disclosure

55. _____ Confrontation

a. Subjective feelings that result from one's thoughts and perceptions
b. Used to center on key elements or concepts of the message
c. Concise review of key aspects of an interaction
d. Subjectively true, personal experiences about self that are intentionally revealed to another
e. Being attentive to what the patient is saying both verbally and nonverbally
f. Strategy that can reduce anxiety and promote positive feelings
g. This technique can help start a conversation with a patient who is quiet or withdrawn
h. Helping the patient become aware of inconsistencies in his or her feelings, attitudes, beliefs, and behaviors
i. Seeking information needed for decision making
j. Restating another's message more briefly using one's own words
k. Restating an unclear or ambiguous message
l. Patients have the right to know about their health status and what is happening in their environment
m. Ability to understand and accept another person's reality
n. Allows a patient to think and gain insight
o. "Sense of possibility"
p. Most potent and personal form of communication

Match the following nontherapeutic communication techniques with the appropriate responses.

56. _____ Asking personal questions

57. _____ Giving personal opinions

58. _____ Changing the subject

59. _____ Autonomic responses

60. _____ False reassurance

61. _____ Sympathy

62. _____ Asking for explanations

63. _____ Approval or disapproval

64. _____ Defensive responses

65. _____ Passive responses

66. _____ Arguing

a. "No one here would intentionally lie to you."
b. "How can you say you didn't sleep a wink? You were snoring all night long."
c. "I'm so sorry about your mastectomy; it must be terrible to lose a breast."
d. "You shouldn't even think about assisted suicide; it is not right."
e. "Why are you so anxious?"
f. "Older adults are always confused."
g. "Why don't you and John get married?"
h. "Don't worry; everything will be all right."
i. "Things are bad, and there's nothing I can do about it."
j. "Let's not talk about your problems with the insurance company. It's time for your walk."
k. "If I were you, I'd put your mother in a nursing home."

Briefly explain how to communicate with patients who have special needs.

67. Cannot speak clearly (aphasia, dysarthria, muteness): _____

_____

68. Cognitive impairment: _____

_____

69. Hearing impairment: _____

_____

70. Visually impaired: _____

_____

71. Unresponsive: _____

_____

72. Does not speak English: _____

_____

Evaluation

73. Identify what the process recording analysis reveals.

a. _____

b. _____

c. _____

d. _____

e. _____

f. _____

g. _____

CASE STUDY

74. A family member angrily tells the nurse, "No one told me that my husband was back in his room after surgery. I have been waiting and worrying for 3 hours!" How might the nurse reply to the wife?

REVIEW QUESTIONS

Select the appropriate answer and cite the rationale for choosing that particular answer.

75. In demonstrating the method for deep breathing exercises, the nurse places his or her hands on the patient's abdomen to explain diaphragmatic movement. This technique involves the use of which communication element?
    1. Referent
    2. Message
    3. Feedback
    4. Tactile channel

    Answer: _____

    Rationale: _____

    _____

    _____

76. Which statement about nonverbal communication is correct?
    1. The nurse's verbal messages should be reinforced by nonverbal cues.
    2. It is easy for a nurse to judge the meaning of a patient's facial expression.
    3. The physical appearance of the nurse rarely influences nurse–patient interaction.
    4. Words convey meanings that are usually more significant than nonverbal communication.

    Answer: _____

    Rationale: _____

    _____

    _____

77. The term referring to the sender's attitude toward the self, the message, and the listener is:
   1. Denotative meaning
   2. Metacommunication
   3. Connotative meaning
   4. Nonverbal communication

   Answer: _____

   Rationale: _____

   _____

   _____

78. The referent in the communication process is:
   1. Information shared by the sender
   2. The means of conveying messages
   3. That which motivates the communication
   4. The person who initiates the communication

   Answer: _____

   Rationale: _____

   _____

   _____

79. A nurse is conducting an admission interview with a patient. To maintain the patient's territoriality and maximize communication, the nurse should sit:
   1. 4 to 12 feet from the patient
   2. 0 to 18 inches from the patient
   3. 12 feet or more from the patient
   4. 18 inches to 4 feet from the patient

   Answer: _____

   Rationale: _____

   _____

   _____

25 Patient Education

PRELIMINARY READING

Chapter 25

COMPREHENSIVE UNDERSTANDING

Purposes of Patient Education

Briefly explain patient education in each phase of health care.

1. Maintenance and promotion of health and illness prevention: _____

   _____

2. Restoration of health: _____

   _____

3. Coping with impaired functions: _____

   _____

Teaching and Learning

Match the following terms.

4. _____ Teaching

5. _____ Learning

6. _____ Learning objective

7. _____ Cognitive learning

8. _____ Affective learning

9. _____ Psychomotor learning

10. _____ Domains of learning

11. _____ Motivation

12. _____ Self-efficacy

a. Cognitive, affective, and psychomotor
b. A person's perceived ability to successfully complete a task
c. Imparting knowledge through a series of directed activities
d. Internal state that helps arouse, direct, and sustain human behavior
e. Integration of mental and muscular activity, ranging from perception to origination
f. Describes what the learner will be able to do after successful instruction
g. Receiving, responding, valuing, organizing, and characterizing
h. Acquisition of new knowledge, behaviors, and skills
i. Knowledge, comprehension, application analysis, synthesis, and evaluation

13. Identify the six ACCESS model components.

   a. _____

   b. _____

   c. _____

   d. _____

   e. _____

   f. _____

14. Identify the factors that affect readiness to learn.

   a. _____

   b. _____

   c. _____

Summarize how each of the following influences the ability to learn.

15. Developmental capability: _____

_____

16. Learning in children: _____

_____

17. Adult learning: _____

_____

18. Physical capability: _____

_____

Nursing Process

19. Explain how the nursing process and the teaching process differ.

   a. The nursing process requires: _____

   _____

   b. The teaching process focuses on: _____

   _____

Assessment

Success in teaching the patient requires the nurse to assess the following factors. List the elements of each factor.

20. Learning needs:

   a. _____

   b. _____

   c. _____

21. Motivation to learn:

   a. _____

   b. _____

   c. _____

   d. _____

   e. _____

   f. _____

   g. _____

   h. _____

22. Ability to learn (cognitive and physical ability):

    a. _____

    b. _____

    c. _____

    d. _____

    e. _____

    f. _____

    g. _____

23. Teaching environment:

    a. _____

    b. _____

    c. _____

24. Resources for learning:

    a. _____

    b. _____

    c. _____

    d. _____

    e. _____

Analysis and Nursing Diagnosis

25. Identify nursing diagnoses that indicate a need for education.

    a. _____

    b. _____

    c. _____

    d. _____

    e. _____

Planning and Outcomes Identification

The principles of teaching are techniques that incorporate the principles of learning. Explain the following principles.

26. Learning outcomes: _____

    _____

27. Setting priorities: _____

    _____

28. Timing: _____

    _____

29. Organizing teaching material: _____

    _____

Implementation

Match the following teaching approaches.

30. _____ Telling

31. _____ Participating

32. _____ Entrusting

33. _____ Reinforcement

34. _____ One-on-one discussion

35. _____ Group instruction

36. _____ Return demonstration

37. _____ Analogies

38. _____ Role-play

39. _____ Simulation

a. Economical way to teach a number of patients at one time
b. The nurse poses a pertinent problem or situation for patients to solve, which provides an opportunity to identify mistakes
c. The nurse outlines the task the patient will perform and gives explicit instructions
d. Supplement verbal instruction with familiar images
e. The nurse and patient set objectives and become involved in the learning process together
f. People play themselves or someone else
g. The chance to practice the skill
h. Most common method of instruction
i. Provides the patient with the opportunity to manage self-care
j. Using a stimulus that increases the probability for a response

Evaluation

40. Identify the nurse's responsibility in evaluating the outcomes of the teaching learning process. _____

_____

_____

CASE STUDY

41. A nurse is teaching an older-adult patient about poststroke seizures. What teaching method would be appropriate to use?

REVIEW QUESTIONS

Select the appropriate answer and cite the rationale for choosing that particular answer.

42. An internal impulse that causes a person to take action is:
    1. Anxiety
    2. Motivation
    3. Adaptation
    4. Compliance

    Answer: _____

    Rationale: _____

    _____

    _____

43. Demonstration of the principles of body mechanics used when transferring patients from bed to chair would be classified under which domain of learning?
    1. Social
    2. Affective
    3. Cognitive
    4. Psychomotor

    Answer: _____

    Rationale: _____

    _____

    _____

44. Which of the following patients is most ready to begin a patient-teaching session?
    1. Ms. Hernandez, who is unwilling to accept that her back injury may result in permanent paralysis.
    2. Mr. Frank, who is newly diagnosed with diabetes, who is complaining that he was awake all night because of his noisy roommate.
    3. Mrs. Brown, a patient with irritable bowel syndrome, who has just returned from a morning of testing in the gastrointestinal laboratory.
    4. Mr. Jones, a patient who had a heart attack 4 days ago and now seems somewhat anxious about how this will affect his future.

    Answer: _____

    Rationale: _____

    _____

    _____

45. The nurse works with pediatric patients who have diabetes. Which is the youngest age group to which the nurse can effectively teach psychomotor skills such as insulin administration?
    1. Toddler
    2. Preschool
    3. School age
    4. Adolescent

    Answer: _____

    Rationale: _____

    _____

    _____

46. Which of the following is an appropriately stated learning objective for Mr. Ryan, who is newly diagnosed with diabetes?
    1. Mr. Ryan will understand diabetes.
    2. Mr. Ryan will be taught self-administration of insulin by 5/2.
    3. Mr. Ryan will know the signs and symptoms of low blood sugar by 5/5.
    4. Mr. Ryan will perform blood glucose monitoring with the EZ-Check Monitor by the time of discharge.

    Answer: _____

    Rationale: _____

    _____

    _____

26 Informatics and Documentation

Chapter 26

COMPREHENSIVE UNDERSTANDING

Define the following term.

1. Documentation: _____

_____

Purposes of the Health Care Record

Match the following purposes of a record.

2. _____ Interprofessional communication

3. _____ Legal documentation

4. _____ Diagnostic-related groups (DRGs)

5. _____ Education

6. _____ Research

7. _____ Auditing

a. Objective, ongoing reviews to determine the degree to which quality improvement standards are met
b. Learning the nature of an illness and the individual patient's responses
c. Means by which patient needs and progress, individual therapies, patient education, and discharge planning are conveyed to others in the health care team
d. Gathering of statistical data of clinical disorders, complications, therapies, recovery, and deaths
e. Describes exactly what happens to the patient and must follow organizational standards
f. Classification system based on patients' medical diagnoses that supports reimbursement

8. The term electronic medical record (**EMR**) refers to: _____

_____

9. The term electronic health record (**EHR**) refers to: _____

_____

10. Meaningful use requires that use of the electronic health record system (**EHRS**) results in:

    a. _____

    b. _____

    c. _____

    d. _____

    e. _____

11. According to HIPAA (Health Insurance Portability and Accountability Act), to eliminate barriers that could delay care, providers are:

    a. _____

    b. _____

106

12. What is the purpose of a firewall? _____

Standards and Guidelines for Quality Nursing Documentation

13. To maintain institutional accreditation, current documentation standards require that all patients admitted to a health care agency be assessed for: _____

_____

Standards and Guidelines for Quality Documentation

Five important guidelines must be followed to ensure quality documentation and reporting. Explain each one.

14. Factual: _____

_____

15. Accurate: _____

_____

16. Complete: _____

_____

17. Current: _____

_____

18. Organized: _____

_____

Methods of Documentation

Match the following documentation systems used for recording patient data.

19. _____ Narrative

20. _____ Focus charting

21. _____ PIE notes

22. _____ Charting by exception

a. Focuses on deviations from the established norm or abnormal findings
b. Uses data, action, and response (DAR)
c. Problem, intervention, and evaluation
d. Storylike format

Common Record Keeping Forms within the Electronic Health Record

Match the following formats used for record keeping.

23. _____ Admission nursing history forms

24. _____ Flow sheets

25. _____ Patient care summary

26. _____ Acuity records

27. _____ Standardized care plans

28. _____ Discharge summary forms

a. Includes medications, diet, community resources, and follow-up care
b. Level is based on the type and number of nursing interventions required over a 24-hour period
c. Provides current information that is accessible to all members of the health care team
d. Provides baseline data to compare with changes in the patient's condition
e. Provides the most current information that has been entered into the EHR
f. Preprinted, established guidelines used to care for the patient

Documenting Communication With Providers and Unique Events

29. List the information that needs to be documented with telephone reports.

    _____

30. List the guidelines the nurse should follow when receiving telephone and verbal orders from health care providers.

    a. _____

    b. _____

    c. _____

    d. _____

    e. _____

    f. _____

31. An incident or occurrence reports are _____. Give some examples
    of incidents.

    _____

    _____

Case Management and Use of Critical Pathways

32. Define case management: _____

33. Define critical pathways: _____

34. When does a variance occur within a critical pathway?

    _____

Informatics and Information Management in Health Care

35. Define health informatic technology (HIT).

    _____

    _____

36. Identify the nursing clinical information systems (NCIS) that are available.

    a. _____

    b. _____

37. Identify the advantages of a nursing clinical information system.

    a. _____

    b. _____

    c. _____

    d. _____

    e. _____

    f. _____

    g. _____

    h. _____

38. Define nursing informatics. _____

CASE STUDY

39. A patient is being discharged to an acute rehabilitation facility. You need to print some information from the patient's health care record and fax it to that facility. What actions would the nurse take to maintain privacy and confidentiality of the patient's information in providing the health record information to the acute rehabilitation facility?

REVIEW QUESTIONS

Select the appropriate answer and cite the rationale for choosing that particular answer.

40. The primary purpose of a patient's medical record is to:
    1. Provide validation for hospital charges
    2. Satisfy requirements of accreditation agencies
    3. Provide the nurse with a defense against malpractice
    4. Communicate accurate, timely information about the patient

    Answer: _____

    Rationale: _____

    _____

    _____

41. Which of the following is correctly charted according to the six guidelines for quality recording?
    1. Was depressed today.
    2. Respirations rapid; lung sounds clear.
    3. Had a good day. Up and about in room.
    4. Crying. States she doesn't want visitors to see her like this.

    Answer: _____

    Rationale: _____

    _____

    _____

42. During a change-of-shift report:
    1. Two or more nurses always visit all patients to review their plan of care.
    2. The nurse should identify nursing diagnoses and clarify patient priorities.
    3. Nurses should exchange judgments they have made about patient attitudes.
    4. Patient information is communicated from a nurse on a sending unit to a nurse on a receiving unit.

    Answer: _____

    Rationale: _____

    _____

    _____

43. An incident report is:
    1. A legal claim against a nurse for negligent nursing care
    2. A summary report of all falls occurring on a nursing unit
    3. A report of an event inconsistent with the routine care of a patient
    4. A report of a nurse's behavior submitted to the hospital administration

    Answer: _____

    Rationale: _____

    _____

    _____

44. You work in a health care agency that uses EHR. Which nursing actions are inappropriate? (Select all that apply.)
    1. Allow a temporary staff member to use your computer user name and password.
    2. Remain logged into a computer when you leave to administer a medication.
    3. Prevent others from seeing a display monitor that contains patient information
    4. Allow a health care provider to quickly enter an order using the computer that you are currently logged into to document patient care.

    Answer: _____

    Rationale: _____

    _____

    _____

27 Patient Safety and Quality

PRELIMINARY READING

Chapter 27

COMPREHENSIVE UNDERSTANDING

1. Identify The Joint Commission 2021 National Patient Safety Goals.

   a. _____

   b. _____

   c. _____

   d. _____

   e. _____

   f. _____

   g. _____

Scientific Knowledge Base

2. Identify Maslow's hierarchy of basic needs that influence a person's safety.

   a. _____

   b. _____

   c. _____

3. List the physical hazards in the environment that threaten a person's safety.

   a. _____

   b. _____

   c. _____

   d. _____

   e. _____

Define the following terms.

4. Pathogen: _____

5. Immunization: _____

6. Pollutant: _____

Nursing Knowledge Base

7. In addition to being knowledgeable about the environment, nurses must be familiar with:

   a. _____

   b. _____

   c. _____

   d. _____

8. Identify the individual risk factors that can pose a threat to safety.

   a. _____

   b. _____

   c. _____

   d. _____

9. List the four major risks to patient safety in the health care environment.

   a. _____

   b. _____

   c. _____

   d. _____

Nursing Process

Assessment

10. Identify the specific patient assessments to perform when considering possible threats to the patient's safety.

    a. _____

    b. _____

    c. _____

    d. _____

Analysis and Nursing Diagnosis

11. Identify actual or potential nursing diagnoses that apply to patients whose safety is threatened.

    a. _____

    b. _____

    c. _____

    d. _____

Implementation

12. Identify the strategies needed to provide safe nursing care.

    a. _____

    b. _____

    c. _____

    d. _____

Give an example(s) of an intervention for the following developmental stages.

13. Infant and toddler: _____

14. Preschooler: _____

15. School-age child: _____

16. Adolescent: _____

17. Adult: _____

18. Older-adult: _____

19. Nursing interventions directed at eliminating environmental threats include:

   a. _____

   b. _____

   c. _____

20. The Joint Commission recommends that hospitals have formal fall-reduction programs, which include a fall risk assessment of every patient conducted:

   a. _____

   b. _____

21. A physical restraint is: _____

22. A chemical restraint is: _____

23. Use of restraints must meet one of the following objectives.

   a. _____

   b. _____

   c. _____

   d. _____

24. Explain the mnemonic RACE to set priorities in case of fire.

   a. R: _____

   b. A: _____

   c. C: _____

   d. E: _____

25. Explain seizure precautions.

   _____

   _____

26. The Joint Commission (2020) requires that hospitals have an emergency management plan that addresses:

   a. _____

   b. _____

   c. _____

27. The nurse finds a 68-year-old woman wandering in the hallway and exhibiting confused behavior. The patient says that she is looking for the bathroom. State some interventions that would be appropriate to ensure the safety of this patient.

REVIEW QUESTIONS

Select the appropriate answer and cite the rationale for choosing that particular answer.

28. Which of the following would most immediately threaten an individual's safety?
    1. 70% humidity
    2. A sprained ankle
    3. Lack of water
    4. Unrefrigerated fresh vegetables

    Answer: _____

    Rationale: _____

    _____

    _____

29. The developmental stage that carries the highest risk of an injury from a fall is:
    1. Preschool
    2. Adulthood
    3. School-age
    4. Older-adulthood

    Answer: _____

    Rationale: _____

    _____

    _____

30. Mrs. Field falls asleep while smoking in bed and drops the burning cigarette on her blanket. When she awakens, her bed is on fire, and she quickly calls the nurse. On observing the fire, the nurse should immediately:
    1. Report the fire
    2. Attempt to extinguish the fire
    3. Assist Mrs. Field to a safe place
    4. Close all windows and doors to contain the fire

    Answer: _____

    Rationale: _____

    _____

    _____

31. Place the following steps for applying a wrist restraint in the correct order.
    1. Pad the skin overlying the wrist
    2. Insert two fingers under secured restraint to be sure it is not too tight
    3. Be sure the patient is comfortable and in correct anatomical alignment
    4. Secure restraint straps to bed frame with quick-release buckle
    5. Wrap limb restraint around wrist or ankle with soft part toward skin and secure snugly

    Answer: _____

    Rationale: _____

    _____

    _____

32. Imagine that you are Mr. Key, the nurse in the care plan in Chapter 27 of your text. Complete the *Assessment phase* of the critical thinking model with these questions in mind.

    a. As you review your assessment, what key areas did you cover?

    _____

    b. In developing Ms. Cohen's plan of care, what knowledge did Mr. Key apply?

    _____

    c. In what way might Mr. Key's previous experience assist in this case?

    _____

    d. What intellectual or professional standards were applied to Ms. Cohen?

    _____

    e. What critical thinking attitudes might have been applied in this case?

    _____

Next Generation NCLEX® Examination-Style Questions

33. For each patient presented, click or highlight to specify the nursing teaching that is most appropriate for the safety of the patient. Each patient presented may have more than one potential nursing teaching. Each patient must have at least one response option selected.

Patient	Potential Nursing Teaching
6-month-old infant weighing 9.5 kg (21 pounds)	Use a three point harness, forward-facing safety seat.
	The infant should remain rear-facing for as long as possible.
	A convertible seat is the only option for your infant.
8-year-old child that is 4 feet 4 inches tall	This child can sit in the front seat with a lap and shoulder restraint.
	Be sure to use a booster seat for your child.
	A forward-facing harness restraint is the safest option.
4-year-old that weighs 20.8 kg (46 pounds)	Use a rear facing convertible safety seat.
	A booster seat with a lab and shoulder restraint is the best option.
	A forward-facing, car safety seat with a harness is recommended.

28 Infection Prevention and Control

PRELIMINARY READING

Chapter 28

COMPREHENSIVE UNDERSTANDING

Scientific Knowledge Base

Match the following terms that are related to the infectious process.

1. _____ Pathogen
2. _____ Colonization
3. _____ Infectious disease
4. _____ Communicable disease
5. _____ pH
6. _____ Portal of exit
7. _____ Major route of transmission
8. _____ Virulence
9. _____ Susceptibility
10. _____ Immunocompromised
11. _____ Reservoir
12. _____ Carriers
13. _____ Aerobic bacteria
14. _____ Anaerobic bacteria
15. _____ Bacteriostasis
16. _____ Bactericidal

a. Individual's degree of resistance to pathogens
b. Persons who show no symptoms of illness but who have the pathogens that are transferred to others
c. Prevention of the growth and reproduction of bacteria by cold temperatures
d. Infectious agent
e. Bacteria that require oxygen for survival
f. Having an impaired immune system
g. Acidity of the environment
h. Bacteria that thrive with little or no free oxygen
i. A temperature or chemical that destroys bacteria
j. A place where a pathogen survives
k. Unwashed hands of a health care worker
l. An infectious disease that is transmitted directly from one person to another
m. Organism that multiplies within a host but without tissue invasion or damage
n. Sites such as blood, mucus membranes, respiratory tract, genitourinary tract, and gastrointestinal tract
o. If pathogens multiply and alter normal tissue function
p. Ability to survive in the host or outside the body

17. Development of an infection occurs in a cycle that depends on the following elements:

a. _____

b. _____

c. _____

d. _____

e. _____

f. _____

18. Explain the most common modes of transmission.

    a. Direct: _____

    b. Indirect: _____

    c. Droplet: _____

    d. Airborne: _____

    e. Vehicles: _____

    f. Vector: _____

The Infectious Process

19. Infections follow a progressive course by four stages. List and explain each stage.

    a. _____

    b. _____

    c. _____

    d. _____

20. Describe the two types of infections.

    a. Localized: _____

    _____

    b. Systemic: _____

    _____

21. Explain the normal body defenses against infection.

    a. Normal flora: _____

    _____

    b. Body system defenses: _____

    _____

    c. Inflammation: _____

    _____

22. Acute inflammation is an immediate response to cellular injury. Explain each briefly.

    a. Vascular and cellular responses: _____

    _____

    b. Inflammatory exudate: _____

    _____

    c. Tissue repair: _____

    _____

23. Health care–associated infections (HAIs) result from the following:

    a. _____

    b. _____

    c. _____

    d. _____

116

24. Identify the sites of health care–associated infections.

   a. _____

   b. _____

   c. _____

   d. _____

25. Define the following types of health care–associated infections (nosocomial).

   a. Exogenous: _____

   _____

   b. Endogenous: _____

   _____

   c. Iatrogenic: _____

   _____

Nursing Knowledge Base

26. The following factors influence a patient's susceptibility to infection. Briefly explain them, giving an example of each.

   a. Age: _____

   _____

   b. Nutritional status: _____

   _____

   c. Stress: _____

   _____

   d. Disease process: _____

   _____

   e. Sex differences: _____

   _____

Nursing Process

Assessment

27. Assess the patient for his or her defense mechanisms, susceptibility, and knowledge of how infections are transmitted. Briefly explain.

   a. Review of risk factors: _____

   b. Possible existing infections: _____

   c. Recent travel history: _____

   d. Medication history: _____

   e. Stressors : _____

28. Fill in the following table.

Laboratory Value	Normal (Adult) Values	Indication of Infection
WBC count		
Erythrocyte sedimentation rate		
Iron level		
Cultures of urine and blood		
Cultures and Gram stain of wound, sputum, and throat		
Neutrophils		
Lymphocytes		
Monocytes		
Eosinophils		
Basophils		

Analysis and Nursing Diagnosis

29. Identify some common nursing diagnoses that apply to patients at risk or who have an actual infection.

   a. _____

   b. _____

   c. _____

   d. _____

   e. _____

Planning and Outcomes Identification

30. List four common goals for a patient with an actual or potential risk for infection.

   a. _____

   b. _____

   c. _____

   d. _____

Implementation

31. List the ways a nurse can teach patients and their families to prevent an infection from developing or spreading in home and community settings.

   a. _____

   b. _____

   c. _____

   d. _____

32. The nurse follows certain principles and procedures to prevent infection and to control its spread. Briefly explain:

   a. Medical asepsis: _____

33. Explain the following methods of controlling or eliminating infectious agents.

   a. Disinfection: _____

   b. Sterilization: _____

34. Identify the factors that influence the efficacy of the disinfecting or sterilizing method.

   a. _____

   b. _____

   c. _____

   d. _____

   e. _____

   f. _____

35. Effective prevention and control of infection requires the nurse to be aware of the following reservoirs of infection:

   a. Bathing: _____

   b. Dressing changes: _____

   c. Contaminated articles: _____

   d. Contaminated sharps: _____

   e. Bedside unit: _____

   f. Bottled solutions: _____

   g. Surgical wounds: _____

   h. Drainage bottles and bags: _____

36. The elements of respiratory hygiene or cough etiquette are:

   a. _____

   b. _____

   c. _____

   d. _____

   e. _____

   f. _____

37. The basic technique in preventing and controlling the transmission of infection is hand hygiene. Identify the four techniques.

   a. _____

   b. _____

   c. _____

   d. _____

119

38. The CDC recommendations for isolation precautions contain two tiers of precautions. Briefly explain each one.

    a. The Standard precautions (tier 1): _____

    _____

    b. Isolation precautions (tier 2): _____

    _____

Briefly explain the following precautions and what they require.

39. Contact precautions: _____

40. Droplet precautions: _____

41. Airborne precautions: _____

Identify the rationale for the following personal protective equipment.

42. Gowns: _____

    _____

43. Masks: _____

    _____

44. Eye protection: _____

    _____

45. Gloves: _____

    _____

46. List the responsibilities of infection control professionals.

    a. _____

    b. _____

    c. _____

    d. _____

    e. _____

    f. _____

    g. _____

    h. _____

    i. _____

    j. _____

    k. _____

47. Identify clinical situations in which a nurse would use surgical asepsis.

    a. _____

    b. _____

    c. _____

120

48. List the seven principles of surgical asepsis.

a. _____

b. _____

c. _____

d. _____

e. _____

f. _____

g. _____

49. List, in order, the steps for performing a sterile procedure.

a. _____

b. _____

c. _____

d. _____

e. _____

f. _____

g. _____

h. _____

i. _____

j. _____

Evaluation

50. The expected outcome is the absence of signs and symptoms of infection. List some ways the nurse can monitor the patient.

a. _____

b. _____

c. _____

d. _____

CASE STUDY

51. A patient that you are caring for has been diagnosed with a multidrug-resistant organism in his surgical wound. He asks you as his nurse what it means to be on isolation. What is the best response to his question?

Select the appropriate answer and cite the rationale for choosing that particular answer.

52. The severity of a patient's illness depends on all of the following except:
   1. Incubation period
   2. Extent of infection
   3. Susceptibility of the host
   4. Pathogenicity of the microorganism

   Answer: _____

   Rationale: _____

   _____

   _____

53. Which of the following best describes an iatrogenic infection?
   1. It results from a diagnostic or therapeutic procedure.
   2. It results from an extended infection of the urinary tract.
   3. It involves an incubation period of 3 to 4 weeks before it can be detected.
   4. It occurs when patients are infected with their own organisms as a result of immunodeficiency.

   Answer: _____

   Rationale: _____

   _____

   _____

54. The nurse sets up a nonbarrier sterile field on the patient's overbed table. In which of the following instances is the field contaminated?
   1. Sterile saline solution is spilled on the field.
   2. The nurse, who has a cold, wears a double mask.
   3. Sterile objects are kept within a 1-inch border of the field.
   4. The nurse keeps the top of the table above his or her waist.

   Answer: _____

   Rationale: _____

   _____

   _____

55. When a patient on respiratory isolation must be transported to another part of the hospital, the nurse:
   1. Places a mask on the patient before leaving the room
   2. Obtains a health care provider's order to prohibit the patient from being transported
   3. Instructs the patient to cover his or her mouth and nose with a tissue when coughing or sneezing
   4. Advises other health team members to wear masks and gowns when coming in contact with the patient

   Answer: _____

   Rationale: _____

   _____

   _____

56. In what order would you prepare to enter the room of a patient in contact and droplet isolation precautions for MRSA?
   1. Put on eyewear
   2. Perform hand hygiene
   3. Put on gloves
   4. Put on mask
   5. Put on gown

   Answer: _____

   Rationale: _____

   _____

   _____

57. The nurse is caring for a 76-year-old patient who is admitted to rule out sepsis. The patient's vital signs are: Temperature 102.3° F (39° C); blood pressure 110/62 mmHg; heart rate 88 beats/min; respiratory rate 20 breaths/min; oxygen saturation 96% on room air. Current laboratory results are shown in the table. **Highlight the assessment data that would be anticipated with sepsis.**

Laboratory Results	Parameter	Result	Reference Range
	WBC	18,000	$5,000 - 10,000/mm^3$
	Neutrophils	45%	55% – 70%
	Lymphocytes	12%	20% – 40%
	Basophils	1%	0.5% – 1.5%

29 Vital Signs

Chapter 29

COMPREHENSIVE UNDERSTANDING

Guidelines for Measuring Vital Signs

1. Identify the guidelines that assist the nurse with incorporating vital sign measurements into practice.

   a. _____

   b. _____

   c. _____

   d. _____

   e. _____

   f. _____

   g. _____

   h. _____

   i. _____

   j. _____

   k. _____

   l. _____

   m. _____

Body Temperature

Match the following terms that address the physiology of body temperature.

2. _____ Core temperature

3. _____ Thermoregulation

4. _____ Hypothalamus

5. _____ Basal metabolic rate (BMR)

6. _____ Shivering

7. _____ Nonshivering thermogenesis

8. _____ Radiation

9. _____ Conduction

10. _____ Convection

11. _____ Evaporation

a. Involuntary body response to temperature differences in the body
b. Transfer of heat from the surface of one object to the surface of another without direct contact
c. Transfer of heat away by air movement
d. Transfer of heat energy when a liquid is changed to a gas
e. The heat produced by the body at absolute rest
f. Controls body temperature
g. Vascular brown tissue is metabolized for heat production in the neonate
h. Temperature of the deep tissues
i. Transfer of heat from one object to another with direct contact
j. Mechanisms that regulate the balance between heat lost and heat produced

12. Diaphoresis is: _____

_____

Chapter **29 Vital Signs**

Copyright © 2023 Elsevier, Inc. All rights reserved.

13. The skin regulates temperature through:

    a. _____

    b. _____

    c. _____

14. The ability of a person to control body temperature depends on:

    a. _____

    b. _____

    c. _____

    d. _____

15. Identify the factors that affect body temperature.

    a. _____

    b. _____

    c. _____

    d. _____

    e. _____

    f. _____

    g. _____

Match the following terms that address temperature alterations.

16. _____ Pyrexia

17. _____ Pyrogens

18. _____ Hyperthermia

19. _____ Malignant hyperthermia

20. _____ Heatstroke

21. _____ Heat exhaustion

22. _____ Hypothermia

23. _____ Frostbite

a. Occurs when the body is exposed to subnormal temperatures
b. The body's inability to promote heat loss or reduce heat production
c. A temperature of 40°C
d. Cold that overwhelms the body's ability to produce heat
e. Fever
f. Hereditary condition of uncontrolled heat production
g. Profuse diaphoresis with excess water and electrolyte loss
h. Bacteria and viruses that elevate body temperature

Nursing Process

Assessment

24. List at least one advantage and one disadvantage of each of the following temperature sites.

    a. Oral: _____

    b. Tympanic membrane: _____

    c. Rectal: _____

    d. Axilla: _____

    e. Skin: _____

    f. Temporal artery: _____

25. State the formulas for the following conversions.

    a. Fahrenheit to Celsius: _____

    b. Celsius to Fahrenheit: _____

Analysis and Nursing Diagnosis

26. Identify the nursing diagnoses related to thermoregulation.

    a. _____

    b. _____

    c. _____

    d. _____

    e. _____

Planning and Outcomes Identification

27. Provide examples of goals for temperature alterations related to the environment.

    a. _____

    b. _____

Implementation

28. Identify the patients who are at risk for hypothermia.

_____

_____

Acute Care

29. Explain the differences related to febrile states in each of the following.

    a. Children: _____

    b. Hypersensitive response to drugs: _____

30. Give an example of each type of fever therapy.

    a. Pharmacologic: _____

    b. Nonpharmacologic: _____

31. First aid treatment for heatstroke is: _____

_____

32. Summarize the treatment for hypothermia.

_____

_____

Evaluation

33. Identify evaluative measures for temperature alterations.

_____

_____

Pulse

34. Identify the two common sites to assess the pulse rate.

   a. _____

   b. _____

35. Identify the measurement criteria for the following pulse sites.

   a. Temporal: _____

   b. Carotid: _____

   c. Apical: _____

   d. Brachial: _____

   e. Radial: _____

   f. Ulnar: _____

   g. Femoral: _____

   h. Popliteal: _____

   i. Posterior tibial: _____

   j. Dorsalis pedis: _____

36. List the characteristics to identify when assessing the following.

   a. Radial pulse: _____

   b. Apical pulse: _____

37. List the acceptable pulse ranges for the following.

   a. Infants: _____

   b. Toddlers: _____

   c. Preschoolers: _____

   d. School-age children: _____

   e. Adolescents: _____

   f. Adults: _____

38. Identify the factors that may increase or decrease the pulse rate.

   a. _____

   b. _____

   c. _____

   d. _____

   e. _____

   f. _____

   g. _____

   h. _____

Define the following terms.

39. Tachycardia: _____

_____

40. Bradycardia: _____

_____

41. Pulse deficit: _____

_____

42. Dysrhythmia: _____

_____

Analysis and Nursing Diagnosis

43. Identify nursing diagnoses related to pulse findings.

   a. _____

   b. _____

   c. _____

   d. _____

   e. _____

Respiration

Define the following terms related to respirations.

44. Ventilation: _____

_____

45. Diffusion: _____

_____

46. Perfusion: _____

_____

47. Hypoxemia: _____

_____

48. Identify which phase of respirations is active and which is passive process.

   a. Inspiration: _____

   b. Expiration: _____

49. Identify factors that influence the character of respirations and the mechanism of each factor.

   a. _____

   b. _____

   c. _____

   d. _____

   e. _____

128

f. _____

g. _____

h. _____

50. Identify the acceptable range for respiratory rates for the following age groups.

a. Newborns: _____

b. Infants: _____

c. Toddlers: _____

d. Children: _____

e. Adolescents: _____

f. Adults: _____

Briefly explain the following alterations in breathing patterns.

51. Bradypnea: _____
_____

52. Tachypnea: _____
_____

53. Hyperpnea: _____
_____

54. Apnea: _____
_____

55. Hyperventilation: _____
_____

56. Hypoventilation: _____
_____

57. Cheyne–Stokes: _____
_____

58. Kussmaul: _____
_____

59. Biot: _____
_____

60. To measure arterial oxygen saturation a pulse oximeter is utilized, briefly explain: _____
_____
_____

61. Capnography is used to: _____

62. Identify nursing diagnoses related to ventilation.

a. _____

b. _____

c. _____

d. _____

Blood Pressure

Define the following terms.

63. Blood pressure: _____

_____

64. Systolic pressure: _____

_____

65. Diastolic pressure: _____

_____

66. Pulse pressure: _____

_____

Blood pressure is reflected by the following. Briefly explain each.

67. Cardiac output: _____

_____

68. Peripheral resistance: _____

_____

69. Blood volume: _____

_____

70. Viscosity: _____

_____

71. Elasticity: _____

_____

72. List eight factors that influence blood pressure.

a. _____

b. _____

c. _____

d. _____

e. _____

f. _____

g. _____

h. _____

73. Identify the average optimal blood pressure for the following ages.

a. Newborn: _____

b. 1 month: _____

c. 1 year: _____

d. 6 years: _____

e. 10 to 13 years: _____

f. 14 to 17 years: _____

g. Older than 18 years: _____

74. List some of the risk factors that are linked to hypertension.

_____

_____

75. Identify some of the risk factors for orthostatic hypotension.

_____

_____

76. Identify the following Korotkoff sounds.

First: _____

Second: _____

Third: _____

Fourth: _____

Fifth: _____

Analysis and Nursing Diagnosis

77. List some nursing diagnoses related to the general state of cardiovascular health.

a. _____

b. _____

c. _____

d. _____

e. _____

78. Identify at least two variations in each vital sign that are unique to older-adults.

a. Temperature: _____

b. Pulse rate: _____

c. Blood pressure: _____

d. Respirations: _____

CASE STUDY

79. A 16-year-old girl with a history of poorly controlled asthma is admitted with dyspnea and fatigue. Her vital signs on admission are HR 118, BP 108/82 mm Hg, RR 28, tympanic temperature 37°C, and oxygen saturation 92%. She is receiving oxygen via nasal cannula at 2 L. How would you expect her vital signs to change to indicate that she was improving following treatment for her asthma?

REVIEW QUESTIONS

Select the appropriate answer and cite the rationale for choosing that particular answer.

80. The skin plays a role in temperature regulation by:
    1. Insulating the body
    2. Constricting blood vessels
    3. Sensing external temperature variations
    4. All of the above

    Answer: _____

    Rationale: _____

    _____

    _____

81. The nurse bathes the patient who has a fever with cool water. The nurse does this to increase heat loss by means of:
    1. Radiation
    2. Convection
    3. Conduction
    4. Condensation

    Answer: _____

    Rationale: _____

    _____

    _____

82. The nurse is assessing a patient whom she suspects has the nursing diagnosis hyperthermia related to vigorous exercise in hot weather. In reviewing the data, the nurse knows that the most important sign of heatstroke is:
    1. Confusion
    2. Excess thirst
    3. Hot, dry skin
    4. Muscle cramps

    Answer: _____

    Rationale: _____

    _____

    _____

83. The nurse is auscultating Mrs. McKinnon's blood pressure. The nurse inflates the cuff to 180 mm Hg. At 156 mm Hg, the nurse hears the onset of a tapping sound. At 130 mm Hg, the sound changes to a murmur or swishing. At 100 mm Hg, the sound momentarily becomes sharper, and at 92 mm Hg, it becomes muffled. At 88 mm Hg, the sound disappears. Mrs. McKinnon's blood pressure is:
    1. 130/88 mm Hg
    2. 156/88 mm Hg
    3. 180/92 mm Hg
    4. 180/130 mm Hg

    Answer: _____

    Rationale: _____

    _____

    _____

84. The nursing instructor is explaining to the student nurse how to use the two-step method of blood pressure assessment to obtain accurate measurements. Place the steps in correct order:
    1. Place stethoscope in ears
    2. Palpate the brachial artery while inflating blood pressure cuff 30 mm Hg over the pulse disappearance
    3. Note point where you hear first Korotkoff sound
    4. Wait 30 seconds
    5. Apply blood pressure cuff 1 inch above brachial artery
    6. Continue to deflate cuff until sound disappears

    Answer: _____

    Rationale: _____

    _____

    _____

85. The nurse is working in an urgent care center and is completing a triage assessment on a 15-year-old male patient. The patient is accompanied by his mother who reports that he has been having abdominal pain and vomiting for the past 12 hours. The patient reports pain as 8 on a scale of 0-10 and indicates the pain is located diffusely in the abdomen. Upon assessment, the patient's oral temperature is 102.4°F (39°C); blood pressure 110/60 mmHg; heart rate 90 beats/min; respirations 20/min; oxygen saturation 96% on room air with clear lung sounds on auscultation. The patient has a history of anxiety, no previous surgeries, no known drug allergies, and no history of chronic illness.

Complete the diagram by dragging from the choices area to specify which condition the patient is most likely experiencing, two actions the nurse should take to address that condition, and two parameters the nurse should monitor to assess the patient's progress.

Highlight correct answers in yellow.

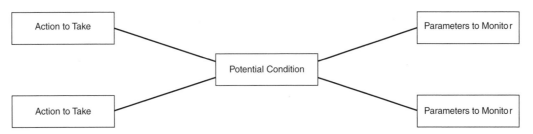

Actions to Take	Potential Condition	Parameters to Monitor
Apply ice packs to the axillae	Pyrexia	Temperature
Administer oxygen at 2 L/min via nasal cannula	Hypothermia	Pain level
Obtain cultures of body fluids (urine, sputum, blood)	Hypoxemia	Capnography
Remove all clothing	Hypotension	Blood glucose
Request an order for acetaminophen	Malignant hyperthermia	Pulse oximetry

30 Health Assessment and Physical Examination

PRELIMINARY READING

Chapter 30

COMPREHENSIVE UNDERSTANDING

Purposes of the Physical Examination

1. List the five nursing purposes for performing a physical assessment.

    a. _____

    b. _____

    c. _____

    d. _____

    e. _____

Preparation for Examination

2. To address cultural diversity, the nurse needs to:

    a. _____

    b. _____

    c. _____

    d. _____

3. Proper preparation for examination should include:

    a. _____

    b. _____

    c. _____

    d. _____

    e. _____

    f. _____

4. List the tips to follow that will help in data collection when examining children.

    a. _____

    b. _____

    c. _____

    d. _____

    e. _____

5. List seven variations in the nurse's individual style that are appropriate when examining older-adults.

a. _____

b. _____

c. _____

d. _____

e. _____

f. _____

g. _____

Organization of the Examination

6. Identify the principles to follow to keep an examination well organized.

a. _____

b. _____

c. _____

d. _____

e. _____

f. _____

g. _____

Techniques of Physical Assessment

7. Define *inspection*.

_____

_____

8. Identify the guidelines to achieve the best results during inspection.

a. _____

b. _____

c. _____

d. _____

e. _____

f. _____

9. Define *palpation*.

_____

_____

10. Explain the difference between:

a. Light palpation: _____

b. Deep palpation: _____

Chapter **30 Health Assessment and Physical Examination**

11. Define *percussion*.

_____

_____

12. Define *auscultation*.

_____

_____

13. The following are sounds that are described when auscultating. Please explain each one.

    a. Frequency: _____

    b. Amplitude: _____

    c. Quality: _____

    d. Duration: _____

General Survey

14. List at least 14 specific observations of the patient's general appearance and behavior that should be reviewed.

    a. _____

    b. _____

    c. _____

    d. _____

    e. _____

    f. _____

    g. _____

    h. _____

    i. _____

    j. _____

    k. _____

    l. _____

    m. _____

    n. _____

15. Identify some signs of patient-abuse.

_____

_____

16. Identify the questions related to the following acronym.

    C _____

    A _____

    G _____

    E _____

136

17. List three actions that should be taken to ensure accurate weight measurement of a hospitalized patient.

a. _____

b. _____

c. _____

Skin, Hair, and Nails

18. Assessment of the skin reveals the patient's health status related to:

a. _____

b. _____

c. _____

d. _____

e. _____

19. Define *pigmentation*.

_____

_____

20. For each skin color variation, identify the mechanism that produces color change, common causes of the variation, and the optimal sites for assessment.

Color	Condition	Causes	Assessment locations
Cyanosis			
Pallor			
Loss of pigmentation			
Jaundice			
Erythema			
Tan-brown			

21. Identify the physical findings of the skin that are indicative of substance-abuse.

a. _____

b. _____

c. _____

d. _____

e. _____

f. _____

g. _____

h. _____

Define the following terms.

22. Indurated: _____

_____

23. Turgor: _____

_____

24. Vascularity: _____

_____

25. Edema: _____

_____

26. Lesions: _____

_____

Briefly describe the following primary skin lesions and give an example of each.

27. Macule: _____

_____

28. Papule: _____

_____

29. Nodule: _____

_____

30. Tumor: _____

_____

31. Wheal: _____

_____

32. Vesicle: _____

_____

33. Pustule: _____

_____

34. Ulcer: _____

_____

35. Atrophy: _____

_____

Explain the following skin malignancies.

36. Basal cell carcinoma: _____

_____

37. Squamous cell carcinoma: _____

_____

38. Melanoma: _____

_____

39. Define the following mnemonic to assess the skin for any type of carcinoma.

A _____

B _____

C _____

D _____

E _____

40. Name the three types of lice.

a. _____

b. _____

c. _____

Briefly describe the following abnormalities of the nail bed.

41. Clubbing: _____
_____

42. Beau lines: _____
_____

43. Koilonychia: _____
_____

44. Splinter hemorrhages: _____
_____

45. Paronychia: _____
_____

Head and Neck

46. Define *hydrocephalus*.

_____
_____

Define the following common eye and visual abnormalities.

47. Hyperopia: _____
_____

48. Myopia: _____
_____

49. Presbyopia: _____
_____

50. Retinopathy: _____
_____

51. Strabismus: _____
_____

52. Cataract: _____

_____

53. Glaucoma: _____

_____

54. Macular degeneration: _____

_____

55. Examination of the eye includes assessment of five areas. Name them.

a. _____

b. _____

c. _____

d. _____

e. _____

56. Identify the structures of the external eye that you would inspect.

a. _____

b. _____

c. _____

d. _____

e. _____

f. _____

g. _____

Define the following terms related to the external eye.

57. Exophthalmos: _____

_____

58. Ectropion: _____

_____

59. Entropion: _____

_____

60. Conjunctivitis: _____

_____

61. Ptosis: _____

_____

62. PERRLA: _____

_____

63. Identify the internal eye structures that an advanced nurse practitioner would examine with an ophthalmoscope.

a. _____

b. _____

c. _____

d. _____

e. _____

f. _____

64. Identify the three parts of the ear canal and list the structures contained within each.

a. _____

b. _____

c. _____

65. The normal tympanic membrane appears: _____

_____

66. Identify the three types of hearing loss and explain how sound is transmitted.

a. _____

b. _____

c. _____

67. Ototoxicity is caused by: _____

_____

Define the following terms that relate to the nose.

68. Excoriation: _____

_____

69. Polyps: _____

_____

Define the following terms that relate to the oral cavity.

70. Leukoplakia: _____

_____

71. Varicosities: _____

_____

72. Exostosis: _____

_____

73. Structures examined during assessment of the neck include:

a. _____

b. _____

c. _____

d. _____

e. _____

f. _____

74. List the sequence for assessing the nodes of the neck.

1. _____

2. _____

3. _____

4. _____

5. _____

6. _____

75. An abnormality of superficial lymph nodes may reveal the presence of a local infection or _____

_____ or _____.

Thorax and Lungs

76. Identify the key landmarks of the chest.

a. _____

b. _____

c. _____

d. _____

e. _____

f. _____

77. Chest excursion is normally:

_____.

Reduced chest excursion may be caused by:

_____.

78. Define *vocal* or *tactile fremitus*.

_____

_____

Define the following normal breath sounds heard over the posterior thorax.

79. Vesicular: _____

_____

80. Bronchovesicular: _____

_____

81. Bronchial: _____

_____

82. Complete the following table of adventitious breath sounds.

Sound	Site Auscultated	Cause	Character
Crackles			
Rhonchi (sonorous wheeze)			
Wheezes (sibilant wheeze)			
Pleural friction rub			

Heart

Explain the following terms related to assessment of the heart.

83. Point of maximal impulse (PMI): _____

_____

84. S1: _____

_____

85. S2: _____

_____

86. S3: _____

_____

87. S4: _____

_____

Identify the appropriate sites for inspection and palpation of the following.

88. Angle of Louis: _____

_____

89. Aortic area: _____

_____

90. Pulmonic area: _____

_____

91. Second pulmonic area: _____

_____

92. Tricuspid area: _____

_____

93. Mitral area: _____

_____

94. Epigastric area: _____

_____

95. Define *murmur*.

_____

_____

96. List the six factors to consider when auscultating a murmur.

a. _____

b. _____

c. _____

d. _____

e. _____

97. Describe the sounds auscultated by the following murmurs.

Grade 1 = _____

Grade 2 = _____

Grade 3 = _____

Grade 4 = _____

Grade 5 = _____

Grade 6 = _____

Vascular System

98. Syncope is caused by: _____.

99. Arterial occlusion is: _____.

100. Stenosis is: _____.

101. A(n) _____ is the blowing sound caused by turbulence in a narrowed section of a blood vessel.

102. Explain the steps the nurse would use to assess venous pressure.

1. _____

2. _____

3. _____

103. Complete the following table by listing the signs of venous and arterial insufficiency.

Assessment criterion	Venous	Arterial
Color		
Temperature		
Pulse		
Edema		
Skin changes		

104. Describe how you would assess for phlebitis.

_____

_____

Breasts

105. The American Cancer Society (2020) recommends preventative screening for the following groups for early detection of breast cancer.

a. Age 40–44: _____

b. Age 45–54: _____

c. Ages 55 and over: _____

d. High-risk groups: _____

106. Identify the three systematic approaches to palpation of the breast.

a. _____

b. _____

c. _____

107. When palpating abnormal masses in the breast, you should note:

a. _____

b. _____

c. _____

d. _____

e. _____

f. _____

g. _____

108. Benign (fibrocystic) breast disease is characterized by: _____

_____

Abdomen

Define the following terms related to the abdomen.

109. Striae: _____

_____

110. Hernias: _____

_____

111. Distention: _____

_____

112. Peristalsis: _____

_____

113. Borborygmi: _____

_____

114. Rebound tenderness: _____

_____

115. Aneurysm: _____

_____

Female Genitalia and Reproductive Tract

116. Chancres are: _____

_____

117. A Papanicolaou specimen is used to: _____

_____

Male Genitalia

118. Identify the common symptoms of testicular cancer.

_____

_____

Rectum and Anus

119. The purpose of digital examination is: _____

_____

Musculoskeletal System

Define the following terms.

120. Kyphosis: _____

_____

121. Lordosis: _____

_____

122. Scoliosis: _____

_____

123. Osteoporosis: _____

_____

124. Goniometer: _____

_____

Identify the correct range of motion for the following terms.

125. Flexion: _____

_____

126. Extension: _____

_____

127. Hyperextension: _____

_____

128. Pronation: _____

_____

129. Supination: _____

_____

130. Abduction: _____

_____

131. Adduction: _____

_____

132. Internal rotation: _____

_____

133. External rotation: _____

_____

134. Eversion: _____

_____

135. Inversion: _____

_____

136. Dorsiflexion: _____

_____

137. Plantar flexion: _____

_____

Define the following terms related to muscle tone and strength.

138. Hypertonicity: _____

_____

139. Hypotonicity: _____

_____

140. Atrophied: _____

_____

Neurological System

141. The purpose of the Mini-Mental State Examination(MMSE) is to measure: _____
_____

142. Delirium is characterized by: _____
_____

143. List the clinical criteria for delirium.

a. _____

b. _____

c. _____

d. _____

e. _____

f. _____

g. _____

h. _____

144. The purpose of the Glasgow Coma Scale is to: _____
_____

145. Briefly explain the two types of aphasia.

a. Receptive: _____

b. Expressive: _____

146. Identify the 12 cranial nerves and their function.

I. _____

II. _____

III. _____

IV. _____

V. _____

VI. _____

VII. _____

VIII. _____

IX. _____

X. _____

XI. _____

XII. _____

147. The sensory pathways of the central nervous system conduct what type of sensations?

    a. _____

    b. _____

    c. _____

    d. _____

    e. _____

148. Identify the functions of the cerebellum.

_____

_____

_____

149. Identify the two types of normal reflexes and provide an example of each.

    a. _____

    b. _____

CASE STUDY

150. You are assessing a patient who has heart failure who is now complaining of shortness of breath. What assessment finding would you be most concerned with?

REVIEW QUESTIONS

Select the appropriate answer and cite the rationale for choosing that particular answer.

151. The component that should receive the highest priority before a physical examination is:
1. Preparation of the equipment
2. Preparation of the environment
3. Physical preparation of the patient
4. Psychological preparation of the patient

Answer: _____

Rationale: _____

_____

_____

152. The nurse assesses the skin turgor of the patient by:
1. Inspecting the buccal mucosa with a penlight
2. Palpating the skin with the dorsum of the hand
3. Grasping a fold of skin on the back of the forearm and releasing
4. Pressing the skin for 5 seconds, releasing, and noting each centimeter of depth

Answer: _____

Rationale: _____

_____

_____

153. While examining Mr. Parker, the nurse notes a circumscribed elevation of skin filled with serous fluid on his upper lip. The lesion is 0.4 cm in diameter. This type of lesion is called a:
    1. Macule
    2. Nodule
    3. Vesicle
    4. Pustule

    Answer: _____

    Rationale: _____

    _____

    _____

154. When assessing the patient's thorax, the nurse should:
    1. Complete the left side and then the right side
    2. Compare symmetrical areas from side to side
    3. Begin with the posterior lobes on the right side
    4. Change the position of the stethoscope between inspiration and expiration

    Answer: _____

    Rationale: _____

    _____

    _____

155. The second heart sound (S_2) occurs when:
    1. Systole begins
    2. There is rapid ventricular filling
    3. The mitral and tricuspid valves close
    4. The aortic and pulmonic valves close

    Answer: _____

    Rationale: _____

    _____

    _____

156. Which statements describe accurate completion of a vascular assessment? (Select all that apply.)
    1. Simultaneously palpate the carotid arteries
    2. Measure blood pressure
    3. Ask about any pain, cramping, or discomfort in the legs
    4. Count an irregular pulse for 30 seconds and multiply by 2
    5. Rate the strength of a pulse on a scale of 0 to 4.

    Answer: _____

    Rationale: _____

    _____

    _____

Next Generation NCLEX® Examination-Style Questions

157. A 72-year-old female presents to the urgent care center with reports of a sore throat and congestion. She states, "I haven't been feeling well and thought I should get checked out."

Highlight in yellow the assessment findings that require followup.

Nurses' Notes:	72-year-old female presents alert and oriented to person, place, and time. Senile keratosis noted on the face near the eyes. The patient is missing two back teeth, oral mucosa is glistening and moist with leukoplakia. The ventral surface of the tongue is pink and smooth with large veins between the frenulum fold. Patient reports no pain when chewing food. Scant amount of yellow exudate along the posterior pharynx. The trachea is midline. Right carotid bruit with auscultation of S_1S_2. Stomach is soft with positive bowels sounds in four quadrants. Skin shows tenting when pinched. Patient reports no difficulty with urination. The patient is able to ambulate with even gate. Vital signs: 98.8°F (37°C), 120/64 mmHg, 88 beats/min, 18 breaths/min, oxygen saturation 98% on room air.

31 Medication Administration

PRELIMINARY READING

Chapter 31

COMPREHENSIVE UNDERSTANDING

Scientific Knowledge Base

1. Briefly summarize the roles of the following in relation to the regulation of medications.

   a. Federal regulations: _____

   b. State and local regulations: _____

   c. Health care agencies: _____

   d. Nurse Practice Act: _____

A single medication may have three different names. Define each one.

2. Chemical name: _____

_____

3. Generic name: _____

_____

4. Trade name: _____

_____

5. A medication classification indicates: _____

_____

6. The form of the medication determines its: _____

_____

7. Pharmacokinetics is: _____

_____

8. Absorption is: _____

_____

9. Identify the factors that influence drug absorption.

   a. _____

   b. _____

   c. _____

   d. _____

   e. _____

151

10. Identify the factors that affect the rate and extent of medication distribution.

   a. _____

   b. _____

   c. _____

   d. _____

   e. _____

11. Explain the role of metabolism.

   _____

   _____

12. Identify the primary organ for drug excretion, and explain what happens if this organ's function declines.

   _____

   _____

Define the following predicted or unintended effects of drugs.

13. Therapeutic effects: _____

   _____

14. Side effects: _____

   _____

15. Adverse effects: _____

   _____

16. Toxic effects: _____

   _____

17. Idiosyncratic reactions: _____

   _____

18. Allergic reactions: _____

   _____

19. Anaphylactic reactions: _____

   _____

20. Medication interaction: _____

   _____

21. Synergistic effect: _____

   _____

22. Medication tolerance: _____

23. Medication dependence: _____

Define the following terms related to medication dose responses.

24. Minimum effective concentration (MEC): _____

_____

25. Peak concentration: _____

_____

26. Trough concentration: _____

_____

27. Biological half-life: _____

_____

28. Identify the three types of oral routes.

    a. _____

    b. _____

    c. _____

29. List the four major sites for parenteral injections.

    a. _____

    b. _____

    c. _____

    d. _____

Define the following advanced techniques of medication administration.

30. Epidural: _____

_____

31. Intrathecal: _____

_____

32. Intraosseous: _____

_____

33. Intraperitoneal: _____

_____

34. Intrapleural: _____

_____

35. Intraarterial: _____

_____

36. Intracardiac: _____

_____

37. Intraarticular: _____

_____

38. Identify five methods for applying medications to mucous membranes.

a. _____

b. _____

c. _____

d. _____

e. _____

39. Identify the benefit of the inhalation route.

_____

_____

40. Identify the two types of measurements used in medication therapy.

a. _____

b. _____

41. A solution is: _____

_____

Nursing Knowledge Base

42. Write out the formula used to determine the correct dose when preparing solid or liquid forms of medications.

_____

_____

43. Medication errors can be prevented in children by:

a. _____

b. _____

c. _____

d. _____

e. _____

f. _____

44. State the guidelines to follow when calculating out pediatric doses.

a. _____

b. _____

c. _____

d. _____

e. _____

f. _____

g. _____

Briefly explain the common types of medication orders.

45. Verbal: _____

_____

46. Standing or routine: _____

_____

47. prn: _____

_____

48. Single (one-time): _____

_____

49. STAT: _____

_____

50. Now: _____

_____

51. List the medication distribution systems.

a. _____

b. _____

52. Identify the common medication errors that can cause patient harm.

a. _____

b. _____

c. _____

d. _____

e. _____

53. Identify the process for medication reconciliation.

a. _____

b. _____

c. _____

d. _____

Critical Thinking

54. List the seven rights of medication administration.

a. _____

b. _____

c. _____

d. _____

e. _____

f. _____

g. _____

55. Briefly summarize *The Patient Care Partnership* related to medication administration and maintaining patient rights.

a. _____

b. _____

c. _____

d. _____

e. _____

f. _____

g. _____

h. _____

Nursing Process

Assessment

56. Identify the areas the nurse needs to assess to determine the need for and potential response to medication therapy.

a. _____

b. _____

c. _____

d. _____

e. _____

f. _____

g. _____

h. _____

i. _____

Analysis and Nursing Diagnosis

57. Identify potential nursing diagnoses used during the administration of medications.

a. _____

b. _____

c. _____

d. _____

e. _____

Planning and Outcomes Identification

58. Identify the outcomes for a patient with newly diagnosed type 2 diabetes.

a. _____

b. _____

c. _____

d. _____

e. _____

Implementation

59. Identify factors that can influence the patient's compliance with the medication regimen.

a. _____

b. _____

c. _____

d. _____

60. Identify the components of medication orders.

a. _____

b. _____

c. _____

d. _____

e. _____

f. _____

g. _____

61. The recording of medication includes:

a. _____

b. _____

c. _____

d. _____

e. _____

62. Explain the reasons why polypharmacy happens to a patient.

_____

_____

Evaluation

63. Identify two goals for safe and effective medication administration.

a. _____

b. _____

Medication Administration

64. Identify the precautions to take when administering any oral preparation to prevent aspiration.

a. _____

b. _____

c. _____

d. _____

e. _____

f. _____

g. _____

h. _____

i. _____

j. _____

k. _____

l. _____

m. _____

n. _____

o. _____

p. _____

65. Identify the guidelines to ensure safe administration of transdermal or topical medications.

a. _____

b. _____

c. _____

d. _____

e. _____

f. _____

66. The most common form of nasal instillation is: _____

_____

67. List four principles for administering eye instillations.

a. _____

b. _____

c. _____

d. _____

68. Failure to instill ear drops at room temperature causes:

a. _____

b. _____

c. _____

69. Vaginal medications are available as:

a. _____

b. _____

c. _____

d. _____

70. Rectal suppositories are used for: _____

71. Explain the following types of inhalation inhalers:

    a. Pressurized metered-dose inhalers (pMDIs): _____

    b. Breath-actuated metered-dose inhalers (BAIs): _____

    c. Dry powder inhalers (DPIs): _____

72. Identify the aseptic techniques to use to prevent an infection during an injection.

    a. _____

    b. _____

    c. _____

    d. _____

73. Identify the factors that must be considered when selecting a needle for an injection.

    a. _____

    b. _____

74. Describe each of the following.

    a. Ampule: _____

    b. Vial: _____

75. List the three principles to follow when mixing medications from two vials.

    a. _____

    b. _____

    c. _____

76. Insulin is classified by: _____

    _____

77. Identify the principles to follow when mixing two types of insulin in the same syringe.

    a. _____

    b. _____

    c. _____

    d. _____

    e. _____

78. List the techniques used to minimize patient discomfort that is associated with injections.

    a. _____

    b. _____

    c. _____

    d. _____

    e. _____

    f. _____

    g. _____

    h. _____

79. Identify the best sites for subcutaneous injections.

    a. _____

    b. _____

    c. _____

80. What is the maximum amount of water-soluble medication given by the subcutaneous route?

    _____

    _____

81. What angles should be used when administering a subcutaneous injection, and with which needle should they be used?

    a. _____

    b. _____

82. What is the angle of insertion for an intramuscular (IM) injection?

    _____

    _____

83. Indicate the maximum volume of medication for an IM injection in each of the following groups.

    a. Well-developed adults: _____

    b. Older children, older-adults, and thin adults: _____

    c. Older infants and small children: _____

Describe the characteristics of the following intramuscular injection sites.

84. Ventrogluteal: _____

    _____

85. Vastus lateralis: _____

    _____

86. Deltoid: _____

    _____

87. Explain the rationale for the Z-track method in IM injections.

    _____

    _____

88. Explain the rationale for intradermal injections.

    _____

    _____

89. List the methods a nurse can use to administer medications intravenously.

a. _____

b. _____

c. _____

90. Identify the advantages of the intravenous (IV) route of administration.

a. _____

b. _____

c. _____

91. List the advantages of using volume-controlled infusions.

a. _____

b. _____

c. _____

92. What is a piggyback set?

_____

_____

93. What is a volume-control administration set?

_____

_____

94. What is a syringe pump?

_____

_____

95. List the advantages of using intermittent venous access devices.

a. _____

b. _____

c. _____

CASE STUDY

96. A patient you are caring for had a stroke 3 days ago and is still hospitalized and receiving oral medications. What techniques can you do as the nurse to reduce the patient's risk for aspiration?

Select the appropriate answer and cite the rationale for choosing that particular answer.

97. The study of how drugs enter the body, reach their sites of action, are metabolized, and exit from the body is called:
    1. Pharmacology
    2. Pharmacopoeia
    3. Pharmacokinetics
    4. Biopharmaceutical

    Answer: _____

    Rationale: _____

    _____

    _____

98. Which statement correctly characterizes drug absorption?
    1. Most drugs must enter the systemic circulation to have a therapeutic effect.
    2. Oral medications are absorbed more quickly when administered with meals.
    3. Mucous membranes are relatively impermeable to chemicals, making absorption slow.
    4. Drugs administered subcutaneously are absorbed more quickly than those injected intramuscularly.

    Answer: _____

    Rationale: _____

    _____

    _____

99. The onset of drug action is the time it takes for a drug to:
    1. Produce a response
    2. Accelerate the cellular process
    3. Reach its highest effective concentration
    4. Produce blood serum concentration and maintenance

    Answer: _____

    Rationale: _____

    _____

    _____

100. Which of the following is not a parenteral route of administration?
    1. Buccal
    2. Intradermal
    3. Intramuscular
    4. Subcutaneous

    Answer: _____

    Rationale: _____

    _____

    _____

101. The nurse is preparing an insulin injection in which both regular and NPH will be mixed. Into which vial should the nurse inject air first?
    1. The vial of regular insulin
    2. The vial of NPH
    3. Either vial, as long as modified insulin is drawn up first
    4. Neither vial; it is not necessary to put air into vials before withdrawing medication

    Answer: _____

    Rationale: _____

    _____

    _____

102. A young-adult patient tells her nurse that she is afraid of injections. The nurse is preparing to administer the patient a flu vaccine. Which of the following techniques can the nurse use to reduce the patient's discomfort? (Select all that apply.)
    1. Ask the patient to think about why the injection is necessary
    2. Position the patient comfortably
    3. Apply a vapocoolant to the skin before giving the injection
    4. Use a large-gauge needle
    5. Carefully use anatomical landmarks to select injection site

    Answer: _____

    Rationale: _____

    _____

    _____

103. The nurse is caring for a 54-year-old patient with Type 1 diabetes mellitus. The patient has orders for 6 units of regular and 5 units of intermediate (NPH) insulin to be administered subcutaneously. To administer the medication as ordered, the nurse will first _____1_____. Then the nurse will ____2_____.

Options for 1	Options for 2
Shake both insulin vials.	Draw 6 units of NPH insulin into a U-100 syringe.
Roll the NPH insulin between the palms.	Inject 5 units of air into the intermediate (NPH) insulin using a U-100 syringe.
Make sure both insulin vials are clear.	Draw 11 units of 70/30 insulin (NPH) into a U-100 syringe.
Roll the regular insulin between the palms.	Draw 5 units of NPH insulin into a U-500 syringe.

PRELIMINARY READING

Chapter 32

COMPREHENSIVE UNDERSTANDING

Complementary and Integrative Therapies

Describe the difference between the following terms.

1. Complementary therapies: _____

    _____

2. Alternative therapies: _____

    _____

3. Explain the following biologically based therapies.

    a. Dietary supplements: _____

    b. Herbal medicines: _____

    c. Macrobiotic diet: _____

    d. Mycotherapies: _____

    e. Orthomolecular medicine: _____

    f. Probiotics: _____

    g. The "zone": _____

4. Explain the following energy therapies.

    a. Acupuncture: _____

    b. Healing touch: _____

    c. Reiki therapy: _____

    d. Therapeutic touch: _____

    e. Magnet therapy: _____

5. Explain the following manipulative and body-based methods.

    a. Acupressure: _____

    b. Chiropractic medicine: _____

    c. Craniosacral therapy: _____

    d. Massage therapy: _____

    e. Simple touch: _____

6. Explain the following mind–body interventions.

   a. Art therapy: _____

   b. Biofeedback: _____

   c. Breathwork: _____

   d. Guided imagery: _____

   e. Meditation: _____

   f. Music therapy: _____

   g. Yoga: _____

   h. Tai chi: _____

7. Explain the following movement therapies:

   a. Dance therapy: _____

   b. Pilates: _____

8. Integrative health care emphasizes the:

   a. _____

   b. _____

   c. _____

   d. _____

Nursing-Accessible Therapies

9. Complementary therapies teach individuals ways to change their behavior to help alter physical responses to stress and improve symptoms such as _____, _____, _____ or _____ .

10. The characteristics of the relaxation response are: _____

    _____

11. Progressive relaxation training helps to: _____

    _____

12. The goal of passive relaxation is: _____

    _____

13. The outcome of relaxation therapy is: _____

    _____

14. Identify the limitations of relaxation therapy.

    _____

    _____

15. Meditation is: _____

    _____

Chapter **32 Complementary, Alternative, and Integrative Therapies**

16. Identify the indications for the use of meditation.

_____

_____

17. Identify the limitations of meditation.

_____

_____

18. Imagery is: _____

_____

19. Creative visualization is: _____

_____

20. Identify the clinical applications of imagery.

_____

_____

Training-Specific Therapies

21. Biofeedback is: _____

_____

22. Identify some clinical applications for the use of biofeedback.

_____

_____

23. Identify the limitations of biofeedback.

_____

_____

24. What is the most important concept of Traditional Chinese medicine (TCM)?

_____

_____

25. Briefly explain the following TCM therapeutic modalities.

   a. Moxibustion: _____

   b. Cupping: _____

   c. Tai chi: _____

   d. Qi gong: _____

26. Describe the clinical applications of TCM.

_____

_____

27. Limitations of TCM:

_____

_____

28. Explain the following terms related to acupuncture.

    a. *Qi*: _____

    b. Meridians: _____

    c. Acupoints: _____

29. Identify the five phases of Therapeutic Touch (TT).

    a. _____

    b. _____

    c. _____

    d. _____

    e. _____

30. Identify the clinical applications of touch therapies.

_____

_____

31. Identify the limitations of touch therapies.

_____

_____

32. Identify the clinical applications of chiropractic therapy. _____

33. Identify the limitations of chiropractic therapy. _____

34. Identify the clinical applications of herbal therapy.

_____

_____

35. Identify the limitations of herbal therapy.

_____

_____

The Integrative Nursing Role

36. Explain what the integrative medicine approach is.

_____

_____

37. You are taking care of a patient who is practicing relaxation techniques. Identify some cognitive skills that this patient can develop while practicing relaxation?

REVIEW QUESTIONS

Select the appropriate answer and cite the rationale for choosing that particular answer.

38. Patients choose to use unconventional therapy because:
    1. They are willing to pay more to feel better.
    2. They are dissatisfied with conventional medicine.
    3. They want religious approval for the remedies they use.
    4. It is now widely accepted by the Food and Drug Administration.

    Answer: _____

    Rationale: _____

    _____

    _____

39. The Dietary Supplement and Health Education Act states that:
    1. The Food and Drug Administration must evaluate all herbal therapies.
    2. Herbs, vitamins, and minerals may be sold with their therapeutic advantages listed on the label.
    3. Herbs, vitamins, and minerals may be sold as long as no therapeutic claims are made on the label.
    4. In conjunction with the Food and Drug Administration, all supplements are considered safe for use.

    Answer: _____

    Rationale: _____

    _____

    _____

40. Which of the following steps should nurses take to be better informed about alternative therapies?
    1. Review herb manufacturers' literature on specific herbs.
    2. Read current books and magazines on alternative therapies.
    3. Familiarize themselves with general principles of phytotherapy.
    4. Familiarize themselves with recent case studies on alternative therapies.

    Answer: _____

    Rationale: _____

    _____

    _____

33 Self-Concept

PRELIMINARY READING

Chapter 33

COMPREHENSIVE UNDERSTANDING

Scientific Knowledge Base

1. Define self-concept.

   _____

   _____

Nursing Knowledge Base

2. Self-concept is a dynamic perception that is based on the following:

   a. _____

   b. _____

   c. _____

   d. _____

   e. _____

   f. _____

   g. _____

   h. _____

   i. _____

Match the following terms.

3. _____ Identity

4. _____ Body image

5. _____ Role performance

6. _____ Self-esteem

a. Attitudes related to physical appearance, structure, and function of the body

b. The way in which individuals perceive their ability to carry out significant roles

c. Individual's overall feeling of self-worth or the emotional appraisal of self-concept

d. Internal sense of individuality, wholeness, and consistency of a person over time and in different situations

7. A self-concept stressor is any: _____

   _____

169

Match the following stressors that affect self-concept.

8. _____ Identity

9. _____ Body image

10. _____ Role performance

11. _____ Role conflict

12. _____ Role ambiguity

13. _____ Role strain

14. _____ Role overload

15. _____ Self-esteem stressors

a. Example: perceived inability to meet parental expectations, harsh criticism, and inconsistent discipline

b. Example: providing care to a family member with Alzheimer disease

c. Example: a middle-aged woman with teenage children assuming responsibility for the care of her older parents

d. Amputation, facial disfigurement, or scars from burns

e. Unsuccessfully attempting to meet the demands of work and family while carving out some personal time

f. Example: people move, marry, divorce, or change jobs

g. An adolescent attempting to adjust to the physical, emotional, and mental changes of increasing maturity

h. Example: parents, peers, and the media pressure adolescents to assume adult-life roles

16. List five areas the nurse must clarify and assess about him- or herself to promote a positive self-concept in patients.

a. _____

b. _____

c. _____

d. _____

e. _____

f. _____

Nursing Process

Assessment

17. Identify the focus of assessing each component of self-concept.

_____

_____

18. Give some examples of behaviors suggestive of altered self-concept.

_____

_____

_____

Analysis and Nursing Diagnosis

19. Identify examples of self-concept nursing diagnoses.

a. _____

b. _____

c. _____

d. _____

Planning and Outcomes Identification

20. State the expected outcomes for the nursing diagnosis Situational Low Self-Esteem related to a recent job layoff.

_____

_____

Implementation

21. List some healthy lifestyle measures that support adaptation to stress.

_____

_____

Evaluation

22. Identify the expected outcomes for a self-concept disturbance.

_____

_____

CASE STUDY

23. You are doing a history and physical exam with an adolescent in the clinic and you are concerned about behaviors that can signal self-esteem disturbances. What specific at-risk behaviors are of concern in this age group?

REVIEW QUESTIONS

Select the appropriate answer and cite the rationale for choosing that particular answer.

24. Which developmental stage is particularly crucial for identity development?
    1. Infancy
    2. Young adult
    3. Adolescence
    4. Preschool-age

    Answer: _____

    Rationale: _____

    _____

    _____

25. Which of the following statements about body image is correct?
    1. Body image refers only to the external appearance of a person's body.
    2. Physical changes are quickly incorporated into a person's body image.
    3. Perceptions by other persons have no influence on a person's body image.
    4. Body image is a combination of a person's actual and perceived (ideal) body.

    Answer: _____

    Rationale: _____

    _____

    _____

26. Robert, who is 2-years-old, is praised for using his potty instead of wetting his pants. This is an example of learning a behavior by:
    1. Imitation
    2. Substitution
    3. Identification
    4. Reinforcement–extinction

    Answer: _____

    Rationale: _____

    _____

    _____

27. Mrs. Watson has just undergone a radical mastectomy. The nurse is aware that Mrs. Watson will probably have considerable anxiety over:
    1. Self-esteem
    2. Body image
    3. Self-identity
    4. Role performance

    Answer: _____

    Rationale: _____

    _____

    _____

28. Imagine that you are the student nurse, Susan, in the care plan in Chapter 33 of your text. Complete the *Assessment phase* of the critical thinking model with these questions in mind.

   a. In developing Mrs. Johnson's plan of care, what knowledge did Susan apply?

   _____

   b. In what way might Susan's previous experience apply in this case?

   _____

   c. What intellectual or professional standards were applied to Mrs. Johnson?

   _____

   d. What critical thinking attitudes did you use in assessing Mrs. Johnson?

   _____

   e. As you review your assessment, what key areas did you cover?

   _____

Next Generation NCLEX® Examination-Style Questions

29. The nurse is caring for 13-year-old female patient who is being seen for a routine physical. The patient's weight is 135 pounds and she is 5 feet, 2 inches tall. The patient states that she is in the 8th grade at a local school and requests medicine to "help lose weight". She states, "I am fat, even my friends tell me that I am." The nurse notes areas of broken skin on the patient's arms and legs. When asked about self-harm, the patient states, "Sometimes I cut myself."

Use Word Choices to complete the sentence(s). Highlight correct answers in yellow.

The patient is demonstrating _____, _____, and _____ issues.

Word Choices		
Body image	Self-esteem	Identity confusion
Self-concept	Role performance	Role Strain

34 Sexuality

PRELIMINARY READING

Chapter 34

COMPREHENSIVE UNDERSTANDING

Scientific Knowledge Base

Match the following terms to the appropriate responses.

1. _____ Sexuality
2. _____ Sexual health
3. _____ Gender roles
4. _____ Gender identity
5. _____ School-age children
6. _____ Adolescents
7. _____ Sexual orientation and identity
8. _____ Dyspareunia
9. _____ Young adulthood
10. _____ Middle adulthood
11. _____ Older-adulthood
12. _____ Contraceptive options

a. Pill, intrauterine device, condoms, diaphragm, tubal ligation, vasectomy
b. Changes in physical appearance lead to concerns about sexual attractiveness
c. Factors that determine sexual activity include present health status, past and present life satisfaction, status of intimate relationships
d. Need accurate information on sexual activity, emotional responses with relationships, sexually transmitted infections, contraception, and pregnancy
e. Have general questions regarding the physical and emotional aspects of sex
f. Part of a person's personality and important for overall health
g. Influenced by culture
h. State of physical, emotional, mental, and social well-being in relation to sexuality
i. Person's private view of maleness and femaleness
j. Heterosexual, lesbian, gay, bisexual, or transgender
k. Painful intercourse
l. Intimacy and sexuality are issues for this group

13. Identify the unique stressors that LGBTQ+ individuals related to their sexual identify and sexual orientation.

   a. _____

   _____

   b. _____

   _____

   c. _____

   _____

14. Sexual dysfunction involves _____, _____ or _____.

15. Erectile dysfunction is generally related to:

   a. Chronic disease –

   b. Medications –

16. Many menopausal woman report the following that require interventions by a health care provider:

a. _____

b. _____

c. _____

Nursing Knowledge Base

17. Identify the sociocultural dimensions of sexuality.

a. _____

b. _____

c. _____

18. Identify three decisional issues that promote or preserve sexual health.

a. _____

b. _____

c. _____

19. List the commonly diagnosed sexually transmitted infections (STIs).

a. _____

b. _____

c. _____

d. _____

e. _____

f. _____

20. Identify four alterations in sexual health.

a. _____

b. _____

c. _____

d. _____

Nursing Process

Assessment

21. What factors that may affect sexuality would the nurse assess?

a. _____

b. _____

c. _____

d. _____

e. _____

f. _____

22. The PLISSIT assessment of sexuality stands for: _____

Analysis and Nursing Diagnosis

23. Identify possible nursing diagnoses related to sexual functioning.

    a. _____

    b. _____

    c. _____

    d. _____

    e. _____

Planning and Outcomes Identification

24. The expected outcomes for the nursing diagnosis Sexual Dysfunction Related to Decreased Sexual Drive are:

    a. _____

    b. _____

Implementation

25. List the sexual health issues that you would include when educating your patient.

    a. _____

    b. _____

    c. _____

    d. _____

    e. _____

26. Identify strategies that enhance sexual functioning.

    a. _____

    b. _____

    c. _____

    d. _____

    e. _____

    f. _____

    g. _____

Acute Care

27. During periods of illness individuals experience situational stressors. Identify them.

    _____

    _____

Evaluation

28. Identify the follow-up discussions to determine whether the goals and outcomes were achieved.

    a. _____

    b. _____

29. You as the nurse are taking a sexual history during the admission process and want to establish a relaxed and matter-of-fact approach to help the patient feel safe. How could you phrase the question to establish this repour?

REVIEW QUESTIONS

Select the appropriate answer and cite the rationale for choosing that particular answer.

30. At what developmental stage is it particularly important for children reared in single-parent families to be exposed to same-sex adults?
    1. Infancy
    2. School-age
    3. Adolescence
    4. Toddlerhood and preschool years

    Answer: _____

    Rationale: _____

    _____

    _____

31. Which statement about sexual response in older-adults is correct?
    1. The resolution phase is slower.
    2. The orgasm phase is prolonged.
    3. The refractory phase is more rapid.
    4. Both genders experience a reduced availability of sex hormones.

    Answer: _____

    Rationale: _____

    _____

    _____

32. The only 100% effective method to avoid contracting a disease through sex is:
    1. Abstinence
    2. Using condoms
    3. Avoiding sex with partners at risk
    4. Knowing the sexual partner's health history

    Answer: _____

    Rationale: _____

    _____

    _____

33. Imagine that you are the nurse in the care plan in Chapter 34 of your text. Complete the *Assessment phase* of the critical thinking model with these questions in mind.

    a. In developing Mr. Clements' plan of care, what knowledge did the nurse apply?

    _____

    b. In what way might the nurse's previous experience assist in this case?

    _____

    c. What intellectual or professional standards were applied to Mr. Clements?

    _____

    d. What critical thinking attitudes did you use in assessing Mr. Clements?

    _____

    e. As you review your assessment, what key areas did you cover?

    _____

Next Generation NCLEX® Examination-Style Questions

34. For each patient, specify the potential developmental assessment data that would be appropriate for the age of the patient.

Each patient may support more than one potential developmental assessment data. Each category must have at least one response option selected. Highlight your answers in yellow.

Patient	Developmental Assessment Data
3-year-old natal male	Knows there are boys and girls.
	Waits to see what peers do in a situation.
	Identifies with his male caregiver.
6-year-old natal female	Prefers to be in group with other females.
	Seems anxious and worried if she fits in with others.
	Asks her mom about how to make friends.
12-year-old natal female	Reports anxiety and asks, "Do you think I am normal?"
	Identifies sexual intimacy as a basic need.
	Reports breast development and body changes.

35 Spiritual Health

PRELIMINARY READING

Chapter 35

COMPREHENSIVE UNDERSTANDING

Scientific Knowledge Base

1. Define *spirituality*.

_____

_____

Nursing Knowledge Base

Match the following terms.

2. _____ Transcendence

3. _____ Connectedness

4. _____ Atheist

5. _____ Agnostic

6. _____ Spiritual well-being

7. _____ Faith

8. _____ Religion

9. _____ Hope

10. _____ Spiritual distress

a. An energizing source that has an orientation to future goals and outcomes
b. Belief that there is no known ultimate reality
c. Allows people to have firm beliefs despite lack of physical evidence
d. Does not believe in the existence of God
e. Belief that there is a force outside of and greater than the person
f. Intrapersonally, interpersonally, and transpersonally
g. Having a vertical and horizontal dimension
h. The system of organized beliefs and worship that a person practices
i. Impaired ability to experience and integrate meaning and purpose in life

11. Briefly explain each of the following causes of spiritual distress.

   a. Acute illness:

_____

_____

   b. Chronic illness:

_____

_____

   c. Terminal illness:

_____

_____

   d. Near-death experience:

_____

_____

178

Nursing Process

Assessment

Various tools are available to assess a patient's spiritual well-being. Briefly summarize the following dimensions.

12. Faith/belief:

_____

_____

13. Life/self-responsibility:

_____

_____

14. Connectedness:

_____

_____

15. Life satisfaction:

_____

_____

16. Culture:

_____

_____

17. Fellowship and community:

_____

_____

18. Ritual and practice:

_____

_____

19. Vocation:

_____

_____

Analysis and Nursing Diagnosis

20. List the nursing diagnoses that pertain to spiritual health.

  a. _____

  b. _____

  c. _____

  d. _____

  e. _____

Planning and Outcomes Identification

21. Identify the outcomes for the patient to achieve personal harmony and connections with members of his or her support system.

    a. _____

    b. _____

    c. _____

    d. _____

Implementation

22. Identify behaviors that establish the nurse's presence.

    _____

    _____

    _____

23. Identify the factors that are evident when a healing relationship develops between a nurse and patient.

    a. _____

    b. _____

    c. _____

Explain how the following interventions are helpful in the patient's therapeutic plan.

24. Support systems:

    _____

    _____

25. Diet therapies:

    _____

    _____

26. Supporting rituals:

    _____

    _____

27. Prayer:

    _____

    _____

28. Meditation:

    _____

    _____

29. Supporting grief work:

    _____

    _____

Evaluation

30. Identify the successful outcomes of spiritual health.

_____

_____

_____

CASE STUDY

31. The nurse is caring for a woman who is recovering from a total hip replacement. During the assessment, the nurse learns that the patient is Roman Catholic. The patient tells the nurse that she is very nervous about starting therapy. Based on this information, what interventions could the nurse implement to enhance the patient's spiritual health?

REVIEW QUESTIONS

Select the appropriate answer and cite the rationale for choosing that particular answer.

32. When planning care to include spiritual needs for a patient of Islamic faith, the religious practices the nurse should understand include all of the following except:
    1. Strength is gained through group prayer.
    2. Family members are a source of comfort.
    3. A priest must be present to conduct rituals.
    4. Faith healing provides psychological support.

    Answer: _____

    Rationale: _____

    _____

    _____

33. When consulting with the dietary department regarding meals for a patient of the Hindu religion, which of the following dietary items would not be included on the meal trays?
    1. Fruits
    2. Meats
    3. Dairy products
    4. Vegetable entrees

    Answer: _____

    Rationale: _____

    _____

    _____

34. If an Islamic patient dies, the nurse should be aware of what religious practice?
    1. Last rites are mandatory.
    2. The body is always cremated.
    3. Muslims wash the body of the patient and wrap it in white cloth with the head turned to the right shoulder.
    4. Members of a ritual burial society cleanse the body.

    Answer: _____

    Rationale: _____

    _____

    _____

35. If a nurse were to use a nursing diagnosis to relate concerns about spiritual health, which of the following would be used?
   1. Lack of faith
   2. Spiritual distress
   3. Inability to adjust
   4. Religious dilemma

   Answer: _____

   Rationale: _____

   _____

   _____

36. Mr. Phillips was recently diagnosed with a malignant tumor. The staff had observed him crying on several occasions, and now he cries as he reads from his Bible. Interventions to help Mr. Phillips cope with his illness would include:
   1. Praying with Mr. Phillips as often as possible
   2. Asking the hospital chaplain to visit him daily
   3. Supporting his use of inner resources by providing time for meditation
   4. Engaging Mr. Phillips in diversional activities to reduce feelings of hopelessness

   Answer: _____

   Rationale: _____

   _____

   _____

CRITICAL THINKING MODEL FOR NURSING CARE PLAN FOR READINESS FOR ENHANCED SPIRITUAL WELL-BEING

37. Imagine that you are the nurse in the care plan in Chapter 35 of your text. Complete the *Planning phase* of the critical thinking model with these questions in mind.

   a. In developing Lisa's plan of care, what knowledge did the nurse apply?

   _____

   b. In what way might the nurse's previous experience assist in developing a plan of care for Lisa?

   _____

   c. When developing a plan of care, what intellectual and professional standards were applied?

   _____

   d. What critical thinking attitudes might have been applied to developing Lisa's plan?

   _____

   e. How will the nurse accomplish the goals?

   _____

36 Loss and Grief

Chapter 36

COMPREHENSIVE UNDERSTANDING

Scientific Knowledge Base

Match the following terms.

1. _____ Maturational losses
2. _____ Situational loss
3. _____ Actual loss
4. _____ Perceived loss
5. _____ Grief
6. _____ Mourning
7. _____ Bereavement
8. _____ Normal grief
9. _____ Complicated grief
10. _____ Disenfranchised grief
11. _____ Delayed grief
12. _____ Ambiguous loss
13. _____ Exaggerated grief
14. _____ Masked grief
15. _____ Anticipatory grief

a. The unconscious process of disengaging before the actual loss or death occurs
b. Captures grief and mourning, emotional responses, and outward behaviors for a person experiencing loss
c. Difficult to process because of the lack of finality and unknown outcomes
d. Marginal or unsupported grief; the relationship may not be socially sanctioned
e. Person is unaware of disruptive behavior as a result of loss
f. Emotional response to a loss, which is unique to the individual
g. May exhibit self-destructive or maladaptive behavior, obsessions, or psychiatric disorders
h. Suppressing or postponing normal grief responses
i. Dysfunctional; the grieving person has a prolonged or significant time moving forward after a loss
j. Complex emotional, cognitive, social, physical, behavioral, and spiritual responses to loss and death
k. Outward social expression of grief and the behavior associated with loss that can be culturally influenced
l. Form of necessary loss, including all normally expected life changes across the life span
m. Can no longer feel, hear, or know a person or object
n. Sudden, unpredictable external event
o. Are uniquely defined by the person experiencing loss and are less obvious to other people

Nursing Knowledge Base

16. Identify the factors that influence loss and grief.

a. _____

b. _____

c. _____

d. _____

e. _____

f. _____

g. _____

h. _____

Nursing Process
Assessment

17. Identify the important areas of assessment.

_____

_____

18. Give an example of the following grief reactions.

a. Feelings _____

_____

b. Cognitions (thought patterns) _____

_____

c. Physical sensations _____

_____

d. Behaviors _____

_____

Analysis and Nursing Diagnosis

19. List the nursing diagnoses that pertain to the patient experiencing grief, loss, or death.

a. _____

b. _____

c. _____

d. _____

e. _____

Planning and Outcomes Identification

20. The expected outcomes for a patient experiencing loss, give some examples:

a. _____

b. _____

c. _____

Implementation

21. Define *palliative care.*

_____

_____

22. The World Health Organization (2018) summarizes palliative care as:

a. _____

b. _____

c. _____

d. _____

e. _____

f. _____

g. _____

h. _____

i. _____

23. Hospice programs are built on the following core beliefs and services:

a. _____

b. _____

c. _____

d. _____

e. _____

f. _____

g. _____

h. _____

24. Identify the psychosocial care and symptom management that the nurse provides.

a. _____

b. _____

c. _____

d. _____

e. _____

f. _____

g. _____

h. _____

i. _____

25. Identify the nursing strategies for the family members to facilitate mourning.

a. _____

b. _____

c. _____

d. _____

e. _____

f. _____

g. _____

Define the following terms that relate to the care of the patient after death.

26. Organ and tissue donation:

_____

_____

27. Autopsy:

_____

_____

28. Postmortem care:

_____

_____

Evaluation

Identify the short- and long-term outcomes that signal a family's recovery from a loss.

29. Short-term:

_____

_____

30. Long-term:

_____

_____

CASE STUDY

31. A patient's husband asks you to explain grief. What points would you include in the teaching?

Select the appropriate answer and cite the rationale for choosing that particular answer.

32. Which statement about loss is accurate?
    1. Loss may be maturational, situational, or both.
    2. The degree of stress experienced is unrelated to the type of loss.
    3. Loss is only experienced when there is an actual absence of something valued.
    4. The more an individual has invested in what is lost, the less the feeling of loss.

    Answer: _____

    Rationale: _____

    _____

    _____

33. A hospice program emphasizes:
    1. Prolongation of life
    2. Hospital-based care
    3. Palliative treatment and control of symptoms
    4. Curative treatment and alleviation of symptoms

    Answer: _____

    Rationale: _____

    _____

    _____

34. Trying questionable and experimental forms of therapy is a behavior that is characteristic of which stage of dying?
    1. Anger
    2. Bargaining
    3. Depression
    4. Acceptance

    Answer: _____

    Rationale: _____

    _____

    _____

35. All of the following are crucial needs of the dying patient except:
    1. Control of pain
    2. Love and belonging
    3. Freedom from decision making
    4. Preservation of dignity and self-worth

    Answer: _____

    Rationale: _____

    _____

    _____

36. A patient's family members ask the nurse what bodily changes they should expect when their relative's death is imminent. Which points does the nurse include in the teaching? (Select all that apply.)
    1. Warm hands and feet
    2. Noisy breathing
    3. Limited intake of food
    4. Consistent shallow breaths
    5. Reduction of urine output
    6. Orientation to person, place, and time

    Answer: _____

    Rationale: _____

    _____

    _____

37. Imagine that you are the student nurse in the care plan in Chapter 36 of your text. Complete the *Evaluation phase* of the critical thinking model with these questions in mind.

a. In evaluating Mrs. Allison's plan of care, what did you apply?

_____

b. In what way might your previous experience influence your evaluation of Mrs. Allison's care?

_____

c. During evaluation, what intellectual and professional standards were applied to Mrs. Allison's care?

_____

d. In what way do critical thinking attitudes play a role in how you approach evaluation of Mrs. Allison's care?

_____

e. How might you adjust Mrs. Allison's care?

_____

Next Generation NCLEX® Examination-Style Questions

38. The nurse is assessing a patient who lost her spouse 2 days ago. The couple had been married for 42 years and the patient presented to the emergency department with chest pain. The patient is tearful. **For each assessment finding, place an "X" to indicate whether findings from this patient's assessment are generally associated with stages of dying theory by Kubler-Ross or Attachment theory by Bowlby.**

Each row must have only one response option selected.

Assessment Finding	Stages of Dying	Attachment Theory	Both Grief Theories
States, "I don't believe he is gone."			
States, "I just don't want to talk about the loss right now. We don't have to think about it all the time."			
States, "I don't want to eat or drink, I have pain in my chest, and I feel sick at my stomach."			
States, "If God would just take me instead of my husband, it would be better."			
The patient is openly sobbing at times and demonstrates acute physical distress.			

37 Stress and Coping

PRELIMINARY READING

Chapter 37

COMPREHENSIVE UNDERSTANDING

Scientific Knowledge Base

Match the following terms.

1. _____ Stress
2. _____ Allostatic load
3. _____ Appraisal
4. _____ Stressors
5. _____ Fight-or-flight response
6. _____ General adaptation syndrome (GAS)
7. _____ Allostasis
8. _____ Alarm stage
9. _____ Resistance stage
10. _____ Exhaustion stage
11. _____ Situational crisis
12. _____ Adventitious crisis
13. _____ Coping
14. _____ Ego-defense mechanisms
15. _____ Crisis
16. _____ Primary appraisal
17. _____ Posttraumatic stress disorder
18. _____ Secondary appraisal
19. _____ Flashbacks
20. _____ Developmental crisis

a. Implies that a person is facing a turning point in life
b. Person is considering possible coping strategies or resources available to help deal with the event
c. Chronic arousal that causes excessive wear and tear on the person
d. Provoked by external source such as a job change
e. Evaluating an event in terms of personal meaning
f. A three-stage set of physiological processes that prepare or adapt the body for danger to survive
g. Arousal of the central nervous system and body defenses are mobilized
h. Begins when a person experiences, witnesses, or is confronted with a traumatic event and responds with intense fear or helplessness
i. Give a person protection from anxiety and stress
j. Actual or alleged hazard to the balance of hemostasis
k. How people interpret the impact of the stressor on themselves
l. Recurrent or intrusive recollections of the event
m. Any physical, psychological, or social stimuli that are capable of producing stress
n. The body will attempt to return to a state of balance
o. Rising hormone levels result in increased blood volume, blood glucose levels, epinephrine and norepinephrine amounts, heart rate, blood flow to the muscles, oxygen intake, and mental alertness
p. Occurs when the body is no longer able to resist the effects of the stressor
q. Caused by a major natural or human-made disaster
r. Body stabilizes and responds in the opposite manner to the alarm reaction
s. Person's cognitive and behavioral efforts to manage psychological stress
t. Occurs as the person moves through life's stages

Nursing Knowledge Base

21. Briefly describe the following models.

    a. Neuman systems model: _____

    b. Pender's health promotion model: _____

The following factors can influence stress and coping. Give some examples.

22. Situational factors: _____

_____

23. Maturational factors: _____

_____

24. Sociocultural factors: _____

_____

25. Compassion fatigue: _____

_____

26. Second victim syndrome: _____

_____

Nursing Process

Assessment

27. Identify subjective areas that are used to assess a patient's level of stress.

    a. _____

    b. _____

    c. _____

    d. _____

    e. _____

28. Identify some objective findings related to stress and coping.

    a. _____

    b. _____

    c. _____

    d. _____

    e. _____

    f. _____

    g. _____

Analysis and Nursing Diagnosis

29. Identify the multiple diagnoses for stress or failure of coping.

    a. _____

    b. _____

    c. _____

    d. _____

    e. _____

Planning and Outcomes Identification

30. The nurse assesses the level and source of the existing stress and determines the appropriate points for interventions; describe each level.

    a. Primary level of prevention: _____

    b. Secondary level of prevention: _____

    c. Tertiary level of prevention: _____

Implementation

31. Identify the three primary modes of intervention to reduce stress.

    a. _____

    b. _____

    c. _____

32. Describe how the following health promotion activities decrease stress:
    a. Regular exercise:

    _____

    _____

    b. Support system:

    _____

    _____

    c. Time management:

    _____

    _____

    d. Guided imagery and visualization:

    _____

    _____

    e. Progressive muscle relaxation therapies:

    _____

    _____

    f. Assertive training:

    _____

    _____

    g. Journal writing:

    _____

    _____

    h. Mindfulness-based stress reduction:

    _____

    _____

Acute Care

33. Crisis intervention is: _____

_____

Evaluation

34. The desired outcomes for a patient recovering from acute stress are: _____

_____

CASE STUDY

35. A young father is in the primary care clinic for a routine appointment for management of his type 2 diabetes. During the assessment he tells you that his wife suddenly left him. They have two children. His wife left without the children, so he is now a single parent to two school-aged children 8 and 10 years of age. You suspect that this man is experiencing a developmental crisis. Identify some questions that are appropriate to ask for providing more information about the impact of this crisis.

REVIEW QUESTIONS

Select the appropriate answer and cite the rationale for choosing that particular answer.

36. Which definition does not characterize stress?
    1. Efforts to maintain relative constancy within the internal environment
    2. A condition eliciting an intellectual, behavioral, or metabolic response
    3. Any situation in which a nonspecific demand requires an individual to respond or take action
    4. A phenomenon affecting social, psychological, developmental, spiritual, and physiological dimensions

    Answer: _____

    Rationale: _____

    _____

    _____

37. Which of the following is an example of the general adaptation syndrome?
    1. Alarm reaction
    2. Inflammatory response
    3. Fight-or-flight response
    4. Ego-defense mechanisms

    Answer: _____

    Rationale: _____

    _____

    _____

38. Crisis intervention is a specific measure used for helping a patient resolve a particular, immediate stress problem. This approach is based on:
    1. An in-depth analysis of a patient's situation
    2. The ability of the nurse to solve the patient's problems
    3. Effective communication between the nurse and patient
    4. Teaching the patient how to use ego-defense mechanisms

    Answer: _____

    Rationale: _____

    _____

    _____

39. Your co-worker tells you that she "no longer cares about her patients." You conclude that she is experiencing compassion fatigue. Which other signs and symptoms do you expect to find? (Select all that apply.)
    1. Hopelessness
    2. Flashbacks
    3. Anxiety
    4. Fatigue
    5. Loss of pleasure in activities
    6. Depression

    Answer: _____

    Rationale: _____

    _____

    _____

40. Imagine that you are the nurse in the care plan in Chapter 37 of your text. Complete the *Evaluation phase* of the critical thinking model with these questions in mind.

a. In evaluating the care of Sandra and John, what knowledge did the nurse apply?

_____

b. In what way might the nurse's previous experience influence the evaluation of Sandra and John's care?

_____

c. During evaluation, what intellectual and professional standards were applied to Sandra and John's care?

_____

d. In what way do critical thinking attitudes play a role in how the nurse approaches the evaluation of Sandra and John's care?

_____

e. How might the nurse adjust their care?

_____

Next Generation NCLEX® Examination-Style Questions

41. The employee health nurse is meeting with a nurse who has been working on the COVID unit for the past 6 months. The nurse states "I am tired. All I do is take care of people who are going to die. I can't keep working all these hours."

Choose the most likely options for the information missing from the statement(s) by selecting from the lists of options provided.

The employee health nurse determines that the nurse working in the COVID unit is most likely experiencing _____1_____. The employee health nurse suggests the most important thing is to _____2_____. The employee health nurse presents several strategies to help the nurse including _____3_____.

Options for 1	Options for 2	Options for 3
Posttraumatic stress disorder	Recognize this is temporary and will get better	Taking PRN benzodiazepines
Anxiety	Take time-off from work	Practicing self-care
Compassion fatigue	Recognize the concern	Moving to a different unit
Second victim syndrome	Attend a support group	Taking medical leave
Dissociation	See a mental health professional	Becoming more informed about current COVID treatment

38 Activity and Exercise

PRELIMINARY READING

Chapter 38

COMPREHENSIVE UNDERSTANDING

Scientific Knowledge Base

Match the following terms.

1. _____ Concentric tension
2. _____ Eccentric tension
3. _____ Body alignment
4. _____ Balance control
5. _____ Coordinated body movement
6. _____ Friction
7. _____ Skeletal system
8. _____ Isotonic contractions
9. _____ Isometric contractions
10. _____ Resistive isometric exercises
11. _____ Fibrous joints
12. _____ Cartilaginous joints
13. _____ Synovial joints
14. _____ Ligaments
15. _____ Tendons
16. _____ Cartilage
17. _____ Antagonistic muscles
18. _____ Synergistic muscles
19. _____ Fixators
20. _____ Proprioception

a. The awareness of the position of the body and its parts
b. Bands of tissue that connect muscle to bone
c. Muscles that are involved with joint stabilization
d. Causes lengthening of a muscle to control the speed and direction of movement
e. Provides attachments for muscles and ligaments and the leverage necessary for mobility
f. Have little movement but are elastic and use cartilage to separate body surfaces
g. Freely movable joints
h. Nonvascular supporting connective tissue
i. Provide precision and control during contraction of prime mover
j. Muscles that contract to accomplish the same movement as primer mover
k. Increased muscle contraction causes muscle shortening
l. Involves the integrated functioning of the musculoskeletal and nervous systems
m. The force that occurs in a direction to oppose movement
n. Without this the center of gravity is displaced; required for static position and moving
o. Static contraction that causes an increase in muscle tension but no shortening or active movement of the muscle
p. An individuals' center of gravity is stable
q. Exercises that cause muscle contraction and change in muscle length (walking, swimming, biking)
r. Bands of fibrous tissue that bind joints and connect bones and cartilage
s. Contraction of muscles while pushing against a stationary object or resisting the movement of the object (e.g., push-ups)
t. Joints that fit closely together and are fixed

21. Identify the steps the nurse uses to achieve balance and alignment.

    a. _____

    b. _____

    c. _____

22. Identify the pathological conditions that influence body alignment, mobility, and activity.

    a. _____

    b. _____

    c. _____

    d. _____

23. Identify the significant risk factors for child obesity.

    a. _____

    b. _____

    c. _____

Nursing Knowledge Base

24. Identify some factors that affect activity and exercise.

    a. _____

    b. _____

    c. _____

    d. _____

    e. _____

    f. _____

Identify the descriptive characteristics of body alignment and mobility related to the following developmental changes.

25. Infants: _____

_____

26. Toddlers: _____

_____

27. Adolescents: _____

_____

28. Young to middle adults: _____

_____

29. Older-adults: _____

_____

Nursing Process

Assessment

30. Identify the stages of change that an individual may go through to change behavior.

    a. _____

    b. _____

    c. _____

    d. _____

    e. _____

31. Identify the objectives for assessing body alignment.

    a. _____

    b. _____

    c. _____

    d. _____

    e. _____

    f. _____

    g. _____

32. Identify the five components to assess mobility.

    a. _____

    b. _____

    c. _____

    d. _____

    e. _____

    f. _____

33. Identify the ways to assess a patient's gait.

    a. _____

    b. _____

    c. _____

34. Briefly describe the physiological changes that occur in the following:

    a. Cardiovascular system _____

    b. Pulmonary system _____

    c. Metabolic system _____

    d. Musculoskeletal system _____

    e. Activity tolerance _____

    f. Psychosocial factors _____

Analysis and Nursing Diagnosis

35. Identify the nursing diagnoses that are related to activity and exercise.

    a. _____

    b. _____

    c. _____

    d. _____

    e. _____

Planning and Outcomes Identification

36. List three outcomes for a patient with deficits in activity and exercise.

    a. _____

    b. _____

    c. _____

Implementation

37. Explain how to calculate the patient's target heart rate (THR).

    _____

    _____

38. An exercise program can consist of the following. Provide examples for each one.

    a. Aerobic exercise: _____

    b. Stretching and flexibility exercises: _____

    c. Resistance training: _____

39. What is the difference between active ROM and passive ROM?

    _____

    _____

40. Walking helps to prevent contractures by: _____

    _____

41. Identify the two types of canes that are available and their use.

    a. _____

    b. _____

42. Explain the four standard crutch gaits.

    a. Four-point gait: _____

    b. Three-point gait: _____

    c. Two-point gait: _____

    d. Swing-through gait: _____

Evaluation

43. Identify the areas to evaluate to determine the effectiveness of the nursing interventions to enhance activity and exercise.

a. _____

b. _____

c. _____

d. _____

e. _____

f. _____

CASE STUDY

44. The nurse is attempting to transfer a patient from bed to chair. Identify the five steps of assessment (in order) for safe and effective transfers.

REVIEW QUESTIONS

Select the appropriate answer and cite the rationale for choosing that particular answer.

45. White, shiny, flexible bands of fibrous tissue binding joints together and connecting various bones and cartilage types are known as:
    1. Joints
    2. Muscles
    3. Tendons
    4. Ligaments

    Answer: _____

    Rationale: _____

    _____

    _____

46. The nurse would expect all of the following physiological effects of exercise on the body systems except:
    1. Change in metabolic rate
    2. Decreased cardiac output
    3. Increased respiratory rate and depth
    4. Increased muscle tone, size, and strength

    Answer: _____

    Rationale: _____

    _____

    _____

47. You are the nurse caring for Ms. McDonnell, a 68-year-old female, with osteoarthritis of the right knee and hands. She was a regularly active skier in her twenties until she injured her right knee and gave up the sport. She has not participated in any regular exercise since that time. Her other medical conditions include hypertension and hyperlipidemia. Select all the factors that influence activity tolerance in Ms. McDonnell (Select all that apply.):
    1. Skeletal abnormalities
    2. Diabetes mellitus
    3. Hypoxemia
    4. Female sex
    5. Motivation
    6. Prior exercise patterns

    Answer: _____

    Rationale: _____

    _____

    _____

48. Imagine that you are the nurse in the care plan in Chapter 38 of your text. Complete the *Planning phase* of the critical thinking model with these questions in mind.

   a. In developing Mrs. Smith's plan of care, what knowledge did the nurse apply?

   _____

   b. In what way might the nurse's previous experience assist in developing a plan of care for Mrs. Smith?

   _____

   c. When developing a plan of care, what intellectual or professional standards were applied to Mrs. Smith?

   _____

   d. What critical thinking attitudes might have been applied in developing Mrs. Smith's plan?

   _____

   e. How will the nurse accomplish the goals of the plan of care?

   _____

Next Generation NCLEX® Examination-Style Questions

49. The nurse is planning an exercise awareness course for a group of older-adult women. Each woman participating is in relatively good health and is 70 years of age or older. Each participant has been cleared for regular exercise by their provider. Which teaching will the nurse include? (Select all that apply.)
   1. To find the target heart rate, multiple your current age by 60%.
   2. Encourage regular stretching and limit periods of long sitting.
   3. It is expected to have some mild dizziness when walking briskly for endurance.
   4. Weight-bearing exercises, like hiking or climbing stairs are encouraged.
   5. High-impact aerobics can help develop balance and muscle strength.
   6. Even exaggerating normal movements can help to build strength.
   7. Once muscle is lost, it is too late to build strength again.
   8. Remember to limit fluids to avoid potential stress on the heart from too much fluid.

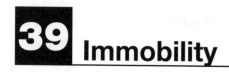 **Immobility**

PRELIMINARY READING

Chapter 39

COMPREHENSIVE UNDERSTANDING

Scientific Knowledge Base

Match the following terms related to the nature of movement.

1. _____ Mobility
2. _____ Body alignment
3. _____ Friction
4. _____ Shear

    a. Force that occurs in a direction to oppose movement
    b. Force exerted against the skin while the skin remains stationary, and the bony structures move
    c. Reduces strain on musculoskeletal structures, aids in maintaining muscle tone, promotes comfort, and contributes to balance
    d. When optimized, correlates with positive patient outcomes

Describe how the following are related to movement.

5. Joints: _____

_____

6. Ligaments: _____

_____

7. Tendons: _____

_____

8. Cartilages: _____

_____

9. Skeletal muscles: _____

_____

10. Nervous system: _____

_____

11. Describe how the following pathological abnormalities affect mobility.

    a. Postural: _____

    b. Muscle: _____

    c. Damage to the central nervous system: _____

    d. Damage to the musculoskeletal system _____

Nursing Knowledge Base

Define the following terms.

12. Mobility: _____

_____

13. Immobility: _____

_____

14. Disuse atrophy: _____

_____

15. Identify the complications of immobility in relation to the metabolic functioning of the body.

_____

_____

16. Explain the following respiratory changes that occur with immobility.

    a. Atelectasis: _____

    b. Hydrostatic pneumonia: _____

17. Explain the following cardiovascular changes that occur with immobility.

    a. Orthostatic hypotension: _____

    b. Thrombus: _____

18. Identify the complications of immobility in relation to the musculoskeletal system.

    a. _____

    b. _____

    c. _____

    d. _____

    e. _____

19. Identify the complications of immobility in relation to the urinary system.

    a. _____

    b. _____

20. Identify the complication of immobility in relation to the integumentary system.

_____

_____

21. Identify the psychosocial effects that occur with immobilization.

    a. _____

    b. _____

    c. _____

201

Briefly explain the negative outcomes of immobility to the following groups.

22. Infants, toddlers, and preschoolers: _____

_____

23. Adolescents: _____

_____

24. Adults: _____

_____

25. Older-adults: _____

_____

Nursing Process

Assessment

26. Briefly describe the four major areas for assessment of patient mobility.

    a. Range of motion: _____

    b. Gait: _____

    c. Exercise pattern: _____

    d. Body alignment: _____

Describe the technique to use to assess the physiological hazards of immobility and cite an abnormal finding of each technique.

27. Metabolic: _____

_____

28. Respiratory: _____

_____

29. Cardiovascular: _____

_____

30. Musculoskeletal: _____

_____

31. Skin: _____

_____

32. Elimination: _____

_____

33. Psychosocial: _____

_____

34. Common risk factors for VTE are:

a. _____

b. _____

c. _____

Analysis and Nursing Diagnosis

35. List the actual or potential nursing diagnoses related to an immobilized or partially immobilized patient.

a. _____

b. _____

c. _____

d. _____

Planning and Outcomes Identification

36. List the expected outcomes for the goal "patient skin remains intact."

a. _____

b. _____

Implementation

37. Identify some examples of health promotion activities that address mobility and immobility.

a. _____

b. _____

c. _____

Identify the nursing interventions that will reduce the impact of immobility on the following body systems.

38. Metabolic system.

a. _____

b. _____

39. Respiratory system.

a. _____

b. _____

c. _____

40. Cardiovascular system.

a. _____

b. _____

c. _____

41. Musculoskeletal system.

    a. _____

    b. _____

42. Integumentary system.

    a. _____

    b. _____

43. Elimination system.

    a. _____

    b. _____

44. Psychosocial system.

    a. _____

    b. _____

45. Give a description of the following positions and the common trouble areas with each.

    a. Fowler: _____

    b. Supine: _____

    c. Prone: _____

    d. Side-lying: _____

    e. Sims: _____

46. Instrumental activities of daily living (IADL) are: _____

_____

47. Describe how you would assist patients with hemiplegia or hemiparesis.

_____

_____

CASE STUDY

48. The nurse is caring for a patient who is receiving 5000 units of heparin subcutaneously every 12 hours to prevent venous thromboembolism while on prolonged bedrest. Because bleeding is a potential side effect of this medication, what should the nurse assess the patient for?

Select the appropriate answer and cite the rationale for choosing that answer.

49. Which of the following is a potential hazard that you should assess when the patient is in the prone position?
    1. Plantar flexion
    2. Increased cervical flexion
    3. Internal rotation of the shoulder
    4. Unprotected pressure points at the sacrum and heels

    Answer: _____

    Rationale: _____

    _____

    _____

50. Which of the following is a physiological effect of prolonged bed rest?
    1. An increase in cardiac output
    2. A decrease in lean body mass
    3. A decrease in lung expansion
    4. A decrease in urinary excretion of nitrogen

    Answer: _____

    Rationale: _____

    _____

    _____

51. The nurse would assess the patient for all of the following to determine deep vein thrombosis except:
    1. Checking for a positive Homan's sign
    2. Asking the patient about the presence of calf pain
    3. Observing the dorsal aspect of lower extremities for redness, warmth, and tenderness
    4. Measuring the circumference of each leg daily, placing the tape measure at the midpoint of the knee

    Answer: _____

    Rationale: _____

    _____

    _____

52. Which of the following is an appropriate intervention to maintain the respiratory system of the immobilized patient?
    1. Turn the patient every 4 hours.
    2. Maintain a maximum fluid intake of 1500 mL/day.
    3. Apply an abdominal binder continuously while the patient is in bed.
    4. Encourage the patient to deep breathe and cough every 1 to 2 hours.

    Answer: _____

    Rationale: _____

    _____

    _____

53. Which of the following are potential nursing diagnoses for an immobilized or partially immobilized patient?
    1. Ineffective airway clearance
    2. Impaired sleep
    3. Risk for constipation
    4. Risk for impaired skin integrity
    5. Social isolation

    Answer: _____

    Rationale: _____

    _____

    _____

54. The nurse has begun assessment of an 81-year-old patient admitted to a medical-surgical floor with generalized weakness. During the assessment, the patient states, "I've been in bed for what seems like forever. I'm just too tired to get up and do anything at all." The nurse notes a reddish area at the base of the spine measuring 2 inches by 2 inches (5.08 cm x 5.08 cm). Crepitus, slight resistance, and hypotonia are noted when passive range of motion is performed on the lower extremities. Joint swelling in the fingers and wrists is observed. Vital signs include blood pressure of 100/70 mm Hg, temperature 97.8° F (36.6° C), respirations 12 per minute, and pulse 64 beats per minute. Laboratory results include a urinalysis (below).

Highlight the finding(s) in the paragraph that the nurse will report to the health care provider.

Component	Value	Standard Range
Color, Urine	Yellow	Yellow
Appearance, Urine	Cloudy	
pH, Urine	6.5	4.5–8.0
Specific Gravity, Urine	1.025	1.005–1.030
Protein, Urine	Negative MG/DL	Negative MG/DL
Glucose, Urine	Negative GM/DL	Negative GM/DL
Ketone, Urine	Negative MG/DL	Negative MG/DL
Bilirubin, Urine	Negative	Negative
Blood, Urine	Negative	Negative
Urobilinogen, Urine	Normal	Normal
Nitrites, Urine	Negative	Negative
Leukocytes, Urine	Negative	Negative

40 Hygiene

PRELIMINARY READING

Chapter 40

COMPREHENSIVE UNDERSTANDING

Scientific Knowledge Base

1. Explain the three primary layers of the skin.

   a. Epidermis: _____

   b. Dermis: _____

   c. Subcutaneous: _____

2. Identify the functions of the skin.

   a. _____

   b. _____

   c. _____

   d. _____

Define the following disorders of the oral cavity:

3. Xerostomia: _____

4. Gingivitis: _____

5. Dentalcaries: _____

Nursing Knowledge Base

6. Identify the factors that influence hygiene.

   a. _____

   b. _____

   c. _____

   d. _____

   e. _____

   f. _____

   g. _____

   h. _____

Nursing Process

Assessment

7. Assessment of the skin includes: _____

8. Common skin problems can affect how hygiene is administered. Describe the hygiene provided for the following.

    a. Dry skin: _____

    b. Acne: _____

    c. Skin rashes: _____

    d. Contact dermatitis: _____

    e. Abrasion: _____

9. Identify the characteristics of the following foot and nail problems.

    a. Calluses: _____

    b. Corns: _____

    c. Plantar warts: _____

    d. Tinea pedis: _____

    e. Ingrown nails: _____

    f. Paronychia: _____

    g. Foot odors: _____

Identify the characteristics of the following mouth problems.

10. Halitosis: _____

11. Cheilitis: _____

12. Glossitis: _____

Identify the characteristics of the following hair and scalp conditions.

13. Dandruff: _____

14. Ticks: _____

15. Pediculosis: _____

16. Pediculosis capitis: _____

17. Pediculosis corporis: _____

18. Pediculosis pubis: _____

19. Alopecia: _____

20. Give examples of patients at risk for hygiene problems.

    a. Oral problems: _____

    b. Skin problems: _____

    c. Foot problems: _____

    d. Eye care problems: _____

Analysis and Nursing Diagnosis

21. List the possible nursing diagnoses that apply to patients in need of hygiene care.

    a. _____

    b. _____

    c. _____

    d. _____

    e. _____

Planning and Outcomes Identification

22. Identify three expected outcomes for a patient who has had a cerebral vascular accident.

    a. _____

    b. _____

    c. _____

Implementation

23. List the educational tips for patients about hygiene practices.

    a. _____

    b. _____

    c. _____

    d. _____

Acute and Restorative Care

24. Briefly explain the following types of baths.

    a. Complete bed bath: _____

    b. Partial bed bath: _____

25. State guidelines that the nurse needs to follow regardless of the type of bath.

    a. _____

    b. _____

    c. _____

    d. _____

    e. _____

26. Identify the risk factors for skin breakdown in the perineal area.

    _____

    _____

27. Identify the benefits of a back rub.

_____

_____

28. List the guidelines in a routine foot and nail care program.

a. _____

b. _____

c. _____

d. _____

e. _____

f. _____

g. _____

Briefly explain the benefits of the following in relation to oral hygiene.

29. Brushing: _____

30. Flossing: _____

31. Denturecare: _____

Briefly describe the rationale for the following interventions.

32. Brushing and combing hair: _____

33. Shampooing: _____

34. Mustache and beard care: _____

35. Explain how shaving should be performed and provide a rationale.

_____

_____

36. Describe basic eye care for a patient.

_____

_____

37. Describe the procedure for removal of impacted cerumen.

_____

_____

38. Describe the following types of hearing aids.

a. Completely-in-canal (CIC) aid: _____

b. In-the-ear (ITE) hearing aid: _____

c. Behind-the-ear (BTE) hearing aid: _____

d. Digital hearing aid: _____

210

39. Describe the following common bed positions.

a. Fowler's: _____

b. Semi-Fowler's: _____

c. Trendelenburg: _____

d. Reverse Trendelenburg: _____

e. Flat: _____

CASE STUDY

40. A nurse is caring for a patient who complains of sore feet but who also has decreased sensation in both feet. What interventions should the nurse do for this patient?

REVIEW QUESTIONS

Select the appropriate answer and cite the rationale for choosing that particular answer.

41. Mr. Gray is a 19-year-old patient in the rehabilitation unit. He is completely paralyzed below the neck. The most appropriate bath for Mr. Gray is a:
1. Partial bed bath
2. Complete bed bath
3. Sitz bath
4. Tepid bath

Answer: _____

Rationale: _____

_____

_____

42. All of the following will help maintain skin integrity in older-adults except:
1. Environmental air that is cold and dry
2. Use of warm water and mild cleansing agents for bathing
3. Bathing every other day
4. Drinking 8 to 10 glasses of water a day

Answer: _____

Rationale: _____

_____

_____

43. When preparing to give complete morning care to a patient, what would the nurse do first?
1. Gather the necessary equipment and supplies.
2. Remove the patient's gown or pajamas while maintaining privacy.
3. Assess the patient's preferences for bathing practices.
4. Lower the side rails and assist the patient with assuming a comfortable position.

Answer: _____

Rationale: _____

_____

_____

44. Assessment of the hair and scalp reveals that John has head lice. An appropriate intervention would be:
1. Shave hair off the affected area.
2. Place oil on the hair and scalp until all of the lice are dead.
3. Shampoo with medicated shampoo and repeat 12 to 24 hours later.
4. Shampoo with regular shampoo and dry with hair-dryer set at the hottest setting.

Answer: _____

Rationale: _____

_____

_____

45. A clinical agency is starting to use chlorhexidine gluconate (CHG) 4% in a bath base basin for certain patients. Which points are important to remember? (Select all that apply.)
    1. Use one wash cloth, only once, for each body part.
    2. Patient's skin may feel sticky after bathing.
    3. Wipe off sticky residue from patient's skin.
    4. Wash patient's face with CHG 4%.

    Answer: _____

    Rationale: _____

    _____

    _____

46. You as the nurse are caring for a patient with the diagnosis of high-risk for impaired skin integrity who has redness over the sacral area, limited mobility, and stool incontinence. Select the appropriate interventions that would apply to this patient (Select all that apply.):
    1. Frequent repositioning
    2. Management of incontinence
    3. Wound care
    4. Specialty support surfaces

    Answer: _____

    Rationale: _____

    _____

    _____

CRITICAL THINKING MODEL FOR NURSING CARE FOR SELF-CARE DEFICIT: IMPAIRED ABILITY TO BATH

47. Imagine that you are the nurse in the care plan in Chapter 40 of your text. Complete the *Planning phase* of the critical thinking model with these questions in mind.

    a. In developing Mrs. White's plan of care, what knowledge did the nurse apply?

    _____

    b. In what way might the nurse's previous experience apply in this case?

    _____

    c. What intellectual or professional standards were applied to Mrs. White?

    _____

    d. What critical thinking attitudes did you use in providing care to Mrs. White?

    _____

    e. As you review your plan, what key areas did you cover?

    _____

Next Generation NCLEX® Examination-Style Questions

48. The nurse has provided orientation and education to a new assistive personnel (AP). Today, after assuring the five rights of delegation, the nurse has delegated the AP to provide a complete bed bath to a 68-year-old patient admitted several days ago with nausea and vomiting following chemotherapy treatment. Although the patient is improving slowly, full assistance is still needed with ADLs due to persistent weakness. Once the AP has communicated an understanding of what is to be done, they gather supplies and enter the patient's room. The nurse walks by the room several minutes later and has an opportunity to witness the AP performing the delegated task.

Select four observations that require the nurse to intervene and provide re-teaching to the AP.

Dons clean gloves prior to beginning care
Offers to clip the patient's toenails that are long
Utilizes drapes over the unexposed parts of the body
Places dentures on a napkin by the sink
Tests water temperature prior to using it for bathing
Raises the bed to a comfortable position
Encourages the patient to wash their face and perineum
Provides commercial mouthwash for rinsing after oral care

212

41 Oxygenation

Chapter 41

COMPREHENSIVE UNDERSTANDING

Scientific Knowledge Base

Match the following key terms that relate to respiratory physiology.

1. _____ Ventilation
2. _____ Work of breathing
3. _____ Inspiration
4. _____ Expiration
5. _____ Compliance
6. _____ Airway resistance
7. _____ Residual volume
8. _____ Deoxyhemoglobin
9. _____ Diffusion
10. _____ Tidal volume

a. Moves the respiratory gases from one area to another according to concentration gradients
b. Hemoglobin and oxygen dissociate
c. Amount of air exhaled after normal inspiration
d. Pressure difference between the mouth and the alveoli in relation to the rate of flow of inspired gas
e. Process of moving gases into and out of the lungs (inhalation and exhalation)
f. Is the amount of air left in the alveoli after a full expiration
g. Effort required to expand and contract the lungs
h. Ability of the lungs to distend or to expand in response to increased interalveolar pressure
i. Active process stimulated by chemical receptors in the aorta
j. Passive process dependent on the elastic recoil properties of the lungs

Match the following cardiopulmonary physiology terms.

11. _____ Frank–Starling law
12. _____ Cardiac output
13. _____ S1 and S2
14. _____ Stroke volume
15. _____ Preload
16. _____ Afterload
17. _____ ECG
18. _____ Normal sinus rhythm

a. Reflects the electrical activity of the conduction system
b. End-diastolic volume
c. As the myocardium stretches, the strength of the contraction increases
d. Normal sequence on the electrocardiogram (ECG)
e. Amount of blood ejected from the left ventricle each minute
f. The amount of blood ejected from the ventricles during systole
g. The resistance to left ventricular ejection
h. Closure of heart valves

Explain what the following waves in the conduction system represent and the normal values for each.

19. P wave: _____

_____

20. PR interval: _____

_____

21. QRS complex: _____

_____

22. QT interval: _____

_____

23. Identify the factors that affect oxygenation.

    a. _____

    b. _____

    c. _____

    d. _____

24. Identify conditions that affect chest wall movement and provide an example.

    a. _____

    b. _____

    c. _____

    d. _____

    e. _____

    f. _____

    g. _____

Explain the following alterations in respiratory functioning.

25. Hyperventilation: _____

_____

26. Hypoventilation: _____

_____

27. Hypoxia: _____

_____

28. Cyanosis: _____

_____

29. Electrical impulses that do not originate for the SA node cause conduction disturbances, and these rhythm disturbances are called: _____

30. Briefly explain the following dysrhythmias.

    a. Tachycardia: _____

    b. Bradycardia: _____

    c. Atrial fibrillation: _____

    d. Paroxysmal supraventricular tachycardia: _____

    e. Ventricular tachycardia: _____

31. Explain the difference between the following types of heart failure.

    a. Left-sided heart failure: _____

    b. Right-sided heart failure: _____

32. Briefly explain the following valvular dysfunctions.

   a. Stenosis: _____

   _____

   _____

   b. Regurgitation: _____

   _____

   _____

Describe the following disorders.

33. Myocardial ischemia: _____

   _____

34. Angina pectoris: _____

   _____

35. Myocardial infarction: _____

   _____

Nursing Knowledge Base

Identify the cardiopulmonary risk factors for the following developmental levels.

36. Infants and toddlers: _____

   _____

37. School-age children and adolescents: _____

   _____

38. Young- and middle-aged adults: _____

   _____

39. Older-adults: _____

   _____

40. List the lifestyle modifications to decrease cardiopulmonary risks.

   a. _____

   b. _____

   c. _____

   d. _____

   e. _____

   f. _____

41. List four occupational pollutants.

   a. _____

   b. _____

   c. _____

   d. _____

Nursing Process

Assessment

42. Explain the following assessment tools.

   a. Pulse oximetry: _____

   _____

   _____

   b. Capnography (end-tidal CO_2) _____

   _____

   _____

43. Explain the focus of the nursing history to meet oxygen needs for the following.

   a. Cardiac function: _____

   _____

   b. Respiratory function: _____

   _____

44. Explain the differences between the following types of chest pain.

   a. Cardiac pain: _____

   _____

   b. Pleuritic chest pain: _____

   _____

   c. Musculoskeletal pain: _____

   _____

Explain how the following affect oxygenation.

45. Fatigue: _____

   _____

46. Dyspnea: _____

   _____

47. Orthopnea: _____

   _____

48. Cough: _____

   _____

49. Wheezing: _____

   _____

Briefly explain what information is gained from the following techniques used during the physical examination to assess tissue oxygenation.

50. Inspection: _____

   _____

51. Palpation: _____

_____

52. Percussion: _____

_____

53. Auscultation: _____

_____

54. Describe the following diagnostic tests used to determine the adequacy of cardiopulmonary function.

　a. Holter monitor: _____

_____

　b. Exercise stress test: _____

_____

　c. Thallium stress test: _____

_____

　d. Electrophysiologic study (EPS): _____

_____

　e. Transthoracic echocardiography: _____

_____

　f. Scintigraphy: _____

_____

　g. Cardiac catheterization and angiography: _____

_____

55. Describe the following tests used to measure the adequacy of ventilation and oxygenation.

　a. Pulmonary function tests: _____

_____

　b. Peak expiratory flow rate (PEFR): _____

_____

　c. Bronchoscopy: _____

_____

　d. Lung scan: _____

_____

　e. Thoracentesis: _____

_____

Analysis and Nursing Diagnosis

56. List the nursing diagnoses that are appropriate for the patient with alterations in oxygenation.

a. _____

b. _____

c. _____

d. _____

e. _____

Planning and Outcomes Identification

57. List the specific outcomes for the goal of an improved breathing pattern.

a. _____

b. _____

c. _____

Implementation

58. Prevention of respiratory infections is a priority for maintaining optimal health. List the teaching strategies to utilize.

a. _____

b. _____

c. _____

59. List the interventions that promote mobilization of pulmonary secretions.

a. _____

b. _____

c. _____

d. _____

60. Describe the following types of cough.

a. Huff: _____

_____

b. Quad: _____

_____

c. Diaphragmatic breathing: _____

_____

61. Postural drainage is a component of pulmonary hygiene and consists of:

a. _____

b. _____

62. Percussion is contraindicated in:

a. _____

b. _____

c. _____

63. Briefly explain positive expiratory pressure (PEP).

_____

64. Briefly explain high-frequency chest wall compression (HFCWC).

_____

65. Nursing interventions that maintain or promote lung expansion include the following noninvasive techniques. Briefly explain each one.

a. Ambulation: _____

_____

b. Positioning: _____

_____

c. Incentive spirometry: _____

_____

66. Briefly explain the following artificial airways:

a. Oral airway _____

b. Endotracheal airway (ET) _____

c. Tracheostomy _____

67. Explain the two types of suctioning:

a. Open method _____

b. Closed method _____

68. List the clinical indications for invasive mechanical ventilation.

a. _____

b. _____

c. _____

d. _____

e. _____

f. _____

69. Noninvasive ventilatory support (NPPV) can be achieved using a variety of modes. List two of them.

a. _____

b. _____

70. List the advantages of noninvasive ventilation (NPPV)

a. _____

b. _____

c. _____

71. Identify the three reasons for inserting chest tubes.

a. _____

b. _____

c. _____

219

72. Define the following.

    a. Hemothorax: _____

    _____

    b. Pneumothorax: _____

    _____

73. The goal of oxygen therapy is: _____

    `_____

74. Describe the following methods of oxygen delivery.

    a. Nasal cannula: _____

    _____

    b. High-flow nasal cannula (HFNC) _____

    _____

    c. Face mask: _____

    _____

    d. Venturi mask: _____

    _____

75. Cardiopulmonary resuscitation (CPR) is: _____

76. In cardiopulmonary resuscitation, CAB stands for: _____

77. The goal of cardiopulmonary rehabilitation for the patient to maintain an optimal level of health focuses on:

    a. _____

    b. _____

    c. _____

    d. _____

Briefly explain the following breathing techniques used to improve ventilation and oxygenation.

78. Pursed-lip breathing: _____

    _____

79. Diaphragmatic breathing: _____

    _____

CASE STUDY

80. The nurse is caring for a patient with an endotracheal tube. What would be some reasons that the nurse would need to suction the patient?

Select the appropriate answer and cite the rationale for choosing that particular answer.

81. Ventilation, perfusion, and exchange of gases are the major purposes of:
    1. Respiration
    2. Circulation
    3. Aerobic metabolism
    4. Anaerobic metabolism

    Answer: _____

    Rationale: _____

    _____

    _____

82. Afterload refers to:
    1. The resistance to left ventricular ejection
    2. The amount of blood in the left ventricle at the end of diastole
    3. The amount of blood ejected from the left ventricle each minute
    4. The amount of blood ejected from the left ventricle with each contraction

    Answer: _____

    Rationale: _____

    _____

    _____

83. The movement of gases into and out of the lungs depends on:
    1. 50% oxygen content in the atmospheric air
    2. The pressure gradient between the atmosphere and the alveoli
    3. The use of accessory muscles of respiration during expiration
    4. The amount of carbon dioxide dissolved in the fluid of the alveoli

    Answer: _____

    Rationale: _____

    _____

    _____

84. Mr. Isaac comes to the emergency department complaining of difficulty breathing. An objective finding associated with his dyspnea might include:
    1. Feelings of heaviness in the chest
    2. Complaints of shortness of breath
    3. Use of accessory muscles of respiration
    4. Statements about a sense of impending doom

    Answer: _____

    Rationale: _____

    _____

    _____

85. The use of chest physiotherapy to mobilize pulmonary secretions involves the use of:
    1. Hydration
    2. Percussion
    3. Nebulization
    4. Humidification

    Answer: _____

    Rationale: _____

    _____

    _____

86. Mrs. Wade is a 74-year-old African-American woman with a 22 year history of chronic obstructive pulmonary disease (COPD). She has been admitted to a medical unit for an acute episode of her disease. She is retired for a plastics factory, lives with her spouse in a 3rd floor apartment located in urban setting. Ms. Wade no longer smokes but had a 42-pack year history. There is no alcohol or illegal drugs. It is her 3rd admission in the past 8 months. Select all the risk factors that apply to Ms. Wade:
    1. urban setting
    2. age
    3. smoking history
    4. use of alcohol and marijuana
    5. living on the 3rd floor

    Answer: _____

    Rationale: _____

    _____

    _____

87. Imagine that you are the student nurse in the care plan in Chapter 41 of your text. Complete the *Assessment phase* of the critical thinking model with these questions in mind.

   a. What knowledge base was applied to Mr. Edwards?

   _____

   b. In what way might your previous experience apply in this case?

   _____

   c. What intellectual or professional standards were applied to Mr. Edwards?

   _____

   d. What critical thinking attitudes did you use in assessing Mr. Edwards?

   _____

   e. As you review your assessment, what key areas did you cover?

   _____

42 Fluid, Electrolyte, and Acid–Base Balance

Chapter 42

COMPREHENSIVE UNDERSTANDING

Scientific Knowledge Base

1. Body fluids are distributed in two distinct compartments. Briefly explain each one.

   a. Extracellular (ECF): _____

   b. Intracellular (ICF): _____

Define the following terms related to the composition of body fluids.

2. Cations: _____

3. Anions: _____

Explain the following types of solution.

4. Isotonic: _____

   _____

   _____

5. Hypotonic: _____

   _____

   _____

6. Hypertonic: _____

   _____

   _____

Define the following terms related to the movement of body fluids.

7. Active transport: _____

8. Osmosis: _____

   _____

9. Osmotic pressure: _____

   _____

10. Diffusion: _____

   _____

11. Filtration: _____

   _____

12. Hydrostatic pressure: _____

13. Colloid osmotic pressure: _____

_____

14. List the three processes that maintain fluid homeostasis.

    a. _____

    b. _____

    c. _____

15. Define how antidiuretic hormone (ADH) regulates fluid balance.

_____

_____

16. Changes in renal perfusion initiate the renin–angiotension–aldosterone (RAAS) mechanism. Explain the mechanism.

_____

_____

17. How does atrial natriuretic peptide (ANP) affect extracellular fluid volume (ECF)?

_____

_____

18. Explain the difference between the two types of fluid imbalances below.

    a. Extracellular fluid volume deficit (ECF deficit): _____

    b. Extracellular fluid volume excess (ECF excess): _____

19. Osmolality imbalances are the following. Briefly explain.

    a. Hypernatremia: _____

    b. Hyponatremia: _____

20. Complete the following table:

Electrolyte	Intake and absorption	Important Function
Potassium		
Ionized calcium		
Magnesium		
Phosphate		

21. For each electrolyte disturbance, identify the diagnostic laboratory finding and list at least four characteristic signs and symptoms in the following table.

Imbalance	Laboratory Finding	Signs and Symptoms
Hypokalemia		
Hyperkalemia		
Hypocalcemia		
Hypercalcemia		
Hypomagnesemia		
Hypermagnesemia		

22. Acid–base homeostasis is the dynamic interplay of three processes. Identify and explain.

a. _____

b. _____

c. _____

23. The four primary types of acid–base imbalances are listed in the following table. For each acid–base imbalance, identify the diagnostic laboratory finding and list the characteristic signs and symptoms.

Acid–Base Imbalance	Laboratory Findings	Signs and Symptoms
Respiratory acidosis		
Respiratory alkalosis		
Metabolic acidosis		
Metabolic alkalosis		

Nursing Process

Assessment

Explain how the following can affect fluid, electrolyte, and acid–base balances.

24. Age: _____
_____

25. Acute illness: _____
_____

26. Recent surgery: _____
_____

27. Burns: _____
_____

28. Cancer: _____
_____

29. Heart failure: _____
_____

30. Gastrointestinal disturbances: _____
_____

31. Environmental factors: _____
_____

32. Diet: _____
_____

33. Lifestyle: _____
_____

34. Medications:

    a. Diuretics: _____

    b. Corticosteroids: _____

    c. ACE inhibitors: _____

    d. Antidepressants: _____

    e. Penicillins: _____

    f. Calcium carbonate: _____

    g. Magnesium hydroxide: _____

    h. Nonsteroidal antiinflammatory drugs: _____

35. Indicate the possible fluid, electrolyte, or acid–base imbalances associated with each physical finding.

Assessment	Imbalances
Loss of 1 kg (2.2 pounds) or more in 24 hours	
Orthostatic hypotension	
Bounding pulse rate	
Full or distended neck veins	
Lung sounds: crackles or rhonchi	
Dark yellow urine	
Dependent edema in ankles	
Dry mucus membranes	
Thirst present	
Restlessness and mild confusion	
Decreased level of consciousness	
Irregular pulse and EKG changes	
Increased rate and depth of respirations	
Muscle weakness	
Decreased deep tendon reflexes	
Hyperactive reflexes, muscle twitching, and cramps	
Tremors	
Abdominal distention	
Decreased bowel sounds	
Constipation	

Analysis and Nursing Diagnosis

36. List potential or actual nursing diagnoses for a patient with fluid, electrolyte, or acid–base imbalances.

    a. _____

    b. _____

    c. _____

    d. _____

    e. _____

Planning and Outcomes Identification

37. List the goals that are appropriate for a patient with dehydration

a. _____

b. _____

Implementation

Briefly describe the rationale for the following interventions.

38. Enteral replacement of fluids: _____

39. Restriction of fluids: _____

_____

40. Parenteral replacement of fluids and electrolytes: _____

_____

41. Total parenteral nutrition (TPN): _____

_____

42. Intravenous (IV) therapy (crystalloids): _____

_____

43. Give an example of the following types of electrolyte solutions.

a. Isotonic: _____

b. Hypotonic: _____

c. Hypertonic: _____

44. What are Vascular access devices (VADs)? _____

45. A venipuncture is: _____

_____

46. Describe the principles to follow for venipunctures in older-adults:

a. _____

b. _____

c. _____

d. _____

e. _____

f. _____

g. _____

h. _____

i. _____

j. _____

47. Electronic infusion devices (EIDs) are necessary for: _____

_____

48. Line maintenance involves:

    a. _____

    b. _____

    c. _____

    d. _____

49. Complete the table below describing complications of IV therapy.

Complication	Assessment Finding	Nursing Action
Infiltration		
Infection		
Phlebitis		
Circulatory overload		
Bleeding		

50. The objectives for blood transfusions are:

    a. _____

    b. _____

    c. _____

51. The ABO system includes: _____

52. The universal blood donor is: _____

53. The universal blood recipient is: _____

54. A transfusion reaction is: _____

    _____

55. Define autotransfusion. _____

    _____

56. Briefly describe the following acute transfusion reactions and their causes.

Reaction	Cause	Clinical Manifestations
Acute intravascular hemolytic		
Febrile, nonhemolytic		
Mild allergic		
Anaphylactic		
Circulatory overload		
Sepsis		

57. List the steps the nurse should follow if a transfusion reaction is suspected.

a. _____

b. _____

c. _____

d. _____

e. _____

f. _____

g. _____

h. _____

CASE STUDY

58. You are taking care of a patient who is receiving IV infusion of 0.9% NaCl, and the patient develops crackles in the lung bases and shortness of breath. What would be your priority nursing action for this patient?

REVIEW QUESTIONS

Select the appropriate answer and cite the rationale for choosing that particular answer.

59. The body fluids constituting the interstitial fluid and blood plasma are:
    1. Hypotonic
    2. Hypertonic
    3. Intracellular
    4. Extracellular

    Answer: _____

    Rationale: _____

    _____

    _____

60. Mrs. Green's arterial blood gas results are as follows: pH, 7.32; $PaCO_2$, 52 mm Hg; PaO_2, 78 mm Hg; HCO_3^-, 24 mEq/L. Mrs. Green has:
    1. Metabolic acidosis
    2. Metabolic alkalosis
    3. Respiratory acidosis
    4. Respiratory alkalosis

    Answer: _____

    Rationale: _____

    _____

    _____

61. Mr. Frank is an 82-year-old patient who has had a 3-day history of vomiting and diarrhea. Which symptom would you expect to find on a physical examination?
    1. Tachycardia
    2. Hypertension
    3. Neck vein distention
    4. Crackles in the lungs

    Answer: _____

    Rationale: _____

    _____

    _____

62. Select all the related causes for a patient to experience respiratory alkalosis? (Select all that apply.)
    1. Steroid use
    2. Fad dieting
    3. Hyperventilation
    4. Chronic alcoholism
    5. Hypoxemia
    6. Stress

    Answer: _____

    Rationale: _____

    _____

    _____

63. You need to discontinue a VAD. Place the steps in the correct order.
    1. Turn off the roller clamp on the IV tubing
    2. Place sterile gauze over the VAD insertion site and apply light pressure while removing the catheter
    3. Document VAD removal
    4. Review the health care provider's order for discontinuing the VAD
    5. Perform hand hygiene and apply clean gloves
    6. Inspect the catheter end for intactness while applying firm pressure with the gauze
    7. Explain to the patient the reason for discontinuing the VAD
    8. Maintain continuous firm pressure with the gauze for 2 to 3 minutes or longer if need
    9. Remove IV site dressings and tape, and clean any secretions

    Answer: _____

    Rationale: _____

    _____

    _____

CRITICAL THINKING MODEL FOR NURSING CARE PLAN FOR DEFICIENT FLUID VOLUME

64. Imagine that you are the nurse in the care plan in Chapter 42 of your text. Complete the *Evaluation phase* of the critical thinking model with these questions in mind.

    a. What knowledge did you apply in evaluating Mrs. Beck's care?

    _____

    b. In what way might your previous experience influence your evaluation of Mrs. Beck?

    _____

    c. During evaluation, what intellectual and professional standards were applied to Mrs. Beck's care?

    _____

    d. In what way do critical thinking attitudes play a role in how you approach the evaluation of Mrs. Beck?

    _____

    e. How might you evaluate Mrs. Beck's care?

    _____

43 Sleep

Chapter 43

COMPREHENSIVE UNDERSTANDING

Scientific Knowledge Base

Match the following terms related to sleep.

1. _____ Sleep
2. _____ Circadian rhythm
3. _____ Biological clock
4. _____ nonrapid eye movement (NREM)
5. _____ rapid eye movement (REM)
6. _____ Dreams
7. _____ Nocturia
8. _____ Hypersomnolence
9. _____ Polysomnogram
10. _____ Insomnia
11. _____ Sleep hygiene
12. _____ Sleep apnea
13. _____ Excessive daytime sleepiness (EDS)
14. _____ Narcolepsy
15. _____ Cataplexy
16. _____ Sleep deprivation
17. _____ Parasomnias

a. Urination during the night, which disrupts the sleep cycle
b. Involves the use of electroencephalogram (EEG), electromyogram (EMG), and electrooculogram (EOG) to monitor stages of sleep
c. Results in impaired waking function, poor work performance, accidents, and emotional problems
d. Most common sleep complaint, signaling an underlying physical or psychological disorder
e. More common in children, an example is sudden infant death syndrome (SIDS)
f. Cyclical process that alternates with longer periods of wakefulness
g. Rapid eye movement (REM) phase at the end of each sleep cycle
h. Synchronizes sleep cycles
i. Influences the pattern of major biological and behavioral functions
j. Sleep that progresses through four stages (light to deep)
k. More vivid and elaborate during REM sleep and are functionally important to learning
l. Characterized by the lack of airflow through the nose and mouth for 10 seconds or longer during sleep
m. Practices that the patient associates with sleep
n. Inadequacies in either the quantity or quality of nighttime sleep
o. Problem patients experience as a result of dyssomnia
p. Sudden muscle weakness during intense emotions at any time during the day
q. Dysfunction of mechanisms that regulate the sleep and wake states (excessive daytime sleepiness)

Nursing Knowledge Base

18. Complete the following table listing the normal sleep patterns of the following developmental stages.

Developmental Stage	Sleep Patterns
Neonates	
Infants	
Toddlers	
Preschoolers	
School-age children	
Adolescents	
Young adults	
Middle adults	
Older-adults	

Describe how each of the following affects sleep and give an example of each.

19. Drugs and illicit substances: _____

20. Lifestyle: _____

21. Usual sleep patterns: _____

22. Emotional stress: _____

23. Environment: _____

24. Exercise and fatigue: _____

25. Food and caloric intake: _____

Nursing Process

Assessment

26. Identify sources for sleep assessment.

_____

27. List the components of a sleep history.

a. _____

b. _____

c. _____

d. _____

e. _____

f. _____

g. _____

h. _____

Analysis and Nursing Diagnosis

28. List the common nursing diagnoses related to sleep problems.

a. _____

b. _____

c. _____

d. _____

e. _____

Planning and Outcomes Identification

29. List the outcomes that you might use for a patient with a sleep disturbance:

a. _____

b. _____

c. _____

d. _____

Implementation

Many factors affect the ability to gain adequate rest and sleep. Briefly give examples of each of the following in relation to health promotion.

30. Environmental controls: _____

31. Promoting bedtime routines: _____

32. Promoting safety: _____

33. Promoting comfort: _____

34. Establishing periods of rest and sleep: _____

35. Stress reduction: _____

36. Bedtime snacks: _____

37. Pharmacologic approaches: _____

Acute Care

For each of the following situations, give two examples of nursing measures that will promote sleep.

38. Environmental controls:

    a. _____

    b. _____

39. Promoting comfort:

    a. _____

    b. _____

40. Establishing periods of rest and sleep:

    a. _____

    b. _____

41. Promoting safety:

    a. _____

    b. _____

42. Stress reduction:

    a. _____

    b. _____

Evaluation

43. With regard to sleep disturbances, the patient is the source for outcomes evaluation. List three outcomes for a patient with a sleep disturbance.

    a. _____

    b. _____

    c. _____

44. Mrs. Wilson is a 70-year-old patient who visits the medical clinic for a routine visit. What nursing interventions would you recommend for this patient to promote a healthy sleeping routine? (Select all that apply.)

   a. Encourage a liberal fluid intake all day.

   b. Ensure room temperature is comfortably warm.

   c. Maintain a regular bedtime and wake-up schedule.

   d. Encourage napping during the day

   e. Use warm bath and relaxation techniques.

   f. Encourage light exercise or watching TV before bedtime.

REVIEW QUESTIONS

Select the appropriate answer and cite the rationale for choosing that particular answer.

45. The 24-hour day–night cycle is known as:
   1. Ultradian rhythm
   2. Circadian rhythm
   3. Infradium rhythm
   4. Non-REM rhythm

   Answer: _____

   Rationale: _____

   _____

   _____

46. Which of the following substances will promote normal sleep patterns?
   1. Alcohol
   2. Narcotics
   3. l-Tryptophan
   4. Beta blockers

   Answer: _____

   Rationale: _____

   _____

   _____

47. All of the following are symptoms of sleep deprivation except:
   1. Irritability
   2. Hyperactivity
   3. Decreased motivation
   4. Rise in body temperature

   Answer: _____

   Rationale: _____

   _____

   _____

48. Mrs. Peterson complains of difficulty falling asleep, awakening earlier than desired, and not feeling rested. She attributes these problems to leg pain that is secondary to her arthritis. What would be the appropriate nursing diagnosis for her?
   1. Fatigue related to leg pain
   2. Insomnia related to arthritis
   3. Deficient knowledge related to sleep hygiene measures
   4. Insomnia related to chronic leg pain

   Answer: _____

   Rationale: _____

   _____

   _____

49. A nursing care plan for a patient with sleep problems has been implemented. All of the following would be expected outcomes except:
   1. Patient reports satisfaction with amount of sleep.
   2. Patient falls asleep within 1 hour of going to bed.
   3. Patient reports no episodes of awakening during the night.
   4. Patient rates sleep as an 8 or above on the visual analogue scale.

   Answer: _____

   Rationale: _____

   _____

   _____

50. Which nursing interventions are appropriate to include in a plan of care to promote sleep for patients who are hospitalized? (Select all that apply.)
   1. Give patient a cup of tea 1 hour before bedtime
   2. Plan vital signs to be taken before patients are asleep
   3. Turn TV on 15 minutes before bedtime
   4. Have patients follow at-home bedtime schedule
   5. Close the door to patients' rooms at bedtime

   Answer: _____

   Rationale: _____

   _____

   _____

CRITICAL THINKING MODEL FOR NURSING CARE PLAN FOR INSOMNIA

51. Imagine that you are the nurse in the care plan in Chapter 43 of your text. Complete the *Evaluation phase* of the critical thinking model with these questions in mind.

   a. What knowledge did you apply in evaluating Julie's care?

   _____

   b. In what way might your previous experience influence your evaluation of Julie's care?

   _____

   c. During evaluation, what intellectual and professional standards were applied to Julie's care?

   _____

   d. In what way do critical thinking attitudes play a role in how you approach the evaluation of Julie's plan?

   _____

   e. How might you evaluate Julie's plan of care?

   _____

235

52. The nurse is performing an initial history and assessment for a patient who has been admitted for shortness of breath and dizziness. In addition to feeling somewhat short of breath on a regular basis, the patient reports having insomnia and being continuously tired, stating, "I feel like I'm never rested no matter how long I sleep." Upon further assessment, the patient admits to taking "a couple of sleeping pills" last night, which were originally prescribed for their partner.

For each finding, place an "X" to indicate whether findings from this patient's assessment are generally associated with sleep apnea or a side effect of medication.

Assessment Finding	Sleep apnea	Medication-induced side effect
Stops breathing for up to 1 minute		
Sleep-walks		
Snores loudly		
Enlarged tonsils		
Excessive daytime sleepiness		
Decreased oxygen saturation		
Eats while asleep		
Respiratory depression		

44 Pain Management

Chapter 44

COMPREHENSIVE UNDERSTANDING

Scientific Knowledge Base

1. The International Association for the Study of Pain (IASP) defines pain as: _____

2. Pain left untreated can lead to serious _____, _____, _____, and _____ consequences.

3. Identify the four physiological processes of normal pain. Briefly explain.

   a. _____

   b. _____

   c. _____

   d. _____

4. Briefly explain gate control theory of pain.

   _____

   _____

5. Define pain tolerance.

   _____

   _____

Match the following physiological reactions to pain to the cause or effect.

6. _____ Dilation of bronchial tubes and increased heart rate

7. _____ Increased heart rate

8. _____ Peripheral vasoconstriction

9. _____ Increased blood glucose level

10. _____ Increased cortisol level

11. _____ Diaphoresis

12. _____ Increased muscle tension

13. _____ Dilation of pupils

14. _____ Decreased gastrointestinal motility

15. _____ Pallor

16. _____ Nausea and vomiting

17. _____ Decreased heart rate and blood pressure

18. _____ Rapid, irregular breathing

a. Provides additional energy
b. Affords better vision
c. Heightened memory functions, a burst of increased immunity
d. Causes blood supply to shift away from periphery
e. Provides increased oxygen intake
f. Elevated blood pressure with shift of blood supply from periphery and viscera to skeletal muscles and brain
g. Vagus nerve sends impulses to chemoreceptor trigger zone in the brain
h. Results from vagal stimulation
i. Prepares muscles for action
j. Controls body temperature during stress
k. Frees energy for more immediate activity
l. Provides increased oxygen transport
m. Causes body defenses to fail under prolonged stress of pain

19. Explain the difference between the following.

a. Acute pain: _____

b. Chronic pain: _____

20. Define the following terms related to pain.

a. Chronic episodic pain: _____

b. Idiopathic pain: _____

Nursing Knowledge Base

21. List some common biases and misconceptions about pain.

a. _____

b. _____

c. _____

d. _____

e. _____

f. _____

g. _____

h. _____

i. _____

22. Identify the physiological factors that influence pain.

a. _____

b. _____

c. _____

d. _____

23. Identify the social factors that can influence pain.

    a. _____

    b. _____

    c. _____

24. Identify the psychological factors that can influence pain.

    a. _____

    b. _____

25. Explain how a person's cultural background factors affect coping with pain.

    _____

    _____

26. List the factors impacted by pain.

    a. _____

    b. _____

    c. _____

    d. _____

Nursing Process

Assessment

27. Identify the ABCDE clinical approach to pain assessment and management.

    a. _____

    b. _____

    c. _____

    d. _____

    e. _____

28. Identify the common characteristics of pain that the nurse would assess.

    a. _____

    b. _____

    c. _____

    d. _____

    e. _____

    f. _____

    g. _____

Analysis and Nursing Diagnosis

29. List potential or actual nursing diagnoses related to a patient in pain.

   a. _____

   b. _____

   c. _____

   d. _____

   e. _____

   f. _____

Planning and Outcomes Identification

30. List the patient outcomes appropriate for the patient experiencing pain.

   a. _____

   b. _____

   c. _____

   d. _____

Implementation

31. Nonpharmacologic interventions include the following. Briefly explain each.

   a. Cognitive behavioral approaches: _____

   b. Physical approaches: _____

32. List the guidelines for an effective pain treatment plan:

   a. _____

   b. _____

   c. _____

   d. _____

   e. _____

Nonpharmacologic interventions such as the following lessen pain. Briefly explain each one.

33. Relaxation: _____

34. Distraction: _____

35. Music: _____

36. Cutaneous stimulation: _____

37. Herbals: _____

38. Reducing pain perception and reception: _____

39. Identify the three types of analgesics used for pain relief.

   a. _____

   b. _____

   c. _____

40. Define adjuvants or coanalgesics.

   _____

   _____

41. Give at least two examples of the following common opioid effects on the following systems.

    a. Central nervous system: _____

    b. Ocular: _____

    c. Respiratory: _____

    d. Cardiac: _____

    e. Gastrointestinal: _____

    f. Genitourinary: _____

    g. Endocrine: _____

    h. Skin: _____

    i. Immunological: _____

42. List the nursing principles for administering analgesics.

    a. _____

    b. _____

    c. _____

    d. _____

43. The main benefit of multimodal analgesia is: _____

44. What is patient-controlled analgesia (PCA)? What is the goal of PCA?

_____

_____

Explain the differences between the following.

45. Local anesthesia:

_____

_____

46. Regional anesthesia:

_____

_____

47. Epidural analgesia: _____

48. List the goals for the care of a patient with epidural infusions. Describe one action for each goal.

    a. _____

    b. _____

    c. _____

    d. _____

    e. _____

    f. _____

49. Identify the following types of breakthrough pain.

a. Incident pain: _____

b. End-of-dose failure pain: _____

c. Spontaneous pain: _____

50. Give some examples of barriers to effective pain management.

a. Patient: _____

b. Health care provider: _____

c. Health care system: _____

51. Define the following terms related to the use of opioids in pain treatment.

a. Physical dependence: _____

b. Drug tolerance: _____

c. Addiction: _____

52. Define *placebo*.

_____

_____

Explain the purpose of the following.

53. Pain clinics: _____

_____

54. Palliative care: _____

_____

55. Hospice: _____

_____

Evaluation

56. Identify some principles to evaluate related to pain management.

_____

_____

CASE STUDY

57. A patient was just admitted to your care after surgery. She states that her pain level is 6 on a 0-to-10 pain scale. She received a dose of IV pain medication 15 minutes ago. What interventions would be beneficial for this patient? (Select all that apply.)

a. reposition for comfort

b. massage her back

c. tell her she cannot have any more pain medication at this time because it is too soon

d. take a few minutes to speak calmly with her to reduce her anxiety

e. return to her room to reassess her pain when it is time for her next dose

Select the appropriate answer and cite the rationale for choosing that particular answer.

58. Pain is a protective mechanism warning of tissue injury and is largely a(n):
    1. Objective experience
    2. Subjective experience
    3. Acute symptom of short duration
    4. Symptom of a severe illness or disease

    Answer: _____

    Rationale: _____

    _____

    _____

59. A substance that can cause analgesia when it attaches to opiate receptors in the brain is:
    1. Endorphin
    2. Bradykinin
    3. Substance P
    4. Prostaglandin

    Answer: _____

    Rationale: _____

    _____

    _____

60. To adequately assess the quality of a patient's pain, which question would be appropriate?
    1. "Is it a sharp pain or a dull pain?"
    2. "Tell me what your pain feels like."
    3. "Is your pain a crushing sensation?"
    4. "How long have you had this pain?"

    Answer: _____

    Rationale: _____

    _____

    _____

61. The use of patient distraction in pain control is based on the principle that:
    1. Small C fibers transmit impulses via the spinothalamic tract.
    2. The reticular formation can send inhibitory signals to gating mechanisms.
    3. Large A fibers compete with pain impulses to close gates to painful stimuli.
    4. Transmission of pain impulses from the spinal cord to the cerebral cortex can be inhibited.

    Answer: _____

    Rationale: _____

    _____

    _____

CRITICAL THINKING MODEL FOR NURSING CARE PLAN FOR ACUTE PAIN

62. Imagine that you are the student nurse in the care plan in Chapter 44 of your text. Complete the *Assessment phase* of the critical thinking model with these questions in mind.

    a. What knowledge base was applied to Mrs. Mays?

    _____

    b. In what way might previous experience assist you in this case?

    _____

    c. What intellectual or professional standards were applied to the care of Mrs. Mays?

    _____

    d. What critical thinking attitudes did you use in assessing Mrs. Mays?

    _____

    e. As you review your assessment, what key areas did you cover?

    _____

243

63. The nurse is caring for a patient who is status-post a left hip replacement and is prescribed patient-controlled analgesia (PCA) for pain. In addition to receiving 2L of oxygen, the patient is also receiving normal saline at 125 cc/minute. Blood glucose monitoring over the past 12 hours has produced normal and expected results. At the last assessment, the patient was very drowsy but could respond to basic commands. Upon documenting the most recent vital signs, the nurse observes these values in the electronic health record:

Date	22-Aug	22-Aug	22-Aug
Time	1630	1700	1730
Blood pressure (mm Hg)	120/94	106/82	98/70
Pulse (beats per minute)	88	74	64
Respirations (per minute)	20	16	12
SpO$_2$	96%	94%	90%
Temperature	98.8°F (37.1°C)	98.8°F (37.1°C)	98.2°F (36.8°C)

Complete the diagram by dragging from the choices area to specify which condition the patient is most likely experiencing, two actions the nurse should take to address that condition, and two parameters the nurse should monitor to assess the patient's progress.

Highlight correct answers in yellow.

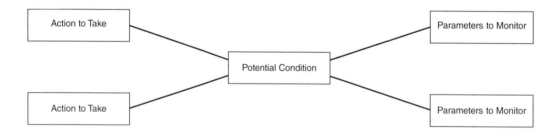

Actions to Take	Potential Conditions	Parameters to Monitor
Administer naloxone immediately	Serotonin syndrome	Urinary output
Notify the health care provider	Sepsis	ALT/AST laboratory values
Ensure oxygen is working properly	Opioid toxicity	SpO$_2$
Request order for fluid bolus	Hypoglycemia	Respiratory rate
Administer PRN oral analgesic		Gait stability

45 Nutrition

PRELIMINARY READING

Chapter 45

COMPREHENSIVE UNDERSTANDING

Match the following biochemical units of nutrition.

1. _____ Basal metabolic rate (BMR)

2. _____ Resting energy expenditure (REE)

3. _____ kcal

4. _____ Nutrient density

5. _____ Saccharides

6. _____ Simple carbohydrates

7. _____ Fiber

8. _____ Proteins

9. _____ Amino acid

10. _____ Indispensable amino acids

11. _____ Dispensable amino acids

12. _____ Nitrogen balance

13. _____ Lipids

14. _____ Triglycerides

15. _____ Saturated fatty acids

16. _____ Unsaturated fatty acids

17. _____ Monounsaturated fatty acids

18. _____ Polyunsaturated fatty acids

19. _____ Water

20. _____ Fat-soluble vitamins

21. _____ Hypervitaminosis

22. _____ Water-soluble vitamins

23. _____ Trace elements

a. Vitamin C and B complex
b. Inorganic elements that act as catalysts in biochemical reactions
c. Energy needed to maintain life-sustaining activities for a specific period of time at rest
d. Simplest form of a protein
e. Made up of three fatty acids attached to a glycerol
f. The intake and output of nitrogen are equal
g. Fatty acids that have two or more double carbon bonds
h. Resting metabolic rate over a 24-hour period
i. Kilocalorie
j. Are found primarily in sugars
k. Polysaccharide that does not contribute calories to the diet
l. Makes up 60% to 70% of total body weight
m. Most calorie-dense nutrient; provides 9 kcal/g
n. The proportion of essential nutrients to the number of kilocalories
o. Carbohydrate units
p. Alanine, asparagine, and glutamic acid
q. Unequal number of hydrogen atoms are attached, and the carbon atoms attach to each other with a double bond
r. Each carbon has two attached hydrogen atoms
s. Histidine, lysine, and phenylalanine
t. Results from megadoses of supplemental vitamins, fortified food, and large intake of fish oils
u. Vitamins A, D, E, and K
v. A source of energy (4 kcal/g)
w. Fatty acids with one double bond

Match the following key terms related to the digestive system.

24. _____ Enzymes

25. _____ Peristalsis

26. _____ Chyme

27. _____ Amylase

28. _____ Alcohol and Aspirin

29. _____ Gastric juice pH level

30. _____ Small intestine pH level

31. _____ Metabolism

32. _____ Anabolism

33. _____ Catabolism

34. _____ Glycogenolysis

35. _____ Glycogenesis

36. _____ Gluconeogenesis

a. Anabolism of glucose into glycogen for storage
b. Acidic, liquefied mass
c. Catabolism of glycogen into glucose, carbon dioxide, and water
d. Building of more complex biochemical substances by synthesis of nutrients
e. Breakdown of biochemical substances into simpler substances, occurring during a negative nitrogen balance
f. Protein like substances that act as catalysts to speed up chemical reactions
g. This enzyme breaks down starches into sugars
h. Wave-like muscular contractions
i. Catabolism of amino acids and glycerol into glucose for energy
j. Alkaline
k. Highly acidic
l. Two substances directly absorbed through the lining of the stomach
m. All biochemical reactions within the cells of the body

37. Explain the four components of the dietary reference intake (DRI).

    a. Estimated average requirement (EAR): _____

    b. Recommended dietary allowance (RDA): _____

    c. Adequate intake (AI): _____

    d. Tolerable upper intake level (UL): _____

Nursing Knowledge Base

38. List the factors to estimate a patient's nutritional requirements.

    a. _____

    b. _____

    c. _____

    d. _____

    e. _____

39. List the benefits of breastfeeding an infant.

    a. _____

    b. _____

    c. _____

    d. _____

    e. _____

    f. _____

    g. _____

Explain why the following should not be used in infant formula.

40. Cow's milk: _____

41. Honey and corn syrup: _____

42. What governs an infant's readiness to begin solid foods?

    a. _____

    b. _____

    c. _____

43. Identify the factors that contribute to childhood obesity.

    a. _____

    b. _____

    c. _____

    d. _____

    e. _____

    f. _____

44. Identify the factors that influence the adolescent's diet.

    a. _____

    b. _____

    c. _____

    d. _____

    e. _____

45. Identify the diagnostic criteria for the following eating disorders.

    a. Anorexia nervosa: _____

    b. Bulimia nervosa: _____

46. Explain the importance of folic acid intake in pregnant women. _____

47. List the factors that influence the nutritional status of older-adults.

    a. _____

    b. _____

    c. _____

    d. _____

    e. _____

Explain the following types of vegetarian diets.

48. Ovolactovegetarian: _____

49. Lactovegetarian: _____

50. Vegan: _____

247

Nursing Process

Assessment

51. List the five components of a nutritional assessment and briefly explain them.

   a. _____

   b. _____

   c. _____

   d. _____

   e. _____

52. Dysphagia is: _____

53. For each assessment area, list at least two signs of poor nutrition.

   a. General appearance: _____

   b. Weight: _____

   c. Posture: _____

   d. Muscles: _____

   e. Nervous system: _____

   f. Gastrointestinal function: _____

   g. Cardiovascular function: _____

   h. General vitality: _____

   i. Hair: _____

   j. Skin: _____

   k. Face and neck: _____

   l. Lips: _____

   m. Mouth, oral membranes: _____

   n. Gums: _____

   o. Tongue: _____

   p. Teeth: _____

   q. Eyes: _____

   r. Neck: _____

   s. Nails: _____

   t. Legs, feet: _____

   u. Skeleton: _____

Analysis and Nursing Diagnosis

54. List the potential or actual nursing diagnoses for altered nutritional status.

   a. _____

   b. _____

   c. _____

   d. _____

   e. _____

Planning and Outcomes Identification

55. List the goals for a patient with impaired low nutritional intake:

    a. _____

    b. _____

    c. _____

Implementation

56. Identify the hospitalized patients who are at high nutritional risk: _____

    _____

57. Identify three ways to promote an appetite.

    a. _____

    b. _____

    c. _____

58. Identify the four levels of the dysphagia diet.

    a. _____

    b. _____

    c. _____

    d. _____

59. Identify the four levels of a liquid diet.

    a. _____

    b. _____

    c. _____

    d. _____

60. Identify the following types of enteral formulas.

    a. Polymeric: _____

    b. Modular: _____

    c. Elemental: _____

    d. Specialty: _____

61. Identify the complications of enteral tube feedings and possible cause.

    a. _____

    b. _____

    c. _____

    d. _____

    e. _____

    f. _____

    g. _____

h. _____

i. _____

j. _____

62. List the three factors on which safe administration of PN depends.

a. _____

b. _____

c. _____

63. Complications of PN include _____ and _____.

64. Intravenous fat emulsions provide: _____

65. Explain the goal of transition from PN to enteral nutrition (EN) or oral feeding.

_____

66. Medical nutrition therapy (MNT) is: _____

67. *Helicobacter pylori* is: _____

Identify the nutritional interventions for the following common disease states.

68. Inflammatory bowel disease: _____

69. Malabsorption syndromes: _____

70. Diverticulitis: _____

71. Diabetes mellitus (DM): _____

72. Cardiovascular disease: _____

73. Cancer: _____

74. Human immunodeficiency virus (HIV): _____

Evaluation

75. Identify the ongoing evaluative measures.

_____

CASE STUDY

76. You are working with a patient that you suspect from your assessment may have dysphagia. What does the nurse need to do next?

Select the appropriate answer and cite the rationale for choosing that particular answer.

77. Which nutrient is the body's most preferred energy source?
    1. Fat
    2. Protein
    3. Vitamin
    4. Carbohydrate

    Answer: _____

    Rationale: _____

    _____

    _____

78. Positive nitrogen balance would occur in which condition?
    1. Infection
    2. Starvation
    3. Pregnancy
    4. Burn injury

    Answer: _____

    Rationale: _____

    _____

    _____

79. Mrs. Nelson is talking with the nurse about the dietary needs of her 23-month-old daughter, Laura. Which of the following responses by the nurse would be appropriate?
    1. "Use skim milk to cut down on the fat in Laura's diet."
    2. "Laura should be drinking at least 1 quart of milk per day."
    3. "Laura needs less protein in her diet now because she isn't growing as fast."
    4. "Laura needs fewer calories in relation to her body weight now than she did as an infant."

    Answer: _____

    Rationale: _____

    _____

    _____

80. All of the following patients are at risk for alteration in nutrition except:
    1. Patient L, whose weight is 10% above his ideal body weight
    2. Patient J, who is 86 years old, lives alone, and has poorly fitting dentures
    3. Patient M, a 17-year-old girl who weighs 90 pounds and frequently complains about her baby fat
    4. Patient K, who has been allowed nothing by mouth (NPO) for 7 days after bowel surgery and is receiving 3000 mL of 10% dextrose per day

    Answer: _____

    Rationale: _____

    _____

    _____

81. Which of the following is the most accurate method of bedside confirmation of placement of a small-bore nasogastric tube?
    1. Assess the patient's ability to speak.
    2. Test the pH of withdrawn gastric contents.
    3. Auscultate the epigastrium for gurgling or bubbling.
    4. Assess the length of the tube that is outside the patient's nose.

    Answer: _____

    Rationale: _____

    _____

    _____

82. A patient who has been hospitalized after experiencing a heart attack will most likely receive a diet consisting of:
    1. Low fat, low sodium, and low carbohydrates
    2. Low fat, low sodium, and high carbohydrates
    3. Low fat, high protein, and high carbohydrates
    4. Liquids for several days, progressing to a soft and then a regular diet

    Answer: _____

    Rationale: _____

    _____

    _____

251

83. Mrs. Williams was admitted to your unit with a chief complaint of difficulties with swallowing. From your assessment you formulate a nursing diagnosis of imbalanced nutrition: less than body requirements. Select the assessment data that supports this diagnosis.

   a. Unable to swallow food or liquids

   b. Wears dentures

   c. Has lost 10 lbs in the last 3 weeks

   d. Diet history reveals inadequate ingestion of proteins, fruits, and vegetables

   e. Lactose intolerance

   f. Serum albumin is level is 3 g/dL

   g. Brittle, dry hair

CRITICAL THINKING MODEL FOR NURSING CARE PLAN FOR IMBALANCED NUTRITION: LESS THAN BODY REQUIREMENTS

84. Imagine that you are the nurse practitioner in the care plan in Chapter 45 of your text. Complete the *Assessment phase* of the critical thinking model with these questions in mind.

   a. In developing Mrs. Cooper's plan of care, what knowledge did Maria apply?

   _____

   b. In what ways might the nurse practitioner's previous experience assist in developing Mrs. Cooper's plan of care?

   _____

   c. When developing a plan of care for Mrs. Cooper, what intellectual and professional standards were applied?

   _____

   d. What critical thinking attitudes might have been applied in developing Mrs. Cooper's plan of care?

   _____

   e. How will the nurse practitioner accomplish these goals?

   _____

Next Generation NCLEX® Examination-Style Questions

85. The nurse has been caring for a 10-year-old patient diagnosed with obesity 6 months ago with a weight of 100 pounds (45.4 kg). At that time, the nurse provided education about healthy food choices, sources of vitamins and minerals necessary for appropriate childhood growth, and multiple ways to incorporate activity into the patient's daily life. Today, the patient has come for a follow-up appointment to evaluate progress toward weight loss and better health.

Highlight in yellow the findings that require the nurse to provide additional teaching to achieve maximum nutrition wellness.

Nurses' Notes:	Patient here for follow-up on weight and general health. Weight today is 92 pounds (41.7 kg). Parent and patient report an increase in daily green vegetable consumption. At school, patient takes part in required physical education classes twice weekly and has joined an after-school marching band program. Breakfast and lunch are provided by the patient's school. Patient reports getting a vending machine snack and soda before each marching band practice. Dinner is usually consumed in the car watching a video between evening appointments while the patient's parent carpools older siblings for sports. No changes in bowel or bladder habits; no chest pain or respiratory difficulties; no headaches reported.

46 Urinary Elimination

PRELIMINARY READING

Chapter 46

COMPREHENSIVE UNDERSTANDING

Scientific Knowledge Base

Match the following terms related to urinary elimination.

1. _____ Nephron

2. _____ Proteinuria

3. _____ Erythropoietin

4. _____ Renin

5. _____ Micturition

6. _____ Urinary reflux

7. _____ Bladder

a. Two portions—trigone and a detrusor
b. Reflux of urine from the bladder into the ureters
c. Presence of large proteins in the urine
d. Functional unit of the kidneys that forms the urine
e. Back flow of urine
f. Enzyme that converts angiotensinogen into angiotensin I
g. Functions within the bone marrow to stimulate red blood cell production

8. List nine factors that influence urination, and give examples of each.

a. _____

b. _____

c. _____

d. _____

e. _____

f. _____

g. _____

h. _____

i. _____

Briefly describe the causes of the following types of incontinence.

9. Transient incontinence: _____

_____

10. Functional incontinence: _____

_____

11. Overflow urinary incontinence: _____

_____

12. Stress incontinence: _____

_____

253

13. Urge/Urgency incontinence: _____

_____

14. Reflex incontinence: _____

_____

15. Urinary tract infection (UTI): _____

_____

Briefly describe the following continent urinary diversions.

16. Continent urinary reservoir: _____

_____

17. Orthotopic neobladder: _____

_____

18. Ureterostomy: _____

_____

19. Nephrostomy: _____

_____

Nursing Process

Assessment

Define the common symptoms of the following urinary alterations.

20. Urgency: _____

21. Dysuria: _____

22. Frequency: _____

23. Hesitancy: _____

24. Polyuria: _____

25. Oliguria: _____

26. Nocturia: _____

27. Dribbling: _____

28. Hematuria: _____

29. Retention: _____

30. List the major factors to be explored during a nursing history in regard to urinary elimination.

a. _____

b. _____

c. _____

Describe the following characteristics of normal urine.

31. Color: _____

_____

32. Clarity: _____

_____

33. Odor: _____

_____

34. Describe the following types of urine specimens collected for testing.

    a. Random: _____

    _____

    b. Clean-voided or midstream: _____

    _____

    c. Sterile: _____

    _____

    d. Timed urine: _____

    _____

Common urine tests include the following. Briefly explain each.

35. Urinalysis: _____

_____

36. Specific gravity: _____

_____

37. Urine culture: _____

_____

38. Briefly explain the purpose of each of the following noninvasive/invasive diagnostic examinations.

    a. Abdominal roentgenogram: _____

    b. Intravenous pyelogram (IVP): _____

    c. Cystoscopy: _____

    d. Computerized axial tomography (CT): _____

    e. Ultrasonography: _____

Analysis and Nursing Diagnosis

39. List the potential or actual nursing diagnoses related to urinary elimination.

    a. _____

    b. _____

    c. _____

    d. _____

    e. _____

Planning and Outcomes Identification

40. List the goals appropriate for a patient with a urinary elimination problem.

    a. _____

    b. _____

    c. _____

255

Implementation

41. List measures that promote normal micturition.

    a. _____

    b. _____

    c. _____

    d. _____

    e. _____

    f. _____

42. State the indications for the following types of catheterizations.

    a. Intermittent: _____

    b. Short- or long-term indwelling: _____

Explain the following nursing measures taken to prevent infection and maintain an unobstructed flow of urine in catheterized patients.

43. Perineal hygiene: _____

    _____

44. Catheter care: _____

    _____

45. Fluid intake: _____

    _____

46. Irrigations and instillations: _____

    _____

Briefly explain the two alternatives to urethral catheterization.

47. Suprapubic catheter: _____

    _____

48. External catheter: _____

    _____

Explain the purpose of the following.

49. Pelvic floor muscle training (PFMT): _____

    _____

50. Bladder retraining: _____

    _____

51. Scheduled toileting: _____

    _____

Evaluation

52. Identify how the nurse would evaluate the effectiveness of the interventions used.

_____

_____

_____

CASE STUDY

53. You are taking care of a patient who requires an insertion of a Foley catheter. In regards to safety considerations with the insertion of a catheter, what should the nurse do?

REVIEW QUESTIONS

Select the appropriate answer and cite the rationale for choosing that particular answer.

54. Mrs. Rantz complains of leaking urine when she coughs and laughs. This is known as:
    1. Urge incontinence
    2. Stress incontinence
    3. Reflex incontinence
    4. Functional incontinence

    Answer: _____

    Rationale: _____

    _____

    _____

55. Ms. Hathaway has a UTI. Which of the following symptoms would you expect her to exhibit? (Select all that apply.)
    1. Dysuria
    2. Oliguria
    3. Polyuria
    4. Proteinuria
    5. Fever and chills
    6. Nausea and vomiting
    7. Malaise

    Answer: _____

    Rationale: _____

    _____

    _____

56. The nurse is working in the radiology department with a patient who is having an intravenous pyelogram. Which of the following complaints by the patient is an abnormal response?
    1. Frequent, loose stools
    2. Thirst and feeling "worn out"
    3. Shortness of breath and audible wheezing
    4. Feeling dizzy and warm with obvious facial flushing

    Answer: _____

    Rationale: _____

    _____

    _____

57. The urinalysis of Ms. Hathaway reveals a high bacteria count. Ampicillin is prescribed for her UTI. When providing education for this patient about managing her UTI for which of the following should the nurse provide education? (Select all that apply.)
    1. Drink at least 2000 mL of fluid daily.
    2. Always wipe the perineum from front to back.
    3. Drink plenty of orange and grapefruit juices.
    4. Explain the possible side effects of medication.

    Answer: _____

    Rationale: _____

    _____

    _____

Chapter **46 Urinary Elimination**

58. Imagine that you are Mrs. Kay, the nurse in the care plan in Chapter 46 of your text. Complete the *Assessment phase* of the critical thinking model with these questions in mind.

   a. What knowledge base was applied to the care of Mrs. Grayson?

   _____

   b. In what way might Mrs. Kay's previous experience assist in this case?

   _____

   c. What intellectual or professional standards were applied to the care of Mrs. Grayson?

   _____

   d. What critical thinking attitudes did you use in assessing Mrs. Grayson?

   _____

   e. As you review the assessment, what key areas did Mrs. Kay cover?

   _____

Next Generation NCLEX® Examination-Style Questions

59. The nurse is caring for a patient who reports several days of increasing frequency and burning upon urination. After the health care provider orders a urinalysis, the nurse reviews the results. **Highlight the laboratory results in the table consistent with a urinary tract infection.**

Laboratory Results	Parameter	Result	Reference Range
	Color	Yellow	Clear or yellow
	Clarity	Cloudy	Clear
	Specific gravity	1.020	1.005–1.030
	pH	7.0	4.5–8.0
	Protein	120 mg/dL	Negative
	Glucose	Negative	Negative
	Ketone	Negative	Negative
	Bilirubin	Negative	Negative
	Blood	Negative	Negative
	Urobilinogen	<2 mg/dL	0–2 mg/dL
	White blood cells (microscope)	6–10 HPF	0–5 HPF
	Red blood cells (microscope)	0–5 HPF	0–5 HPF
	Bacteria	Present	Absent

47 Bowel Elimination

PRELIMINARY READING

Chapter 47

COMPREHENSIVE UNDERSTANDING

Scientific Knowledge Base

Summarize the functions of the following.

1. Mouth: _____

_____

2. Esophagus: _____

_____

3. Stomach: _____

_____

4. Small intestine: _____

_____

5. Large intestine: _____

_____

6. Anus: _____

_____

7. List the physiological factors essential to bowel function and defecation.

    a. _____

    b. _____

    c. _____

    d. _____

8. Identify 12 factors that can influence bowel elimination. Briefly explain the factors.

   a. _____

   b. _____

   c. _____

   d. _____

   e. _____

   f. _____

   g. _____

   h. _____

   i. _____

   j. _____

   k. _____

   l. _____

9. List conditions that may result in painful defecation.

   a. _____

   b. _____

   c. _____

   d. _____

10. List four factors that place a patient at risk for constipation.

   a. _____

   b. _____

   c. _____

   d. _____

11. List the signs of constipation.

   a. _____

   b. _____

12. Define *fecal impaction*.

   _____

   _____

13. List signs and symptoms of fecal impaction.

   a. _____

   b. _____

   c. _____

   d. _____

   e. _____

14. Define *diarrhea*.

_____

_____

15. Name the two complications associated with diarrhea.

    a. _____

    b. _____

16. Explain *Clostridium difficile* infection. _____

_____

17. Explain the following.

    a. Fecal incontinence: _____

    _____

    b. Flatulence: _____

    _____

18. Hemorrhoids are: _____

_____

Define the following bowel diversions.

19. Stoma: _____

_____

20. Ileostomy: _____

_____

21. Colostomy: _____

_____

Nursing Process

Assessment

22. List 14 factors that affect elimination that need to be included in a nursing history for patients with altered elimination status.

    a. _____

    b. _____

    c. _____

    d. _____

    e. _____

    f. _____

    g. _____

    h. _____

i. _____

j. _____

k. _____

l. _____

m. _____

n. _____

Summarize the following steps for assessing the abdomen.

23. Inspection: _____

_____

24. Auscultation: _____

_____

25. Palpation: _____

_____

26. Percussion: _____

_____

27. Define *fecal occult blood testing (FOBT)*.

_____

_____

28. List the common radiologic and diagnostic tests used with a patient with altered bowel elimination.

a. _____

b. _____

c. _____

d. _____

e. _____

f. _____

g. _____

h. _____

Analysis and Nursing Diagnosis

29. List the potential or actual nursing diagnoses for a patient with alteration in bowel elimination.

a. _____

b. _____

c. _____

d. _____

e. _____

Planning and Outcomes Identification

30. List the overall outcomes that are appropriate for patients with elimination problems.

a. _____

b. _____

c. _____

d. _____

e. _____

Implementation

31. List the factors to consider to promote normal bowel elimination.

a. _____

b. _____

c. _____

d. _____

e. _____

Identify the primary action of the following.

32. Cathartics and laxatives: _____

_____

33. Antidiarrheals: _____

_____

34. Enemas: _____

_____

Briefly describe the following types of enemas.

35. Cleansing enema: _____

_____

36. Tap water enema: _____

_____

37. Normal saline: _____

_____

38. Hypertonic solution: _____

_____

39. Soapsuds: _____

_____

40. Oil retention: _____

_____

41. Explain the purpose of a carminative enema.

_____

_____

_____

263

42. List the complications of excessive rectal manipulation.

    a. _____

    b. _____

    c. _____

43. List the purposes of nasogastric (NG) intubation.

    a. _____

    b. _____

    c. _____

    d. _____

44. Explain how the nurse would provide comfort to a patient with an NG tube.

    _____

    _____

    _____

45. List the measures included for a successful bowel training program.

    a. _____

    b. _____

    c. _____

    d. _____

    e. _____

    f. _____

    g. _____

    h. _____

    i. _____

Evaluation

46. Identify some positive outcomes for a patient with alterations in bowel elimination.

    _____

    _____

CASE STUDY

47. The nurse is developing a teaching plan for a patient that reports occasional constipation. What specific lifestyle changes would the nurse include in the plan? (Select all that apply.)

    a. Increase fluid intake

    b. Low fiber diet

    c. Regular exercise

    d. Decrease fruits and increase carbohydrates

    e. Increase vegetables in the diet

Select the appropriate answer and cite the rationale for choosing that particular answer.

48. Most nutrients and electrolytes are absorbed in the:
    1. Colon
    2. Stomach
    3. Esophagus
    4. Small intestine

    Answer: _____

    Rationale: _____

    _____

    _____

49. Which of the following should be included in the teaching plan for the patient who is scheduled for an upper GI series?
    1. The patient will be allowed nothing by mouth (NPO) after midnight.
    2. General anesthetic is usually used for the procedure.
    3. Moderate abdominal pain is common after the procedure.
    4. A cleansing enema will be given the evening before the procedure.

    Answer: _____

    Rationale: _____

    _____

    _____

50. Mrs. Anthony is concerned about her breastfed infant's stool, stating that it is yellow instead of brown. The nurse explains to Mrs. Anthony that:
    1. The stool is normal for an infant.
    2. A change to formula may be necessary.
    3. It will be necessary to send a stool specimen to the laboratory.
    4. Her infant is dehydrated, and she should increase his fluid intake.

    Answer: _____

    Rationale: _____

    _____

    _____

51. After positioning a patient on the bedpan, the nurse should:
    1. Leave the head of the bed flat.
    2. Raise the head of the bed 30 degrees.
    3. Raise the bed to the highest working level.
    4. Raise the head of the bed to a 90-degree angle.

    Answer: _____

    Rationale: _____

    _____

    _____

52. The health care provider has ordered a cleansing enema for 7-year-old Michael. The nurse realizes the maximum volume to be given would be:
    1. 100 to 150 mL
    2. 150 to 250 mL
    3. 300 to 500 mL
    4. 600 to 700 mL

    Answer: _____

    Rationale: _____

    _____

    _____

265

53. Imagine that you are Javier, the home care nurse in the care plan in Chapter 47 of your text. Complete the *Planning phase* of the critical thinking model with these questions in mind.

   a. In developing Mr. Johnson's plan of care, what knowledge did Javier apply?

   _____

   b. In what way might Javier's previous experience assist in developing a plan of care for Mr. Johnson?

   _____

   c. When developing a plan of care, what intellectual and professional standards were applied?

   _____

   d. What critical thinking attitudes might have been applied in developing a plan for Mr. Johnson?

   _____

   e. How will Javier accomplish the goals?

   _____

Next Generation NCLEX® Examination-Style Questions

54. The nurse is caring for a patient who just had a total open abdominal hysterectomy. The patient is prescribed opioid medication for pain relief via a patient-controlled analgesia (PCA) pump and will be discharged with an opioid medication to manage pain at home while continuing to recover.

Use Word Choices to complete the sentence(s). Highlight correct answers in yellow.

The patient is at risk for developing _____, _____, and _____.

Word Choices		
Ileus	Fecal incontinence	Constipation
Diarrhea	*C. difficile* infection	Decreased peristalsis

48 Skin Integrity and Wound Care

PRELIMINARY READING

Chapter 48

COMPREHENSIVE UNDERSTANDING

Scientific Knowledge Base

Match the following key terms related to skin integrity.

1. _____ Epidermis
2. _____ Dermis
3. _____ Collagen
4. _____ Pressure injury
5. _____ Blanching
6. _____ Darkly pigmented skin

a. Tough, fibrous protein
b. Localized injury to the skin and underlying tissue over a body prominence
c. Does not blanch
d. Normal red tones of light-skinned patients are absent
e. Top layer of the skin
f. Inner layer of the skin that provides tensile strength and mechanical support

7. Identify the pressure factors that contribute to pressure injury development.

a. _____

b. _____

c. _____

8. Identify and explain the risk factors that predispose a patient to pressure injury formation.

a. _____

b. _____

c. _____

d. _____

e. _____

f. _____

9. Staging systems for pressure injuries are based on the depth of tissue destroyed. Briefly describe each stage.

I. _____

II. _____

III. _____

IV. _____

10. Explain what a deep tissue pressure injury (**DTPI**) is. _____

Define the following terms related to wound healing.

11. Granulation tissue: _____

12. Slough: _____

13. Eschar: _____

14. Exudate: _____

Describe the physiological process involved with wound healing.

15. Primary intention: _____

16. Secondary intention: _____

_____

17. Identify the three components involved in the healing process of a partial-thickness wound.

    a. _____

    b. _____

    c. _____

18. Explain the four phases involved in the healing process of a full-thickness wound.

    a. Hemostasis: _____

    b. Inflammatory phase: _____

    c. Proliferative phase: _____

    d. Remodeling and maturation: _____

19. Briefly explain the following complications of wound healing.

    a. Hemorrhage: _____

    b. Hematoma: _____

    c. Wound infection: _____

    d. Dehiscence: _____

    e. Evisceration: _____

Nursing Knowledge Base

20. The Braden Scale was developed for assessing pressure injury risks. Identify the subscales of this tool.

    a. _____

    b. _____

    c. _____

    d. _____

    e. _____

    f. _____

21. List and explain the factors that influence pressure injury formation and wound healing.

    a. _____

    b. _____

    c. _____

    d. _____

    e. _____

Nursing Process

Assessment

22. Explain the following factors that place a patient at risk for a pressure injury development.

    a. Mobility: _____

    b. Nutritional status: _____

    c. Body fluids: _____

    d. Pain: _____

23. Identify the following types of emergency setting wounds.

    a. Abrasion: _____

    b. Laceration: _____

    c. Puncture: _____

Explain how the nurse assesses the following.

24. Wound appearance: _____

25. Character of wound drainage: _____

26. Complete the table below describing the characteristics of wound drainage.

Typet	Appearance
Serous	
Purulent	
Serosanguineous	
Sanguineous	

27. A nurse's responsibility with assessing drains is: _____

28. Types of surgical wound closures are: _____

29. Palpation of a wound includes: _____

Analysis and Nursing Diagnosis

30. List the potential or actual nursing diagnoses related to impaired skin integrity.

    a. _____

    b. _____

    c. _____

    d. _____

Planning and Outcomes Identification

31. List possible goals to achieve wound improvement.

    a. _____

    b. _____

    c. _____

    d. _____

Implementation

32. Identify the three major areas of nursing interventions for preventing pressure injuries.

    a. _____

    b. _____

    c. _____

Acute Care

33. List the principles to address to maintain a healthy wound environment.

    a. _____

    b. _____

    c. _____

    d. _____

    e. _____

    f. _____

    g. _____

    h. _____

34. Explain the rationale for debriding a wound.

    _____

    _____

35. Identify the four methods of debridement.

    a. _____

    b. _____

    c. _____

    d. _____

First aid for wounds includes the following. Briefly explain each one.

36. Hemostasis: _____

37. Cleansing: _____

38. Protection: _____

39. List the purposes of dressings.

    a. _____

    b. _____

    c. _____

    d. _____

    e. _____

    f. _____

40. List the clinical guidelines to use when selecting the appropriate dressing.

a. _____

b. _____

c. _____

d. _____

e. _____

f. _____

g. _____

h. _____

41. List the advantages of a transparent film dressing.

a. _____

b. _____

c. _____

d. _____

e. _____

42. List the functions of hydrocolloid dressings.

a. _____

b. _____

c. _____

d. _____

e. _____

f. _____

g. _____

43. List the advantages of the hydrogel dressing.

a. _____

b. _____

c. _____

d. _____

44. List the guidelines to follow during a dressing change procedure.

a. _____

b. _____

c. _____

45. Summarize the principles of packing a wound.

_____

_____

46. Briefly describe how the wound vacuum-assisted closure (wound VAC) device works.

_____

_____

47. Identify three principles that are important when cleaning an incision.

a. _____

b. _____

c. _____

48. Summarize the principles of wound irrigation.

_____

_____

49. Explain the purpose for drainage evacuation.

_____

_____

50. Explain the benefits of binders and bandages.

a. _____

b. _____

c. _____

d. _____

e. _____

f. _____

51. List the nursing responsibilities when applying a bandage or binder.

a. _____

b. _____

c. _____

d. _____

52. Describe the physiological responses to the following.

a. Heat applications: _____

b. Cold applications: _____

53. List the factors that influence heat and cold tolerance.

a. _____

b. _____

c. _____

d. _____

e. _____

f. _____

g. _____

Explain the rationale for the following types of applications.

54. Warm, moist compresses: _____

55. Warm soaks: _____

56. Sitz baths: _____

57. Commercial hot packs: _____

58. Cold, moist, and dry compresses: _____

59. Cold soaks: _____

60. Ice bags or collars: _____

Evaluation

61. List the questions to ask if the identified outcomes were not met.

    a. _____

    b. _____

    c. _____

CASE STUDY

62. You are taking care of a patient who is experiencing frequent fecal and urinary incontinence. What specific nursing interventions could you institute to help manage this patient?

REVIEW QUESTIONS

Select the appropriate answer and cite the rationale for choosing that particular answer.

63. Mr. Post is in a Fowler position to improve his oxygenation status. The nurse notes that he frequently slides down in the bed and needs to be repositioned. Mr. Post is at risk for developing a pressure injury on his coccyx because of:
1. Friction
2. Maceration
3. Shearing force
4. Impaired peripheral circulation

Answer: _____

Rationale: _____

_____

_____

64. Which of the following is not a subscale on the Braden Scale for predicting pressure injury risk?
1. Age
2. Activity
3. Moisture
4. Sensory perception

Answer: _____

Rationale: _____

_____

_____

65. Which of these patients has a nutritional risk for pressure injury development?
    1. Patient A has an albumin level of 3.5.
    2. Patient B has a hemoglobin level within normal limits.
    3. Patient C has a protein intake of 0.5 g/kg/day.
    4. Patient D has a body weight that is 5% greater than his ideal weight.

    Answer: _____

    Rationale: _____

    _____

    _____

66. Mr. Perkins has a stage II ulcer of his right heel. What would be the most appropriate treatment for this ulcer?
    1. Apply a heat lamp to the area for 20 minutes twice daily.
    2. Apply a hydrocolloid dressing and change it as necessary.
    3. Apply a calcium alginate dressing and change when strikethrough is noted.
    4. Apply a thick layer of enzymatic ointment to the ulcer and the surrounding skin.

    Answer: _____

    Rationale: _____

    _____

    _____

67. Place the following steps in correct order for performing a wound irrigation.
    1. Use slow continuous pressure to irrigate the wound
    2. Attach 19-gauge angiocatheter to syringe
    3. Fill syringe with irrigation fluid
    4. Assess wound
    5. Position angiocatheter over wound

    Answer: _____

    Rationale: _____

    _____

    _____

CRITICAL THINKING MODEL FOR NURSING CARE PLAN FOR IMPAIRED SKIN INTEGRITY

68. Imagine that you are the nurse in the care plan in Chapter 48 of your text. Complete the *Assessment phase* of the critical thinking model with these questions in mind.

    a. What knowledge base was applied to Mrs. Stein?

    _____

    b. In what way might your previous experience assist you in this case?

    _____

    c. What intellectual or professional standards were applied to Mrs. Stein?

    _____

    d. What critical thinking attitudes did you use in assessing Mrs. Stein?

    _____

    e. As you review your assessment, what key areas did you cover?

    _____

69. Mr. Montoya is a 70-year-old Hispanic male with a history of type II diabetes mellitus (DM). He has been admitted to the medical-surgical unit for stabilization of his blood sugar. Mr. Montoya has lived in the US for 40 years., and shares in a two-story house with his wife. His son, daughter, and son in law and their three children also live in the home. Mr. Montoya had a below the knee amputation (BKA) of the right leg 2 years ago, after he developed gangrene in his right foot.

Mr. Montoya states for 3 weeks, he has had frequent urination and blurry vision. In addition, he has lost 12 lbs in the last month. Since his surgery has been less physically active. He has seen a dietician, self-monitors his BS occasionally. He takes Glucophage 500 mg BID. He drinks 8 ounces of beer with dinner each evening and smokes ½ pack of cigarettes per day.

His peripheral pulses are 2 + radial, left dorsalis pedis 1 +. His left foot is cool, with capillary refill of 5 seconds. BP 158/98, HR, 84 and respirations 20.

Highlight the areas in the paragraph that indicate Mr. Montoya is at risk for the development of pressure injuries.

70. The nurse is caring for a patient who had bowel resection surgery earlier today. While performing a routine assessment, the nurse notes that the surgical wound is compromised and does not look as expected. **For each assessment finding, indicate whether findings from this patient's assessment are generally associated with evisceration, dehiscence, or are related to both conditions.**

Assessment Finding	Evisceration	Dehiscence	Both evisceration and dehiscence
Wound layers separated			
Opening noted after light coughing			
Reports a sensation of "something giving way"			
Portion of incision line minimally open			
Blood pressure 70/30 mm Hg			
Visceral organs visible			
Partial opening in surgical wound			
Pulse 150 beats per minute			

49 Sensory Alterations

PRELIMINARY READING

Chapter 49

COMPREHENSIVE UNDERSTANDING

Scientific Knowledge Base

Match the following key terms related to sensations.

1. _____ Auditory
2. _____ Tactile
3. _____ Olfactory
4. _____ Gustatory
5. _____ Kinesthetic
6. _____ Stereognosis

a. Enables a person to be aware of position and movement of body parts
b. Taste
c. Hearing
d. Smell
e. Recognition of an object's size, shape, and texture
f. Touch

Match the following terms related to the common sensory deficits.

7. _____ Presbyopia
8. _____ Cataract
9. _____ Dry eyes
10. _____ Glaucoma
11. _____ Diabetic retinopathy
12. _____ Macular degeneration
13. _____ Presbycusis
14. _____ Cerumen accumulation
15. _____ Disequilibrium
16. _____ Xerostomia
17. _____ Peripheral neuropathy
18. _____ Stroke

a. Numbness and tingling of the affected area, stumbling gait
b. Results from vestibular dysfunction, vertigo
c. Gradual decline in the ability of the lens to accommodate or focus on close objects
d. Blurring of reading matter, distortion or loss of central vision and vertical lines
e. Caused by clot, hemorrhage, or emboli to the brain
f. Opaque areas of the lens that cause glaring and blurred vision
g. Decrease in salivary production, leading to thicker mucus and dry mouth
h. Decreased tear production that results in itching and burning
i. Progressive hearing disorder in older-adults
j. Increase in intraocular pressure resulting in peripheral visual loss, halo effect around lights
k. Buildup of earwax, causing conduction deafness
l. Blood vessel changes of the retina, decreased vision, and macular edema

19. Describe what causes sensory overload: _____

_____

Nursing Knowledge Base

20. Identify the factors that influence the capacity to receive or perceive stimuli.

    a. _____

    b. _____

    c. _____

    d. _____

    e. _____

    f. _____

Nursing Process

Assessment

21. Identify the groups that are at high risk for sensory alterations.

    _____

    _____

22. List the two questions that a nurse could ask the family to assess any recent changes in a patient's behavior.

    a. _____

    b. _____

23. Complete the following table by describing at least one assessment technique for the identified sensory function and the behaviors for an adult and child that would indicate a sensory deficit.

Sense	Assessment Technique	Child Behavior	Adult Behavior
Vision			
Hearing			
Touch			
Smell			
Taste			

24. Identify some common home hazards.

    a. _____

    b. _____

    c. _____

    d. _____

    e. _____

    f. _____

    g. _____

25. Explain the following types of aphasia.

    a. Expressive: _____

    b. Receptive: _____

26. Factors other than sensory deprivation or overload cause impaired perception. Give two examples of how medications impair perception.

    a. _____

    b. _____

277

Analysis and Nursing Diagnosis

27. List the actual or potential nursing diagnoses for a patient with sensory alterations.

a. _____

b. _____

c. _____

d. _____

e. _____

Planning and Outcomes Identification

28. List outcomes that would be appropriate for patients with alteration in hearing acuity.

a. _____

b. _____

c. _____

Implementation

29. List the recommended screening interventions to prevent visual impairment.

a. _____

b. _____

c. _____

d. _____

30. The most common visual problem is: _____

_____

31. Risk factors for children at risk for hearing impairment include:

a. _____

b. _____

c. _____

d. _____

e. _____

32. Complete the following table by filling in the sensory deficits that occur, and explain how the nurse can minimize the loss.

Senses	Common Sensory Deficits	Interventions to Minimize Loss
Vision		
Hearing		
Taste and Smell		
Touch		

33. Identify methods to promote communication in the following.

a. Patients with aphasia: _____

b. Patients with an artificial airway: _____

c. Patients with a hearing impairment: _____

Acute Care

34. Identify the approaches to maximize sensory function, and give an example of each.

    a. _____

    b. _____

    c. _____

    d. _____

35. List the principles for reducing loneliness.

    a. _____

    b. _____

    c. _____

    d. _____

    e. _____

    f. _____

    g. _____

    h. _____

Evaluation

36. Explain how the nurse would evaluate whether the measures improved the patient's ability to interact within the environment.

    _____

    _____

CASE STUDY

37. You, as the nurse, are caring for a patient with a visual impairment. Identify the guidelines you would follow in caring for this patient.

Select the appropriate answer and cite the rationale for choosing that particular answer.

38. Mr. Green, a 62-year-old farmer, has been hospitalized for 2 weeks for thrombophlebitis. He has no visitors, and the nurse notices that he appears bored, restless, and anxious. The type of alteration occurring because of sensory deprivation is:
    1. Affective
    2. Cognitive
    3. Receptual
    4. Perceptual

    Answer: _____

    Rationale: _____

    _____

    _____

39. Which of the following would provide meaning-ful stimuli for a hospitalized patient? (Select all that apply.)
    1. Interesting magazines and books
    2. Lights on continuously in the room
    3. A clock or calendar with large numbers
    4. Family pictures and personal possessions
    5. A television that is kept on all day at a low volume
    6. A talkative roommate

    Answer: _____

    Rationale: _____

    _____

    _____

40. Patients with existing sensory loss must be protected from injury. What determines the safety precautions taken?
    1. The existing dangers in the environment
    2. The financial means to make needed safety changes
    3. The nature of the patient's actual or potential sensory loss
    4. The availability of a support system to enable the patient to exist in his or her present environment

    Answer: _____

    Rationale: _____

    _____

    _____

41. A patient who is unable to name common objects or express simple ideas in words or writing has:
    1. Global aphasia
    2. Receptive aphasia
    3. Mental retardation
    4. Expressive aphasia

    Answer: _____

    Rationale: _____

    _____

    _____

42. A patient in the intensive care unit is experiencing sleeplessness, irritability, and difficulty concentrating. Which interventions should the nurse implement to decease stimulation? (Select all that apply.)
    1. Establish a routine
    2. Move the patient to a semiprivate room
    3. Teach self-stimulation methods such as singing
    4. Provide a quiet environment to allow optimal sleep
    5. Coordinate lighting with a normal day and night cycle

    Answer: _____

    Rationale: _____

    _____

    _____

43. Imagine that you are the community health nurse in the care plan in Chapter 49 of your text. Complete the *Planning phase* of the critical thinking model with these questions in mind.

    a. In developing Ms. Long's plan of care, what knowledge did you apply?

    _____

    b. In what way might your previous experience assist in developing a plan of care for Ms. Long?

    _____

    c. When developing a plan of care, what intellectual and professional standards were applied?

    _____

    d. What critical thinking attitudes might have been applied in developing Ms. Long's plan?

    _____

    e. How will you accomplish the goals?

    _____

Next Generation NCLEX® Examination-Style Questions

44. The nurse is caring for a 90-year-old patient who resides in an assisted living facility. The patient is cognitively intact and able to perform most ADLs independently. She has mild visual changes due to cataracts, is hard of hearing, and sometimes doesn't like to eat because "most things don't taste good anymore". **For each sense, highlight the potential nursing intervention that would be appropriate for the care of the patient.**

Each sense may support more than one potential nursing intervention. Each category must have at least one response option selected.

Sense	Potential Nursing Interventions
Sight (visual)	Remove all throw rugs in the living area
	Remind to use eyeglasses to overcome clouded vision
	Ensure adequate lighting in rooms and hallways
	Decrease clutter in the living environment
Hearing (auditory)	Face the patient when speaking
	Encourage regular use of hearing aids
	Write all directions for patient to read
	Assess for presence of cerumen in the ear canal
Taste (gustatory)	Ask which foods are favorites
	Increase seasonings in foods to enhance flavor
	Remove environmental distractors before meals
	Provide foods that are separated and not mixed together

50 Perioperative Nursing Care

PRELIMINARY READING

Chapter 50

COMPREHENSIVE UNDERSTANDING

Scientific Knowledge Base

1. List the types of care that perioperative nursing includes.

   a. _____

   b. _____

   c. _____

Match the following descriptions to the surgical procedure classifications.

2. _____ Major

3. _____ Minor

4. _____ Elective

5. _____ Urgent

6. _____ Emergency

7. _____ Diagnostic

8. _____ Ablative

9. _____ Palliative

10. _____ Restorative

11. _____ Procurement

12. _____ Constructive

13. _____ Cosmetic

a. Restores function lost or reduced as result of congenital anomalies
b. Excision or removal of diseased body part
c. Not necessarily emergency
d. Extensive reconstruction, poses great risks to well-being
e. Performed to improve personal appearance
f. Restores function or appearance to traumatized tissues
g. Must be done immediately to save life or preserve function of body part
h. Involves minimal risks compared with major procedures
i. Exploration that allows diagnosis to be confirmed
j. Is not essential and is not always necessary for health
k. Removal of organs or tissues from a dead person for transplantation into another
l. Relieves or reduces the intensity of disease symptoms; will not produce cure

Nursing Knowledge Base

14. Define the following physical status (PS) classifications and give an example of each.

ASA Class	Definition	Characteristics
ASA I		
ASA II		
ASA III		
ASA IV		
ASA V		
ASA VI		

15. List the surgical risk factors that can affect a patient at any point in the perioperative experience.

a. _____

b. _____

c. _____

d. _____

e. _____

f. _____

g. _____

h. _____

i. _____

j. _____

16. Identify the physiological factors that place the older-adult at risk during surgery, and give an example of each.

a. Cardiovascular system: _____

b. Integumentary system: _____

c. Pulmonary system: _____

d. Gastrointestinal system: _____

e. Renal system: _____

f. Neurologic system: _____

g. Metabolic system: _____

Preoperative Surgical Phase
Assessment

17. The goal of the preoperative assessment is to: _____

_____

18. Pressure injuries are a result of the following. Briefly explain.

a. Intrinsic risks: _____

b. Extrinsic risks: _____

c. OR risk: _____

19. Give an example of how the following medical conditions increase risks of surgery.

a. Thrombocytopenia: _____

_____

b. Diabetes: _____

_____

c. Heart disease: _____

_____

d. Hypertension: _____

_____

283

e. Obstructive sleep apnea: _____

_____

f. Upper respiratory infection: _____

_____

g. Liver disease: _____

_____

h. Fever: _____

_____

i. Chronic respiratory disease: _____

_____

j. Immunologic disorders: _____

_____

k. Alcohol and street drugs: _____

_____

l. Chronic pain: _____

_____

20. Explain how the following drug classes affect the patient during surgery.

a. Antibiotics: _____

_____

b. Antidysrhythmics: _____

_____

c. Anticoagulants: _____

_____

d. Anticonvulsants: _____

_____

e. Antihypertensives: _____

_____

f. Corticosteroids: _____

_____

g. Insulin: _____

_____

h. Diuretics: _____

_____

i. Nonsteroidal antiinflammatory drugs (NSAIDs): _____

_____

j. Herbal therapies: _____

_____

21. Explain how the following habits affect the patient.

    a. Smoking: _____

    _____

    b. Alcohol and substance use and abuse: _____

    _____

22. A comprehensive pain assessment includes:

    a. _____

    b. _____

    c. _____

Briefly explain each of the following factors that need to be assessed in order to understand the impact of surgery on a patient's and family's emotional health.

23. Self-concept: _____

24. Body image: _____

25. Coping resources: _____

26. The physical examination of the patient before surgery includes:

    a. _____

    b. _____

    c. _____

    d. _____

    e. _____

    f. _____

    g. _____

27. Complete the following table of common lab tests for surgical patients.

Test	Normal Values	Low (Significance)	High (Significance)
Hgb			
Hct			
Platelet count			
WBC count			
Na			
K			
Cl			
CO_2			
BUN			
Glucose			
Creatinine			
INR			
PT			
PTT			
Activated PT			

Analysis and Nursing Diagnosis

28. List the potential or actual nursing diagnoses appropriate for the preoperative patient.

a. _____

b. _____

c. _____

d. _____

e. _____

Planning and Outcomes Identification

29. Identify the expected outcomes relevant for a surgical patient:

a. _____

b. _____

c. _____

d. _____

e. _____

Implementation

30. Identify what the informed consent for surgery involves.

_____

_____

31. Structured teaching throughout the perioperative period influences the following. Briefly explain how.

a. Ventilatory function: _____

b. Physical functional capacity: _____

c. Sense of well-being: _____

d. Length of hospital stay: _____

e. Anxiety about pain: _____

32. List the topics that should be covered to ensure comprehensive preoperative instruction.

a. _____

b. _____

c. _____

d. _____

e. _____

f. _____

g. _____

h. _____

i. _____

j. _____

k. _____

Acute Care

33. Identify the interventions to physically prepare the patient for surgery.

    a. _____

    b. _____

    c. _____

34. List the responsibilities of a nurse caring for a patient on the day of surgery.

    a. _____

    b. _____

    c. _____

    d. _____

    e. _____

    f. _____

    g. _____

    h. _____

    i. _____

    j. _____

Intraoperative Surgical Phase

35. Explain the responsibilities for the following operating room nurses.

    a. Circulating nurse: _____

    b. Scrub nurse: _____

36. Identify the nursing diagnosis for the patient during the intraoperative period.

    a. _____

    b. _____

    c. _____

    d. _____

    e. _____

Explain the following four types of anesthesia.

37. General: _____

    _____

38. Regional: _____

    _____

39. Local: _____

    _____

40. Moderate (conscious) sedation: _____

    _____

287

Postoperative Surgical Phase

41. Identify the three phases of the anesthesia recovery.

    a. _____

    b. _____

    c. _____

42. Identify the responsibilities of the nurse in the postanesthesia care unit (PACU).

    _____

    _____

43. Identify the outcomes for discharge from the PACU.

    _____

    _____

Postoperative Recovery and Convalescence

Assessment

44. Describe the frequency of vital sign assessment in the immediate postoperative period.

    _____

    _____

45. Identify the symptoms of respiratory depression in phase III recovery:

    a. _____

    b. _____

    c. _____

    d. _____

46. List the areas the nurse would assess to determine a postoperative patient's circulatory status.

    _____

    _____

47. List the complications of malignant hyperthermia.

    _____

    _____

48. List the areas the nurse assesses to determine fluid and electrolyte alterations.

    a. _____

    b. _____

    c. _____

    d. _____

    e. _____

49. List the areas of assessment that help to determine a postoperative patient's neurologic status.

    a. _____

    b. _____

    c. _____

    d. _____

50. Explain the following complications related to the skin postoperatively.

a. Rash: _____

b. Abrasions or petechiae: _____

c. Burns: _____

51. Explain the reasons why distention of the abdomen may occur.

a. _____

b. _____

Analysis and Nursing Diagnosis

52. List the potential nursing diagnoses that are common in a postoperative patient.

a. _____

b. _____

c. _____

d. _____

e. _____

Planning and Outcomes Identification

53. List the typical postoperative orders prescribed by surgeons.

a. _____

b. _____

c. _____

d. _____

e. _____

f. _____

g. _____

h. _____

i. _____

j. _____

k. _____

54. Identify the expected outcomes for the postoperative patient.

a. _____

b. _____

c. _____

Implementation

55. List the measures that the nurse would use to promote expansion of the lungs.

a. _____

b. _____

c. _____

d. _____

e. _____

f. _____

g. _____

h. _____

i. _____

j. _____

56. Define the following complications and give the cause of each.

a. Atelectasis: _____

b. Pneumonia: _____

c. Hypoxemia: _____

d. Pulmonary embolism: _____

e. Hemorrhage: _____

f. Hypovolemic shock: _____

g. Thrombophlebitis: _____

h. Thrombus: _____

i. Embolus: _____

j. Paralytic ileus: _____

k. Abdominal distention: _____

l. Nausea and vomiting: _____

m. Urinary retention: _____

n. Urinary tract infection: _____

o. Wound infection: _____

p. Wound dehiscence: _____

q. Wound evisceration: _____

r. Skin breakdown: _____

s. Intractable pain: _____

t. Malignant hyperthermia: _____

57. List the measures the nurse would use to prevent circulatory complications.

a. _____

b. _____

c. _____

d. _____

e. _____

f. _____

g. _____

h. _____

58. Identify possible sources of a surgical patient's pain.

_____

_____

59. List the measures the nurse would provide to promote the return of normal elimination.

a. _____

b. _____

c. _____

d. _____

e. _____

f. _____

g. _____

h. _____

i. _____

60. Identify the measures the nurse would provide to promote normal urinary elimination.

a. _____

b. _____

c. _____

d. _____

61. Identify the measures the nurse would use to promote the patient's self-concept.

a. _____

b. _____

c. _____

d. _____

e. _____

f. _____

CASE STUDY

62. A patient who has returned from surgery 3 hours ago following a kidney transplant is reporting pain at a 7 on a scale of 0 to 10. You have tried to reposition the patient, but there has been no improvement in the patient's report of pain. What are some problems that this patient can have with unmanaged surgical pain?

Select the appropriate answer and cite the rationale for choosing that particular answer.

63. Mrs. Young, a 45-year-old patient with diabetes, is having a hysterectomy in the morning. Because of her history, the nurse would expect:
    1. Impaired wound healing
    2. Fluid and electrolyte imbalances
    3. An increased risk of hemorrhaging
    4. Altered elimination of anesthetic agents

    Answer: _____

    Rationale: _____

    _____

    _____

64. The purposes of the nursing history for the patient who is to have surgery include all of the following except:
    1. Deciding whether surgery is indicated
    2. Identifying the patient's perception and expectations about surgery
    3. Obtaining information about the patient's past experience with surgery
    4. Understanding the impact surgery has on the patient's and family's emotional health

    Answer: _____

    Rationale: _____

    _____

    _____

65. Which of the following patients are at risk for developing serious fluid and electrolyte imbalances during and after surgery? (Select all that apply.)
    1. Patient F, who is 1-year-old and having a cleft palate repair
    2. Patient H, who is 79-years-old and has a history of congestive heart failure
    3. Patient G, who is 55-years-old and has a history of chronic respiratory disease
    4. Patient E, who is 81-years-old and having emergency surgery for a bowel obstruction after 4 days of vomiting and diarrhea

    Answer: _____

    Rationale: _____

    _____

    _____

66. What are the purposes of postoperative leg exercises?
    1. Maintain muscle tone
    2. Promote venous return
    3. Assess range of motion
    4. Promote joint mobility
    5. Exercise fatigued muscles

    Answer: _____

    Rationale: _____

    _____

    _____

67. The PACU nurse notices that the patient is shivering. This is most commonly caused by:
    1. Cold irrigations used during surgery
    2. Side effects of certain anesthetic agents
    3. Malignant hypothermia, a serious condition
    4. The use of a reflective blanket on the operating room table

    Answer: _____

    Rationale: _____

    _____

    _____

68. Communication between a nurse caring for a patient in the preoperative holding area and the circulating nurse in the operating room (OR) can best be enhanced by which of the following? (Select all that apply.)
    1. Documenting assessment findings in the medical record
    2. Using a standardized SBAR tool
    3. Being responsive in using nonverbal communication techniques
    4. Giving specific information to a transportation technician to convey to the OR nurse
    5. Listening to OR nurses' questions

    Answer: _____

    Rationale: _____

    _____

    _____

CRITICAL THINKING MODEL FOR NURSING CARE PLAN FOR DEFICIENT KNOWLEDGE

69. Imagine that you are the nurse in the care plan in Chapter 50 of your text. Complete the *Evaluation phase* of the critical thinking model with these questions in mind.

a. What knowledge did you apply in evaluating Mrs. Campana's care?

_____

b. In what way might your previous experience influence your evaluation of Mrs. Campana's care?

_____

c. During evaluation, what intellectual and professional standards were applied to Mrs. Campana's care?

_____

d. In what way do critical thinking attitudes play a role in how you approach evaluation of Mrs. Campana's care?

_____

e. How might you adjust Mrs. Campana's care?

_____

Next Generation NCLEX® Examination-Style Questions

70. The surgical nurse is present while a patient undergoes surgery for a knee replacement. While undergoing anesthesia induction, a change in physical assessment is noted.

Which finding indicates that this patient may have malignant hyperthermia? (Select all that apply.)

Temperature 104.2° F (40° C)

Heart rate 140 beats/minute

Muscular flaccidity

Respirations 28/minute

Ventricular fibrillation

Pulse 50 beats/minute

Skin mottling

Blood pressure 70/50

Answer Key

CHAPTER 1

1. a. Novice
   b. Advanced beginner
   c. Competent
   d. Proficient
   e. Expert
2. a. Assessment
   b. Diagnosis
   c. Outcome identification
   d. Planning
   e. Implementation
   f. Evaluation
3. Nursing incorporates the art of and science of caring and focuses on the protection, promotion, and optimization of health and abilities; prevention of illness and injury; facilitation of healing and alleviation of suffering through compassionate presence.
4. a. Ethics
   b. Advocacy
   c. respect and equitable practice
   d. communication
   e. collaboration
   f. leadership
   g. Education
   h. scholarly inquiry
   i. quality of practice
   j. professional practice evaluation
   k. resource stewardship
   l. environmental health
5. The nursing code of ethics is the philosophical ideals of right and wrong that define the principles you will use to provide care to your patients.
6. b
7. d
8. n
9. g
10. c
11. f
12. m
13. i
14. k
15. j
16. l
17. h
18. e
19. a
20. She saw the role of nursing as being in charge of a patient's health, based on the knowledge of how to put the body in such a state as to be free of disease or to recover from disease.
21. d
22. c
23. b
24. a
25. a. Nurse's self-care
   b. Health care reform and costs
   c. Demographic changes of the population
   d. Human rights
   e. Increased number of medically underserved
26. A term to describe burnout and secondary traumatic stress, which impact the health and wellness of nurses and the quality of care provided to patients
27. a. Patient-Centered Care
   b. Teamwork and collaboration
   c. Evidence-based practice
   d. Quality improvement
   e. Safety
   f. Informatics
28. *Genomics* describes the study of all the genes in a person, as well as interactions of those genes with each other and with that person's environment.
29. c
30. d
31. b
32. e
33. a
34. g
35. f
36. The purpose is to regulate the scope of nursing practice and protect public health, safety, and welfare.
37. A standardized minimum knowledge base for nurses
38. That the nurse may choose to be certified in a specific area of practice by meeting the practice requirements
39. To improve the standards of practice, expand nursing roles, and foster the welfare of nurses within the specialty areas
40. This is an example of teamwork and collaboration, which function effectively when nursing and interprofessional teams foster open communication, mutual respect, and shared decision making to achieve quality patient care.
41. 3. Nurse educators are revising practice and school curricula to meet the ever-changing needs of society.
42. 1. Candidates are eligible to take the NCLEX-RN to become registered nurses in the state in which they will practice.
43. 2. The ANA's works for the improvement of health standards and the availability of health care services for all, fosters high standards of nursing, and promotes development of nurses.

CHAPTER 2

1. a. Diagnosis and treatment of common illnesses, prenatal and well-baby care, nutrition counseling, and family planning
   b. Blood pressure, cholesterol, tobacco use, and cancer screening for the adult; hearing, vision, autism and developmental screening for pediatrics; HIV screening, wellness visits, immunizations, diet counseling, mental health counseling and crisis prevention; community legislation

c. Urgent care, emergency care, acute medical-surgical care, ambulatory care, outpatient surgery, radiological procedures
d. Intensive care, psychiatric facilities, specialty care
e. Rehabilitation programs, sports medicine, spinal cord injury programs, home care
f. Continuing care (assisted living, nursing centers), psychiatric, and older-adult day care

2. a. Health promotion and disease prevention (primary prevention)
   b. Curing of disease (secondary prevention)
   c. Reducing complication (tertiary prevention)

3. A network of organizations that provides or arranges to provide a continuum of services to a defined population and is willing to be held clinically and fiscally accountable for the outcomes and health status of the population served

4. To deliver the right care, at the right time, in the right setting

5. a. Intensive care: patients receive close monitoring and intensive medical care; the health care providers need to have specialized knowledge and skills.
   b. Mental health facilities: patients with emotional and behavioral problems receive special counseling and treatment.

6. a. Improve access to services, including urgent care services, and meet unmet health needs
   b. Engage rural communities in developing rural health care systems
   c. Develop collaborative delivery systems in rural communities as the hubs
   d. Create protocols for coordinating care transition by aligning urban health care systems
   e. Be the subject matter experts and coordinators of the health care environment of providers, patients, and staff

7. Discharge planning is a coordinated, interdisciplinary process that develops a plan for continuing care after a patient leaves a health care agency.

8. The focus is to ensure that a patient transitions to the setting in which his or her health care needs can be appropriately met.

9. a. Emphasizes the role of transition coach in managing/facilitating discharge of the patient to home or a rehab center. Based on four pillars that have different interventions depending on the stage of the hospitalization
   b. Emphasizes comprehensive discharge planning for chronically ill, high-risk, older patients, which contains six key components
   c. Headed by both a nurse practitioner and a social worker; the focus is to help patients manage their health conditions, coordinate their health care, and achieve optimal health

10. a. Discharge medications
    b. Follow-up care (if needed)
    c. List of all medications changed or discontinued
    d. Dietary needs
    e. Follow-up tests or procedures

11. a. Engage the patient and family in the process
    b. Make a referral as soon as possible
    c. Give the care provider receiving the referral as much information as possible about the patient
    d. The care provider will make recommendations for the patients care and incorporate them into the treatment plan as soon as possible.

12. The goal of restorative care is to help individuals regain maximal functional status and to enhance quality of life through promotion of independence and self-care.

13. Helping patients and their family members achieve independence. It addresses recovery from and stabilization of illness in the home. The agencies employ skilled and intermittent professional services.

14. Rehabilitation

15. b		22. b	
16. c		23. e	
17. a		24. c	
18. d		25. g	
19. e		26. d	
20. f		27. a	
21. g		28. f	

29. Inpatient prospective payment system (IPPS)

30. a. Relational communication techniques
    b. Hourly rounding
    c. Nursing staffing patterns
    d. Bedside shift report

31. a. Baby Boomers aging and the need for health care growing
    b. Nursing schools struggle to expand their capacity to meet the rising demands

32. a. Patient-centered care
    b. Teamwork and collaboration
    c. Evidence-based practice
    d. Quality improvement
    e. Safety
    f. Informatics

33. Care that is respectful of and responsive to individual patient preferences, needs, and values and ensures that patient values guide all clinical decisions

34. a. Respect for patient's values, preferences and expressed needs
    b. Coordination and integration of care
    c. Information and education
    d. Physical comfort
    e. Emotional support and alleviation of fear and anxiety
    f. Involvement of family and friends
    g. Continuity and transition
    h. Access to care

35. a. Quality patient care
    b. Nursing excellence
    c. Innovations in professional practice

36. a. Transformational leadership
    b. Structural empowerment
    c. Exemplary professional practice
    d. New knowledge, innovations, and improvements
    e. Empirical quality outcomes

37. Nurse-sensitive outcomes are patient outcomes and se-lect nursing workforce characteristics that are directly related to nursing. Examples include changes in patient symptom experiences, functional status, safety, psycho-logical distress, Registered Nurse (RN) job satisfaction, total nursing hours per patient day, and costs.

38. Telemedicine is a technology that relies on interac-tive video and uses medical information gathered and reviewed at one site and transmits treatment rec-ommendations to another site to improve a patients clinical health status.

39. Health care disparities are differences in health care outcomes and dimensions of health care, including ac-cess, quality, and equity, between population groups.

40. a. Availability of resources to meet daily needs
    b. Access to educational, economic, and job opportunities
    c. Access to health care services
    d. Quality of education and job training
    e. Availability of community-based resources
    f. Transportation options
    g. Public safety
    h. Social support
    i. Social norms and attitudes
    j. Exposure to crime, violence, and social disorder
    k. Socioeconomic conditions
    l. Residential segregation
    m. Language/literacy
    n. Access to mass media and emerging technologies
    o. Culture

41. The level of support the parents offer when the stu-dent completes homework; the level of violence in the family's neighborhood; the cultural values about education held by the family

42. 4. Reduce the incidence of disease, minimize com-plications, and reduce the need to use more ex-pensive health care resources

43. 1. Initially focuses on the prevention of complica-tions related to the illness or injury. After the con-dition stabilizes, rehabilitation helps to maximize the patient's level of independence.

44. 2. Where they receive supportive care until they are able to move back into the community

45. 1. Family-centered care is provided that allows the patient to live with comfort, independence, and dignity while easing the pains of terminal illness.

CHAPTER 3

1. Health promotion, disease prevention, and restor-ative care

2. Reaching everyone in the community, focusing on primary rather than institutional or acute care, and providing knowledge about health and health promo-tion and models of care to the community

3. Political policy, social determinants of health, in-creases in health disparities, and economics

4. a. Assessment
   b. Development and implementation of public health policies
   c. Improved access to care

5. Biological, socioeconomic, psychosocial, behav-ioral, or social factors

6. Health disparities are preventable differences in population's ability to achieve optimal health. Populations can be disadvantaged by the burden of disease , injury, violence or opportunities to achieve optimal health due to social , political, or environ-mental resources.

7. a. Focus requires understanding the needs of a popu-lation or a collection of individuals who have one or more personal or environmental characteristics in common.
   b. Nursing practice in the community, with the pri-mary focus on the health care of individuals, fam-ilies, and groups in the community

8. a. Health promotion
   b. Disease prevention
   c. Improving the quality of life of the population

9. Community settings such as the home or a clinic, where the focus is on the needs of the individual or family

10. a. Are more likely to develop health problems as a result of excess risks
    b. Have limits in access to health care services
    c. Are dependent on others for care

11. Access to health care is limited because of lack of ben-efits, resources, language barriers, and transportation.

12. They live in hazardous environments, work at high-risk jobs, eat less nutritious foods, and have multiple stressors in their lives, and lack adequate transportation.

13. Mental health problems, substance abuse, socioeco-nomic stressors, lack of understanding of child develop-ment or parenting skills, and dysfunctional relationships

14. Homeless or live in poverty and lack the ability to maintain employment or to care for themselves on a daily basis

15. Suffer from chronic diseases and have a greater de-mand for health care services

16. Together with the family, you develop a caring part-nership to recognize actual and potential health care needs and identify community resources.

17. The ability to establish an appropriate plan of care based on assessment of patients and families and to coordinate needed resources and services for the pa-tient's well-being across a continuum of care

18. Acts to empower individuals and their families to creatively solve problems or become instrumental in creating change within a health care agency

19. Provides the information necessary for patients to make informed decisions in choosing and using ser-vices appropriately

20. Mutual trust and respect for each professional's abil-ities and contributions

21. Assists patients in identifying and clarifying health problems and in choosing appropriate courses of action to solve problems
22. Establishes relationships with community service organizations and assesses patients' learning needs and readiness to learn within the context of the individual, the systems with which the individual interacts, and the resources available for support
23. May be involved in case finding, health teaching, and tracking incident rates of illness
24. a. Structure (geographical boundaries, emergency services, housing, economic status)
    b. Population (age and sex distribution, growth trends, education level, ethnic and religious groups)
    c. Social (education and communication systems, government, volunteer programs, welfare system)
25. The nurse would educate the community leaders as to the need for immunizations for illness prevention and would educate them about the location of the clinic and the process for assessing health care resources, which will improve the health care of the children in the community.
26. 1. They are usually jobless and do not have the advantage of shelter and cope with finding a place to sleep at night and finding food.
27. 4. The coordinating of activities of multiple providers and payers in different settings throughout a patient's continuum of care
28. 3. Observe the community's design, location of services, and locations where the residents meet

CHAPTER 4

1. e	10. b
2. f	11. c
3. a	12. d
4. d	13. e
5. h	14. g
6. i	15. f
7. j	16. a
8. c	17. b
9. g	

18. A phenomenon specific to the discipline that developed the theory
19. a. Input: The data that come from a patient's assessment
    b. Output: End product of a system (whether the patient's health improves, declines, or remains stable)
    c. Feedback: The outcomes reflect the patient's responses to nursing interventions
    d. Content: The product and information obtained from the system

20. d	24. c
21. e	25. b
22. g	26. f
23. a	27. h

28. a. Uses logic to explore relationships between phenomena
    b. Determines how accurately a theory describes a nursing phenomenon

29. a. Would focus Bob's care on the need for a clean environment, good water, and light as necessary for health
    b. The nurse would assist Bob in coping and adapting to his diagnosis of pneumonia, self-concept, role function, and interdependence.
30. 1. See Table 4.2.
31. 4. Person: (the recipient of nursing care), level of health, and environment are all possible causes.

CHAPTER 5

1. Evidence-based practice (EBP) is a problem-solving approach to clinical practice that combines the deliberate use of best evidence in combination with a clinician's expertise, patient preferences, and available health care resources in making decisions about patient care.
2. a. Cultivate a spirit of inquiry
   b. Ask a clinical question in PICOT format
   c. Search for the most relevant and best evidence
   d. Clinically appraise the evidence you gather
   e. Integrate all the evidence with one's clinical expertise, patient preferences, and values
   f. Evaluate the outcomes of practice decision or change using evidence
   g. Communicate the outcomes of EBP decision or changes
3. a. P = Patient population of interest
   b. I = Intervention of interest
   c. C = Comparison of interest
   d. O = Outcome
   e. T = Time
4. a. Agency policy and procedure manuals
   b. Quality improvement data
   c. Existing clinical practice guidelines
   d. Computerized databases
5. Accuracy, validity, and rigor are approved for publication by experts before it is published.
6. Randomized controlled trial (RCT)
7. a. What is the level of evidence?
   b. How well was the study (if research) conducted?
   c. How useful are the findings to practice?
8. Summarizes the purpose of the article, the major themes or findings, and the implications for nursing practice
9. Contains more information about its purpose and the importance of the topic for the reader
10. A detailed background of the level of science or clinical information that exists about the topic
11. The population, the health alteration, how patients are affected, or a new therapy or technology
12. a. Purpose statement: The intent or focus of the study; contains research questions of hypothesis
    b. Methods or design: How it was organized and conducted to answer the research question or hypothesis
    c. Analysis: How the data collected are analyzed
    d. Results or conclusions: Summary section

e. Clinical implications: Explains how the generalizability or how to apply the findings in a practice setting

13. Nursing research is a way to identify new knowledge, improve professional education and practice, and use nursing and health care resources effectively.

14. Focuses on testing implementation interventions to improve uptake and use of evidence to improve patient outcomes and population health

15. Outcomes research typically focuses on the benefits, risks, costs, and holistic effects of treatment on patients.

16. The scientific method is a systematic step-by-step process that ensures that the study supports the validity, reliability, and generalizability of the data.

17. a. The research identifies the problem area or area of interest to study.
    b. The steps of planning and conducting the study are systematic and orderly.
    c. External factors that may influence a relationship between the phenomena that are being studied are controlled.
    d. Empirical data are gathered through the use of observations and assessments.
    e. The goal is to apply the knowledge from a study to a broader group of patients.

18. a. The conditions are tightly controlled to eliminate bias and to ensure that findings can be generalizable to similar subjects.
    b. Describe, explain, or predict phenomena; a case-control study
    c. Information is obtained from populations regarding the frequency, distribution, and interrelation of variables among the subjects.
    d. Determines why a program, or some components of the program, are successful or unsuccessful

19. The study of phenomena that are difficult to quantify or categorize, such as patients' perceptions of illness or quality of life

20. a. Assessment
    b. Diagnosis
    c. Planning
    d. Implementation
    e. Evaluation

21. a. Informed consent is when research subjects are given full and complete information about the purpose of the study, procedures, data collection, harms, and benefits.
    b. Are capable of fully understanding the research and implications of participation
    c. Have the power of free choice to voluntarily consent or decline
    d. Understand how the researcher maintains confidentiality or anonymity

22. Guarantees that any information a subject provides will not be reported in any manner that identifies the subject and will not be accessible to people outside the research team

23. Case study: The nurse would meet with all the disciplines to develop a multidisciplinary approach for reducing pressure injuries.

24. 5,2,4,1,6,3,8,7. This is the correct order for the EBP process.

25. 3. Together, the abstract and introduction tell you if the topic of the article is similar to your PICOT question or related closely enough to provide you with useful information.

26. 3. The summary details the results of the study and explains whether a hypothesis is supported. The results of other studies are not presented.

CHAPTER 6

1. Promotes a society in which all people live long, healthy lives. It identifies leading health indicators which are high priority in the United States.

2. Health is a state of complete physical, mental, and social well-being, not merely the absence of disease or infirmity.

3. a. Positive: Immunizations, proper sleep patterns, adequate exercise, stress management, and nutrition
   b. Negative: Smoking, drug or alcohol abuse, poor diet, refusal to take necessary medications

4. a. An individual's perception of susceptibility to an illness
   b. An individual's perception of the seriousness of the illness
   c. The likelihood that a person will take preventive action

5. a. The individual characteristics and experiences
   b. Behavior-specific knowledge and affect
   c. Behavioral outcomes

6. Nursing promotes a patient's optimal level of health by considering the dynamic interaction between the emotional, spiritual, social, cultural, and physical aspects of an individual's wellness.

7. a. Developmental stage (consider a patient's growth and development stage helps you predict a patient's response to an actual illness of the threat of a future illness)
   b. Intellectual background (a person's beliefs about health are shaped in part by the person's knowledge, lack of knowledge, or incorrect information about body functions and illnesses, educational background, and past experiences)
   c. Perception of functioning (subjective data about the way the patient perceives physical functioning such as level of fatigue, shortness of breath, or pain; also obtain objective data about actual functioning, such as blood pressure, height measurements, and lung sound assessment)
   d. Emotional (the patient's degree of stress, depression, or fear can influence health beliefs and practices)
   e. Spiritual factors (how a person lives his or her life, including the values and beliefs exercised, the relationships established with family and friends, and the ability to find hope and meaning in life)

8. a. Family practice (the roles and organization of a family influence how each member defines health and illness and values health practices)
   b. Social determinants (the stability of the person's marital or intimate relationship, lifestyle habits, and occupational environment)
   c. Cultural background (influences beliefs, values, and customs that influence their personal health practices, their approach to the system, and the nurse–patient relationship)
9. Health promotion helps individuals maintain or enhance their resent health; includes activities such as routine exercise and good nutrition.
10. Helps people develop a greater understanding of their health and how to better manage their health risks; physical awareness, stress management, and self-responsibility
11. Illness prevention includes activities that motivate people to avoid declines in health or functional levels; immunizations and blood pressure screening.
12. In passive strategies, individuals gain from the activities of others without acting themselves. In active strategies, individuals are motivated to adopt specific health programs.
13. a. Is true prevention; goal is to reduce the incidence of disease
    b. Focuses preventing the spread of disease, illness, or infection once it occurs
    c. Occurs when a defect or disability is permanent and irreversible; it involves minimizing the effects of long-term disease or disability
14. A risk factor is any attribute, quality, or environmental situation or trait that increases the vulnerability of an individual or group to an illness or accident.
15. a. Pregnant or overweight, diabetes mellitus, cancer, heart disease, kidney disease, or mental illness
    b. Premature infant, heart disease, and cancer with increased age
    c. Industrial workers are exposed to certain chemicals or when people live near toxic waste disposal sites.
    d. Habits that have risk factors (sunbathing, overweight)
16. a. No intent to make changes within the next 6 months
    b. Considering a change within the next 6 months
    c. Making small changes in preparation for a change in the next month
    d. Actively engaged in strategies to change behavior; lasts up to 6 months
    e. Sustained change over time
17. Illness is a state in which a person's physical, emotional, intellectual, social, developmental, or spiritual functioning is diminished or impaired.
18. a. Usually has a short duration and is severe; symptoms appear abruptly, are intense, and often subside after a relatively short period
    b. Usually lasts longer than 6 months; can also affect functioning in any dimension

19. People who are ill often adopt cognitive, affective, and behavioral reactions that are influenced by sociocultural and psychological factors.
20. a. Their perceptions of symptoms and the nature of their illness, such as a person experiencing chest pain in the middle of the night seeking assistance
    b. The visibility of symptoms, social group, cultural background, economic variables, accessibility of the system, and social support
21. a. Depend on the nature of the illness, the patient's attitude toward it, the reaction of others to it, and the variables of the illness behavior
    b. Reaction to the changes in body image depends on the type of changes, their adaptive capacity, the rate at which changes take place, and the support services available.
    c. Depends in part on body image and roles but also includes other aspects of psychology and spirituality
    d. Role reversal can lead to stress, conflicting responsibilities for the adult or child, or direct conflict over decision making.
    e. Is the process by which the family functions, makes decisions, gives support to individual members, and copes with everyday changes and challenges
22. The nurse needs to consider the patient and family may grieve the loss of the leg; the patient may have difficulty coping with the change in the appearance of his body; the patient may experience a change in self-concept that will lead to conflict within the family.
23. 2,3,5
24. 4. Internal variables include all of the ones cited.
25. 1. Any situation, habit, or social or environmental condition that increases the vulnerability of the individual to an illness
26. 1. The health belief model helps nurses understand factors influencing patients' perceptions, beliefs, and behavior.

CHAPTER 7

1. Caring is a universal phenomenon influencing the ways in which people think, feel, and behave in relation to one another.
2. Leininger's concept of care defines care as the domain that distinguishes nursing from other health disciplines. Care is the essential human need and is necessary for the health and survival of all individuals.
3. Watson's transpersonal caring: the nurse looks for deeper sources of inner healing to protect, enhance, and preserve a person's dignity, humanity, wholeness, and inner harmony.
4. This takes place during a single caring moment between nurse and patient when a connection forms; the relationship influences both the nurse and the patient for better or worse.

299

5. a. Knowing: Striving to understand an event as it has meaning in the life of the other
   b. Being with: Being emotionally present to the other
   c. Doing for the other as he or she would do for him- or herself if it were at all possible
   d. Enabling: Facilitating the other's passage through life transitions
   e. Maintaining belief: Sustaining faith in the other's capacity to get through an event or transition and face a future with meaning
6. a. Human interaction or communication
   b. Mutuality
   c. Understanding the context of a person's life and illness
   d. Improving the welfare of patients and their families
7. An ethic of care is concerned with relationships between people and with a nurse's character and attitude toward others. It places the nurse at the patient's advocate, solving ethical dilemmas by attending relationships and giving priority to each patient's unique personhood.
8. Having presence in a person-to-person encounter conveys a closeness and a sense of caring. Presence involves both "being there" and "being with."
9. a. Alleviating suffering
   b. Decreasing a sense of isolation and vulnerability
   c. Personal growth
10. a. Task-oriented touch: When performing a task or a procedure, the skillful and gentle performance of a nursing procedure conveys security and a sense of competence.
    b. Caring touch: A form of nonverbal communication, which successfully influences the patient's comfort and security, enhances self-esteem, and improves reality orientation
    c. Protective touch: Used to protect the nurse, patient, or both, it can be positively or negatively viewed
11. Listening involves paying attention to an individual's words and tone of voice and entering his or her frame of reference.
12. a. Continuity of care
    b. Clinical expertise
13. a. Provide honest, clear, and accurate information
    b. Listen to patient and family concerns, complaints, and fears
    c. Assisting family with implementing advanced directives
    d. Advocating for the patient's care preferences and end-of-life decisions
    e. Involving family in care and teaching the family how to keep the relative physically comfortable
    f. Informing the patient and family about the types of nursing service and the people who may enter the personal care area
    g. Provide comfort
    h. Reading the patient passages from religious texts, favorite books, cards, or mail

i. Assure the patient that nursing services will be available
j. Help patients do as much for themselves as possible
14. Today's health care system: nurses have less time to spend with patients, making it harder to know who they are. The reliance on technology and cost-effective health care strategies and efforts to standardize and refine work processes all undermine the nature of caring.
15. The nurse can sit on the patient's bed and listen to his story and then summarize an interpretation of the patients' story.
16. 1,3
17. 2. Even though human caring is a universal phenomenon, the expressions, processes, and patterns of caring vary among cultures.
18. 4. There is a mutual give and take that develops as nurse and patient begin to know and care for one another.
19. 3. Listening involves paying attention to the individual's words and the tone of his or her voice.
20. 4. It depends on the family's willingness to share information about the patient, their acceptance and understanding of therapies, whether the interventions fit the family's daily practices, and whether the family supports and delivers the therapies recommended.

CHAPTER 8

1. Physical, psychosocial, and economic
2. Pathophysiologic condition that lasts more than one year, requires ongoing medical care, and often limits a person's usual activities of daily living
3. Refers to a patient and family's subjective experience of and response to a chronic disease
4-10. See Table 8.1.
11. Abnormality in inherited genetic material that causes autosomal disorders
12. a. Huntington's chorea, familial hypercholesterolemia, and neurofibromatosis
    b. cystic fibrosis and sickle cell
13. The combination of genetics, environment, and lifestyle leads to the development of chronic disease.
14. a. Multigeneration examination for patterns of the same disease
    b. The age of onset of the disease
    c. Generational frequency of the disorder
15. a. Clarification of the risk of disease development based on family history
    b. Answer questions about the process
    c. Recommend screening tests for the disorder if necessary
    d. Discuss available genetic testing
    e. Recommend life style changes that may decrease the risk of developing the disease
16. a. Smoking cigarettes and exposure to second-hand smoke

b. Poor nutrition
c. Excessive alcohol consumption
d. Lack of exercise
e. Obesity
17. a. Severity and duration of the illness
b. Treatment plan
c. Socioeconomic status
d. Patient characteristics (motivation, personal beliefs about health, treatment plan, health literacy mental health)
e. Characteristics of the health care delivery system (relationships and accessibility)
18. a. Assess: determine a patient's beliefs, behaviors, knowledge
b. Advise: provide specific information regarding health risks and benefits of changing behaviors
c. Agree: collaborate with the patient to set realistic goals
d. Assist: help the patient identify barriers, strategies, problem-solving skills, and available support
e. Arrange: determine a follow-up plan (return visits, phone calls, text messages)
19. Disease process, treatments required
20. Economic, functional, occupational, psychological, sexual, social, and spiritual
21. Frustration, fear of the future, loss of control over one's life
22. Higher levels of pain, fatigue, social isolation, and withdrawing from daily activities
23. a. Their illness becomes more difficult to manage
b. Has a greater impact on the ability to function
c. Symptoms a patient considers to be embarrassing
24. a. Being persistent, having a positive outlook, being kind and caring, positive emotions, kind toward oneself, reconciling oneself with the situation, and having courage
b. Support from family, friends, peers, and health care providers
c. Active planning, reducing stress, goal setting, seeking knowledge and help
25. a. Controlling symptoms
b. Maintain comfort
c. Preventing crisis
26. a. Providing care for more than a year
b. Being 65 years or older
c. A family member who has significant needs
d. Alzheimer disease or dementia
e. Living with the recipient
27. The model considers the complex nature of factors that affect the care delivery needs of persons with chronic illnesses; it illustrates how the community and health care systems influence patient outcomes.
28. a. Health system
b. Delivery system design
c. Decision support
d. Clinical information system
e. Self-management support
f. Community

29. See Table 8.4.
30. a. Learn about their illness (treatments, medications, diet, activity)
b. How to manage symptoms an emotions
c. Make life style changes
31. Improves patient outcomes for patients and their families by offering small, highly interactive group workshops that are facilitated by highly trained leaders who have health challenges of their own. Workshops provide disease-specific information and include the elements of action-planning, decision making, and problem solving.
32. A positive result indicates that the genetic mutation exists in her DNA, placing her at increased risk for developing cancer, but does not mean she will develop it. This information helps the woman makes informed decisions about her health care treatment. Decisions then can be made about life style changes, frequency of screenings, and early preventative therapy such as surgery before the cancer develops.
33. 1. Genetic factors are nonmodifiable, people are born with genetic material from their parents.
34. 1, 3, 4, 5. The other answer should be agree (collaborate with the patient to set realistic goals)
35. 3. You need to first assess what the patient's illness means to the wife, assessing internal and external resources. The wife is at risk for poor health outcomes as a caregiver due to her age, length of illness and diagnosis, and living with him.

CHAPTER 9

1. A particular type of health difference that is closely linked with social, economic, and/or environmental disadvantage
2. The conditions in which people are born, grow, live, work, and age shaped by money, power, and resources at global, national, and local levels
3. A particular type of health difference that is closely linked with social, economic, and/or environmental disadvantage
4. c
5. f
6. a
7. h
8. b
9. e
10. i
11. g
12. j
13. d
14. Is based on one's self-identification with one or more social groups in which a common heritage with a particular racial group is shared
15. The frame in which individuals identify consciously or unconsciously with those with whom they feel a common bond because of similar traditions, behaviors, values, and beliefs
16. Occurs when an individual or group transitions from one culture and develops traits of another culture
17. Is the process in which the individual adapts to the host's cultural values and no longer prefers the components of the origin culture

18. A set of evidence-based, scientifically researched standards of care, they are key quality indicators that help health care institutions improve performance, increase accountability, and reduce costs.
19. a. conducting a self-exam of one's own biases toward other cultures
    b. The professional seeks and obtains sound educational base about culturally diverse groups.
    c. Ability to conduct a cultural assessment of a patient to collect relevant cultural data and conduct a culturally based physical assessment
    d. The process that encourages professionals to directly engage in face-to-face cultural interactions
    e. Is the motivation of the professional to "want to" engage in the process
20. (see Box 9.4)
    a. health beliefs and practices
    b. faith-based influences and special rituals
    c. language and communication
    d. parenting styles and family roles
    e. sources of support beyond the family
    f. dietary practices
21. (see Box 9.5)
    a. culturally unique individual
    b. communication—voice quality, pronunciation, use of silence, nonverbal, touch
    c. space – degree of comfort, distance in conversations, definition of space
    d. social organization – normal state of health, marital status, number of children, parents live or deceased
    e. time – orientation, view of, physicochemical reaction to time
    f. environmental control -locus-of-control, value orientation
    g. biological variations – physical assessment
    h. nursing assessment – cultural assimilation, incorporate data into nursing plan
22. Linguistic competence is the ability to communicate effectively and convey information in a manner that is easily understood by diverse audiences.
23. a. Provide language assistance resources for individuals who have limited English proficiency and/or communication needs
    b. Inform all individuals of the availability of language services clearly and in their preferred language verbally and in writing
    c. Ensure that interpreters are competent in providing language assistance
    d. Provide easy-to-understand print material in language commonly use in the service area
24. Health literacy is the degree to which individuals have the capacity to obtain, process, and understand basic health information and the services needed to make health decisions.
25. is an ongoing process of asking patients for feedback thru explanation or demonstration and of presenting information in a new way until you feel confident that you communicated clearly and that your patient understands the information presented.

26. a. L = listen to the patient's perception of the problem
    b. E = explain your perception of the problem
    c. A = acknowledge not only the differences between the two perceptions of the problem
    d. R = recommendations must involve the patient
    e. N = negotiate a treatment plan
27. Medicaid insurance, lack of transportation, woman's age
28. 2. Nurses need to determine how much an individual's life patterns are consistent with his or her heritage.
29. 2. Caused by the changing demographic profile of the United States in relation to immigration and significant culturally diverse populations
30. 1. Because different cultural groups have distinct linguistic and communication patterns
31. 2,3,5

CHAPTER 10

1. a. Durability is a system of support and structure that extends beyond the walls of the household.
   b. Resiliency is the ability of the family to cope with expected and unexpected stressors.
   c. Diversity is the uniqueness of each family unit; each person has specific needs, strengths, and important developmental considerations.
2. A family: a set of relationships that a patient identifies as family or a network of individuals who influence one another/s lives, whether there are actual biological or legal ties.
3. a. A nuclear family consists of two adults (and perhaps one or more children).
   b. An extended family includes relatives in addition to the nuclear family.
   c. In a single-parent family, one parent leaves the nuclear family because of death, divorce, or desertion, or a single person decides to have or adopt a child.
   d. In a blended family, parents bring unrelated children from prior or foster-parenting relationships into a new, joint living situation.
   e. Alternative families include multiadult households, grand families, and communal groups with children, nonfamilies, and cohabitating partners.
4. a. Increase in people living with chronic illnesses and the older-adult population have created a greater need for family caregiving. Older-adult caregivers have special needs—risk factors for poor health and emotional distress.
   b. Poverty—female single-parent families and families with unrelated individuals are especially vulnerable
   c. Homelessness severely affects the functioning, health, and well-being of the family and its members. Children of homeless families are often in fair or poor health and have higher rates of asthma, ear infections, stomach problems, and mental illness.

d. Domestic violence—Emotional, physical, and sexual abuse occurs toward spouses, children, and older-adults across all social classes. Factors are complex and may include stress, poverty, social isolation, psychopathology, and learned family behavior.

5. a. Structure—each family has a unique structure and way of functioning; each of the relationships has different demands, roles, and expectations

   b. Function—what family does, such as how a family interacts to socialize younger family members, cooperates to meet economic needs, and relates to the larger society.

6. a. A rigid structure dictates who is able to accomplish a task and may limit the number of persons outside the immediate family who assumes these tasks.

   b. An open or extremely flexible structure and consistent patterns of behavior that lead to automatic action do not exist, and enactment of roles is overly flexible.

7. As context—the primary focus is on the health and development of an individual member existing within a specific environment.

8. As patient—family needs, processes, and relationships are the primary focus of nursing care.

9. As system—you care for each family member (context), family unit (patient) using all resources available

10. a. Hardiness—the internal strengths and durability of the family unit.

    b. Resiliency—the family's ability to return to a previous, healthy level of functioning after a disruptive or stressful event has occurred

11. a. Genetics—may or may not result in actual development of a disease. Sometimes identification of genetic factors and counseling help family members decide whether to test for the presence of a disease and/or to have children.

    b. Chronic illness—influences an entire family economically, emotionally, socially, and functionally. It also affects a family's decision making and coping resources.

    c. End-of-life care—the families need for information, support, assurance, and presence is great. Each family approaches and copes with end-of-life decisions differently.

12. a. assess all individuals within their family context

    b. assess the family as patient

    c. assess the family as a system

13. a. family structure—determines members of the family, relationship among family members, and the context of the family

    b. developmental assessment—determines how the families adapt during predictable and unpredictable changes and difficult times

    c. family functioning—addresses how individuals behave in relation to one another; includes instrumental aspects that are routine activities

14. a. Understand the family life
    b. Understand the current changes within it
    c. Understand the family's overall goals
    d. Understand the family's expectations

15. a. Conflicting caregiver attitude
    b. Impaired family coping
    c. Risk for caregiver stress
    d. Impaired family process
    e. Risk for parent-child attachment
    f. Family able to participate in care planning
    e. Family knowledge of disease

16. need to be concrete and realistic, compatible with the family members developmental stages and acceptable to family members and their lifestyle.

17. a. Health promotion: Interventions to improve or maintain the physical, social, emotional, and spiritual well-being of the family unit and its members

    b. Acute care: be aware of the implications of early discharge for patients and their families

    c. Discharge planning: be sure the family caregiver is prepared for discharge and knows where to obtain necessary supplies.

    d. Communication: help the family members to maintain open lines of communication with you and the interprofessional health care team to anticipate your patient's and family member's needs

    e. Restorative care: to maintain patients' functional abilities within the context of the family

18. Patient/family will adopt two interventions to reduce caregiver role strain, explain to all family caregivers the signs and symptoms of caregiver role strain, discuss situations in which caregivers role strain may intensify, describe the importance of having family members set up alternating schedules to give the primary caregiver some rest, provide information about community resources for transportation, respite care, and support groups, offer an opportunity to ask questions, provide family with contact information of the provider.

19. 3,4

20. 3. Ongoing membership of the family and the pattern of relationships, which are often numerous and complex

21. 4. Is critical in forming an understanding of family life, current changes in family life, overall goals and expectations, and planning family-centered care

22. 3. Very rigid structures impair functioning.

CHAPTER 11

1. Gesell's theory of development is that although each child's pattern of growth is unique, this pattern is directed by gene activity; the pattern of maturation follows a fixed developmental sequence.

2. The theory explains development as primary unconscious and influenced by emotion. These unconscious conflicts influence development through universal stages experienced by all individuals.

303

3. a. (oral) Sucking and oral satisfaction are not only vital to life but also pleasurable.
   b. (anal) Children become increasingly aware of the pleasurable sensations of this body region with interest in the products of their effort.
   c. (phallic) The genital organs become the focus of pleasure.
   d. (latency) Sexual urges are repressed and channeled into productive activities that are socially acceptable.
   e. (genital) Earlier sexual urges reawaken and are directed to an individual outside the family circle.
4. b
5. d
6. a
7. e
8. c
9. g
10. f
11. h
12. Temperament is a behavioral style that affects the individual's emotional interactions with others.
13. a. Easy child (regular and predictable)
   b. Slow-to-warm-up child (reacts negatively with mild intensity to new stimuli)
   c. Difficult child (highly active, irritable, and has irregular habits)
14. A contemporary life-span approach considers the individual's personal circumstances, how the person views and adjusts to changes, and the current social and historical context in which the individual is living.
15. a. Period I: Sensorimotor (birth to 2 years) develops a schema or action pattern for dealing with the environment.
   b. Period II: Preoperational (2 to 7 years) learn to think with the use of symbols and mental images.
   c. Period III: Concrete operations (7 to 11 years) now are able to perform mental operations.
   d. Period IV: Formal operations (11 years to adulthood) transition from concrete to formal thinking occurs.
16. Level I: The person reflects on moral reasoning based on personal gain.
   a. Stage 1: Punishment and obedience orientation (in terms of absolute obedience to authority and rules); physical consequences guide right and wrong choices.
   b. Stage 2: Instrumental relativist orientation (more than one right view); the child perceives punishment not as proof of being wrong but as something that one wants to avoid.
17. Level II: Sees moral reasoning based on his or her own personal internalization of societal and others' expectations
   a. Stage 3: Good boy–nice girl orientation (good motives, showing concern for others, and keeping mutual relationships)
   b. Stage 4: Society-maintaining orientation (expand their focus from a relationship with others to societal concerns)
18. Level III: Balance between human rights and obligations and societal rules and regulations

a. Stage 5: Social contract orientation (follows the societal law but recognizes the possibility of changing the law to improve society)
   b. Stage 6: Universal ethical principle orientation (right by the decision of conscience in accord with self-chosen ethical principles)
19. Case Study:
   a. Stage—Industry versus inferiority
   b. Connor appears to be a shy boy and is likely to agree to his mother's presence in the room. However, doing so may cause feelings of embarrassment.
   c. Connor appears to be a slow-to-warm-up child due to his discomfort of a new environment and provider. The nurse needs to individualize his or her care to improve the quality of interactions between the parent, provider, and the child
20. 1. Children achieve the ability to perform mental operations.
21. 2. Puberty, marked preoccupation with appearance and body image
22. 2. The adult focuses on supporting future generations and the ability to expand one's personal and social involvement.
23. 4. Level I: Preconventional reasoning
   Stage 1: Punishment and obedience orientation

CHAPTER 12

1. a. Preembryonic stage (first 14 days)
   b. Embryonic stage (day 15 until the eighth week)
   c. Fetal stage (end of the eighth week until birth)
2. Nausea and vomiting, breast tenderness, urinary frequency, heartburn, constipation, ankle edema, and backache
3. a. Heart rate
   b. Respiratory effort
   c. Muscle tone
   d. Reflex irritability
   e. Color
4. Open airway, stabilizing and maintaining body temperature, protecting the newborn from infection
5. Close body contact, often including breastfeeding, is a satisfying way for most families to start bonding.
6. d
7. c
8. h
9. e
10. f
11. b
12. g
13. a
14. 1 month, 1 year of age
15. Size increases rapidly during the first year of life; birth weight doubles (5 months) and triples (12 months). Height increases an average of 1 inch every 6 months until 12 months.
16. The infant learns by experiencing and manipulating the environment (sensorimotor period). Developing motor skills and increasing mobility expand an infant's environment and with developing visual and auditory skills enhance cognitive development.

17. By age 1 year, infants not only recognize their own names but are also able to say three to five words and understand 100 words. The nurse can promote language development by encouraging parents to name objects on which the infant is focusing.

18. a. Infants are unaware of the boundaries of self, but they learn where the self ends and the external world begins.
    b. Much of the play is solitary and exploratory as they use their senses to observe and examine their own bodies and objects of interest in their surroundings.

19. a. Injury prevention focuses on MVA, suffocation, falls, and poisoning.
    b. Children of any age can experience maltreatment, but the youngest are the most vulnerable. A combination of signs and symptoms or a pattern of injury should arouse suspicion.

20. a. Breastfeeding is recommended for infant nutrition because breast milk contains the essential nutrients of protein, fats, carbohydrates, and immunoglobulins that bolster the ability to resist infection. If breastfeeding is not possible or if the parent does not desire it, an acceptable alternative is iron-fortified commercially prepared formula.
    b. After 6 months, iron-fortified cereal is generally an adequate supplemental source in breastfed infants. Because iron in formula is less readily absorbed than that in breast milk, formula-fed infants need to receive iron-fortified formula throughout the first year.
    c. It is recommended that the administration of the primary series begin after birth and be completed during early childhood.
    d. By 6 months infants demonstrate nocturnal sleep patterns, sleeping between 9 and 11 hours at night.

21. 12 months (1 year), 36 months (3 years)

22. The rapid development of motor skills allows the child to participate in self-care activities such as feeding, dressing, and toileting.

23. Toddlers possess an increased ability to remember events and begin to put thoughts into words (2 years).

24. An 18-month-old child uses approximately 10 words. A 24-month-old child has a vocabulary of up to 300 words and is generally able to speak in two-word sentences.

25. Toddlers develop a sense of autonomy; strong wills are frequently exhibited in negative behavior.

26. Children continue to engage in solitary play during toddlerhood but also begin to participate in parallel play; playing beside rather than with another child.

27. Newly developed locomotion abilities and insatiable curiosity increase injury risks for toddlers. Poisoning, drowning, and MVA are all risks.

28. a. Nutrition: To prevent obesity and its associated chronic illnesses, toddlers need a balanced daily intake of bread and grains, vegetables, fruit, dairy products, and proteins. Limit milk intake to two to three cups per day.
    b. Toilet training: Recognizing the urge to urinate and/or defecate is crucial in determining the child's mental readiness.

29. 3 years and 5 years

30. Children gain about 5 lb per year. Preschoolers grow 2.5 to 3 inches per year, double their birth length around 4 years, and stand an average of 43 inches tall by their fifth birthday.

31. Preschoolers demonstrate their ability to think in a more complex manner by classifying objects, increased social interaction, cause-and-effect relationships; the world remains closely linked to concrete experiences; their greatest fear is bodily harm.

32. a. Their curiosity and development of initiative lead them to actively explore the environment, develop new skills, and make new friends.
    b. Preschoolers' vocabularies continue to increase rapidly, and by the age of 6 years, children have 8000 to 14,000 words.
    c. The greatest fear of this age-group is bodily harm, evident by fear of the dark, animals, thunderstorms, and medical personnel.

33. Play shifts from parallel to associative play, and children engage in similar if not identical activity; there is no division of labor or rigid organization or rules.

34. a. The quality of food is more important than the quantity.
    b. Preschoolers average 12 hours of sleep a night. They take infrequent naps.
    c. Vision should be checked at regular intervals; early detection and treatment of strabismus is essential by age 6 years.

35. 6 years to 12 years

36. Around the age of 12; this signals the end of middle childhood.

37. Rate of growth is slow and consistent; average height is 2 inches per year; weight increase is 4 to 7 lb; many children double their weight during this time.

38. School-age children have the ability to think in a logical manner about the here and now and to understand the relationship between things and ideas. The thoughts of school-age children are no longer dominated by their perceptions; thus, their ability to understand the world greatly expands.

39. a. Psychosocial changes: industry versus inferiority; they begin to define their self-concept and develop self-esteem through ongoing self-evaluation.
    b. Peers: become more important; play involves peers and the pursuit of group goals; prefer same-sex peers
    c. Sexual: are curios about their sexuality; this is the time for them to have exposure to sex education
    d. Stress: from parental expectations, peer expectations, school environment, violence in the family, school, or in the community

40. Accidents and injuries (MVAs and bicycle injuries), infections

41. a. Perception of wellness is based on readily observable facts such as presence or absence of illness and adequacy of eating or sleeping; nurses need to provide for privacy and offer explanations of common procedures.
    b. Promotion of good health practices; teaching children about their bodies and the choices such as nutrition and routine exercise impact their health
    c. Immunizations, screenings, and dental care; parents need to be encouraged to discuss pubertal changes (10 years); routine vaccination for human papilloma virus (HPV) in girls and boys 11 to 12 years of age.
    d. At this age, encourage children to take responsibility for their own safety
    e. Promoting healthy lifestyle habits including nutrition and exercise
42. 13 years to 20 years
43. a. Increased growth rate of skeleton, muscle, and viscera
    b. Sex-specific changes such as changes in shoulder and hip width
    c. Alteration in distribution of muscle and fat
    d. Development of the reproductive system and secondary sex characteristics
44. Adolescents possess the ability to determine possibilities, rank and solve problems, and make decisions through logical operations. They can think abstractly and deal effectively with hypothetical problems. They can move beyond the physical or concrete properties of a situation and use reasoning powers to understand the abstract.
45. a. Provide privacy and a nonthreatening environment
    b. Ensure confidentiality and explain its limitations
    c. Be nonjudgmental
    d. Ask open-ended questions
    e. Start with less sensitive topics and then move to more sensitive issues
46. a. Puberty enhances sexual identity; physical evidence of maturity encourages the development of masculine and feminine behaviors.
    b. Similarity in dress or speech and popularity are major concerns.
    c. Movement toward stronger peer relationships is contrasted with adolescents' movement away from their parents.
    d. They evaluate their own health according to feelings of well-being, ability to function normally, and absence of symptoms.
47. a. Motor vehicle accidents
    b. Violence and homicide
    c. Suicide
48. a. Decrease in school performance
    b. Withdrawal
    c. Loss of initiative
    d. Loneliness, sadness, and crying
    e. Appetite and sleep disturbances
    f. Verbalization of suicidal thought

49. a. Anorexia nervosa is a clinical syndrome with both physical and psychosocial components that involve the pursuit of thinness through starvation.
    b. Bulimia nervosa is most identified with binge eating and behaviors to prevent weight gain (vomiting, laxatives, exercise).
50. a. Screen for use and inform of the risks for use. Those who are at higher risk are from dysfunctional families.
    b. All sexually active adolescents need to be screened for STIs even if they have no symptoms.
    c. Pregnant teens need special attention to nutrition, as well as health supervision, and psychological support.
51. Minority adolescents are at greater risk for learning or emotional difficulties, death related to violence, unintentional injuries, an increased rate of adolescent pregnancy, poverty, and limited access to health care services.
52. The nurse may help the adolescent construct a safety plan before telling his or her family or friends in case the response is not supportive.
53. Case Study
    a. Jordynn is transitioning from childhood to adulthood; the hormonal changes of puberty will result in changes in her appearance. Jordynn will have alterations in distribution of muscle and fat. Increased fat deposits are normal during this stage of development.
    b. Education to promote healthy development; reassurance about their change in appearance that weight gain and body changes with fat deposits are normal; need to perform further individual assessments before determining a weight problem exists.
    c. Dieting and efforts to lose weight can threaten the health of adolescents. Unless an actual or potential disease process exists, a balanced diet is most appropriate.
54. 4. Toddlers often develop food jags or the desire to eat one food repeatedly; continue to offer a variety of nutritious foods.
55. 1. Do not understand what is right or wrong, but they do understand positive and negative reinforcement, thus learning self-control
56. 2. The school and home influence growth and development. If they are positively recognized for success, they feel a sense of worth.

CHAPTER 13

1. Late teens to mid−20
2. Young adults usually complete physical growth by age 20 years. An exception to this is pregnant or lactating women. They are active, experience less severe illnesses, ignore physical symptoms, and often postpone seeking health care.

3. Formal and informal educational experiences, general life experiences, and occupational opportunities (which is a major task) increase the individual's conceptual, problem solving, and motor skills

4. a. The person refines self-perception and ability for intimacy.
   b. The person directs enormous energy toward achievement and mastery of the world.
   c. This is a time of vigorous examination of life goals and relationships.

5. a. Identification of modifiable factors that increase the risk for health problems and provide gender - and culturally specific patient education and support to reduce unhealthy lifestyle behaviors
   b. Successful employment offers economic security as well as fulfillment, friendships, social activities, support, and respect from coworkers.
   c. Young adults who have failed to achieve the developmental task of personal integration sometimes develop relationships that are superficial and stereotyped; encourage young adults to assess their sexual activity and practice safe sex.
   d. Conception, pregnancy, birth, and the puerperium are the major phases that have complex phases.

6. a. Many young adults do not marry until their late 20s or early 30s, or they remain single. Parents and siblings become the nucleus of the family. Close friends and associates may be considered family.
   b. Availability of contraception, social pressures, economic considerations, general health status, and age all factor into the decision of when and if the young adult wishes to start a family.
   c. There is greater acceptance of cohabitation without marriage. Recent research demonstrates that there is no difference in child health outcomes between same-sex and different-sex parent households.

7. A family history of a disease puts a young adult at risk for developing it in the middle-or-older-adult years. Genomic science identifies people at risk for disease through the use of genetic testing.

8. Poor hygiene (sharing utensils, poor dental hygiene) is a risk factor.

9. Mortality or health risks can be attributable to poverty, family breakdown, child abuse and neglect, opioid and other drug use, repeated exposure to violence, and access to guns.

10. Substance abuse health risks include intoxicated MVAs, dependence on stimulant or depressive drugs, opioid abuse crisis, and large amounts of caffeine.

11. Human trafficking, runaways, and homeless youth, and nurses in a variety of settings are the first line of health professionals to identify victims

12. Unplanned pregnancies are a continued source of stress that may result in adverse health outcomes for the mother, infant, and family.

13. Sexually transmitted infections can lead to major health problems, chronic disorders, infertility, or death.

14. Exposure to work-related hazards or agents, which can cause disease and cancer

15. Job assessment includes a description of the usual work performed, changes in sleep or eating habits, and evidence of increased irritability or nervousness.

16. Family assessment includes a review of environmental and familial factors, including support and coping mechanisms commonly used by family members.

17. Comprehensive history of both the male and female partners to determine factors that affect fertility as well as pertinent physical findings

18. Obesity assessment involves a review of diet and physical activity and counsel about the benefits of a healthful diet and physical activity.

19. Conduct a thorough musculoskeletal assessment and exercise history to develop a realistic exercise plan

20. Prenatal care is routine through physical examination of the pregnant woman during regular scheduled intervals.

21. a. Women commonly have morning sickness, breast enlargement and tenderness, and fatigue.
    b. Growth of the uterus and fetus results in some of the physical signs of pregnancy.
    c. Increases in Braxton Hicks contractions (irregular, short contractions), fatigue, and urinary frequency occur.

22. 35 to 64

23. The most visible changes are graying of the hair, wrinkling of the skin, thickening of the waist, and decreases in hearing and visual acuity, which may have an impact on self-concept and body image.

24. a. Perimenopause is the period during which ovulation declines, resulting in a diminished number of ova and irregular menstrual cycles, which usually lasts for 1 to 3 years.
    b. Menopause is the disruption of this cycle, primarily because of the inability of the neurohormonal system to maintain its periodic stimulation of the endocrine system.
    c. Climacteric occurs in men in their late 40s or early 50s because of decreased levels of androgens. Penile erection is less firm, ejaculation is less frequent, and the refractory period is longer.

25. Middle adults having the responsibility of raising their own children while caring for aging parents

26. Changes occur by choice or as a result of changes in the workplace or society (limited upward mobility, decreasing availability of jobs, seeking an occupation that is more challenging).

27. Couples redefine their relationships and find increased marital and sexual satisfaction. The onset of menopause and the climacteric affect sexual health.

28. Choice and freedom; delayed marriage and delayed parenthood, adoption

29. Death of a spouse, separation, divorce, and the choice of remarrying or remaining single; need to assess the level of coping

30. Departure of the last child is a stressor, leading to a readjustment phase. Empty nest syndrome describes the sadness and loneliness that accompany children leaving home.

31. Culturally appropriate stress management programs focusing on wellness guide patients to evaluate health behaviors, lifestyle, and environment.

32. Continued focus on the goal of wellness assists patients in evaluating health behaviors and lifestyle that contribute to obesity during the middle-adult years. Research shows that the type of diet is not as important as caloric restriction, which is associated with better weight outcomes.

33. a. Anxiety can be related to change, conflict, and perceived control of environment, which may motivate the adult to rethink his or her life goals and stimulate creativity or precipitate psychosomatic illness and preoccupation with death.

    b. Depression is a mood disorder that manifests itself in many ways. Although the most frequent age of onset is between ages 25 and 44 years, it is common among adults in the middle years and has many causes.

34. a. Ask Bill if he has ever participated in any workplace health fairs or screenings. Young adults need regular dental care—does he have a dentist? When was the last time he saw a dentist? Ask him about his diet; it should have adequate protein, iron, fruits, and vegetables. Perform a thorough psychosocial assessment including history of physical and substance abuse, education, work history, and social support systems to detect personal and environmental risk factors for violence. Need to investigate his intake of alcohol—amount, frequency, and signs of abuse.

    b. Because Bill is sexually active, you need to explain the rationale for asking questions that he may find embarrassing or intrusive. In a nonjudgmental way, the nurse should ask him at what age he became sexually active, how many sexual partners he has had, and were they women, men, or both. How many partners does he currently have and does he use condoms?

    c. Bill should have a comprehensive physical exam every 5 years, with testicular exam, hearing and vision assessment, and needed immunizations. Personal hygiene habits are risk factors—instruct Bill to not share utensils with someone who has a contagious disease. Visit the dentist annually; poor dental hygiene increases the risk of periodontal disease. Assist Bill in identifying and using personal coping strategies. Identify modifiable behaviors such as smoking, substance abuse, binge drinking, and increased unprotected sexual activity and provide gender- and culturally specific education and support to reduce unhealthy lifestyle behaviors.

35. 1. Factors that predispose include poverty, family breakdown, child abuse and neglect, repeated exposure to violence, and access to guns.

36. 3. The most visible changes are the graying of hair, wrinkling of the skin, and thickening of the waist.

37. 1. Menopause is the disruption of the menstrual cycle primarily because of the inability of the neurohormonal system to maintain its periodic stimulation of the endocrine system.

CHAPTER 14

1. 65
2. a. Ill, disabled, and physically unattractive
   b. Forgetful, confused, rigid, bored, and unfriendly
   c. Unable to understand and learn new information
3. Discrimination against people because of increasing age, which undermines self-confidence of older-adults, limits their access to care, and distorts caregivers' understanding of the uniqueness of each older-adult
4. a. Adjusting to decreasing health and physical strength
   b. Adjusting to retirement and reduced or fixed income
   c. Adjusting to the death of a spouse, children, siblings, friends
   d. Accepting self as an aging person
   e. Maintaining satisfactory living arrangements
   f. Redefining relationships with adult children and siblings
   g. Maintaining a quality of life
5. a. It is a home, a place where people live, privacy is respected
   b. Is Medicare and Medicaid certified
   c. Has adequate, qualified staff members who have passed criminal background checks
   d. Provides quality care, assistance with ADLs, social and recreational activities
   e. Offers quality food and mealtimes
   f. Welcomes family when they visit the facility
   g. Is clean
   h. Active communication from staff to patient
   i. Attends quickly to resident requests
6. a. The interrelation between physical and psychosocial aspects of aging
   b. The effects of disease and disability on functional status
   c. Tailoring the assessment to an older person
7. a. Change in mental status
   b. Falls
   c. Dehydration
   d. Decrease in appetite
   e. Loss of functional ability

8. d
9. f
10. g
11. b
12. i
13. j
14. h
15. e
16. a
17. c

18. Functional status refers to activities of daily living involving physical, psychological, cognitive, and social domains.

19. a. Delirium is an acute confusional state that is potentially reversible, occurs suddenly, and worsens at night. Often has a psychological cause (electrolyte imbalances, untreated pain, infection, cerebral anoxia, hypoglycemia, medication effects, tumors, CVA).
    b. Dementia is a generalized impairment of intellectual functioning that interferes with social and occupational functioning; gradual, progressive, and irreversible decline in cerebral function.
    c. Depression is not a normal part of aging. It is treatable with medication, psychotherapy, or a combination of both. The 85 years and older group has the second-highest suicide rate of all groups.

20. a. The stage of life characterized by transitions and role that require letting go of certain habits and structures and developing new ones. The age varies, but it is the major turning point in life.
    b. By choice (desire not to interact with others) or a response to conditions (impaired sensory function, functional impairment, chronic illness, reduced mobility, and cognitive changes) that inhibit the ability or the opportunity to interact with others
    c. Whether a person is healthy or frail, there is a need to express intimacy and sexual feelings (love, warmth, sharing, and touching).
    d. The ability to live independently determines housing choices (social roles, family responsibilities, health status). Consider resources that promote safety, independence, and functional ability.
    e. Older people have a wide variety of attitudes and beliefs about death, but fear of their own death is uncommon. Rather they fear being a burden, experiencing suffering, being alone, and the use of life-prolonging measures.

21. a. understanding the health services provided to older-adults
    b. chronic disease management
    c. injury prevention
    d. caregivers in the home

22. a. Regular primary care, dental, vision, and hearing visits
    b. Participation in screening activities as indicated by age
    c. Immunizations
    d. Regular exercise, smoking sensation, stress management
    e. Attaining and maintain target weight
    f. Low-fat, well-balanced diet
    g. Moderate alcohol use
    h. Socialization
    i. Good handwashing

23. c
24. h
25. e
26. g
27. k
28. i
29. l
30. m
31. a
32. f
33. b
34. d
35. j
36. c
37. e
38. d
39. b
40. f
41. a

42. Intentional actions that cause harm or create serious risk of harm (whether harm is intended) to a vulnerable elder by a caregiver or other person who is in a trusting relationship to the elder

43. Physical abuse, emotional abuse, financial exploitation, sexual abuse, neglect (intentional and unintentional), and abandonment

44. Provides sensory stimulation, induces relaxation, provides physical and emotional comfort, and conveys warmth

45. Restores a sense of reality, improves the level of awareness, promotes socialization, elevates independent functioning, and minimizes physical regression

46. Accepts the description of time and place as stated by the adult; you do not challenge or argue with statements or behaviors

47. Recalling the past to bring meaning and understanding to the present and resolve current conflicts

48. The risk for delirium increases when hospitalized patients experience immobilization, sleep deprivation, infection, dehydration, pain, sensory impairment, drug interactions, anesthesia, and hypoxia.

49. The risk for dehydration and malnutrition can increase as a result of limiting food and fluids in preparation for diagnostic tests and medications that decrease appetite.

50. The risk for health-associated infections can increase because of age-related reductions in immune system responses, most commonly urinary catheter–related bacteriuria.

51. Causes of transient urinary incontinence include delirium, untreated UTIs, excessive urine production, medications, depression, restricted mobility, and constipation.

52. Older-adults face an increased risk for skin breakdown related to changes in aging and to immobility, incontinence, and malnutrition.

53. Older-adults face an increased risk for falls because of intrinsic factors (gait and balance problems, weakness, fear of falling, impaired vision, postural hypotension, medications, and chronic conditions) and extrinsic factors (polypharmacy, poor lighting, cluttered environment, slippery surfaces, improper use of assistive devices, inappropriate footwear).

54. a. The continuation of the recovery from acute illness or surgery that began in the acute care setting
    b. The support of chronic conditions that affect day-to-day functioning

55. Case study:
    a. When a person has a hearing impairment move to a quiet area to reduce background noise and face the patient and speak directly in clear, low-pitched tones. Make sure the patients wear their hearing aid and that it is working properly.

309

b. You may need to supplement your assessment by information that is contributed by a family member or other caregiver. But remember that the older-adult should remain the primary source of information whenever possible. Information that would be important is self-care habits, medication adherence, allergies, and immunizations.

56. 4. It is a potentially reversible cognitive impairment that often has physiological causes.

57. 1. Often the result of retinal damage, reduced pupil size, development of opacities in the lens, or loss of lens elasticity

58. 4. It is the stage of life characterized by transitions and role changes.

CHAPTER 15

1. Is a conclusion about a patient's needs or health problems that leads to a decision to take or avoid action, use or modify standard approaches or create new approaches based on the patient's response.

2. Evidence-based knowledge is knowledge based on research or clinical expertise.

3. a. Why does the patient have this condition?
   b. How does the condition normally affect a patient physically and psychologically?
   c. Are the signs and symptoms shown by the patient what I would expect for the condition or situation?
   d. Are the signs and symptoms associated with worsening of the condition?
   e. What do I really know about this patient's situation?
   f. What other ways can I collect data to help me understand the problem more fully?
   g. Do I require more information?
   h. What care options do I have?

4. a. recognize cues
   b. analyze cues
   c. prioritize problems/diagnoses
   d. generate solutions
   e. take actions
   f. evaluate outcomes

5. c   9. b
6. d   10. f
7. a   11. e
8. g

12. a. Inductive reasoning moves from reviewing specific data elements to make an inference by forming a conclusion about the related pieces of evidence.
    b. Deductive reasoning moves from the general to the specific.

13. a. Critical thinking competence – diagnostic reasoning and clinical decision-making ability
    b. Specific knowledge base – patient data, basic and nursing science, nursing and healthcare theory
    c. Experience personal, clinical practice, skill competence.

d. Environment – time pressure, setting, task complexity
e. Attitudes: confidence, independence, fairness, responsibility, risk taking, discipline, perseverance, creativity, curiosity, intellectual integrity, humility
f. Standards: intellectual standards is a guideline or principle for rational thought; professional standards refer to the standard of practice, ethical criteria for nursing judgments, criteria for evaluation, professional responsibility.

14. c   20. d
15. g   21. f
16. j   22. b
17. a   23. i
18. e   24. k
19. h

25. R–recall the events
    E–examine your responses
    F–acknowledge your feelings
    L–learn from the experiences
    E–explore options
    C–create a plan of action
    T–set a time

26. a. What did I learn from the experience?
    b. Did I respond appropriately in this situation?
    c. What were the consequences of my actions?
    d. How might I act differently in the future?
    e. Was I working from tradition or evidence-based practices?

27. a. Reflective journaling which helps to clarify concepts
    b. Meeting with colleagues to discuss and examine work experiences and validate decisions
    c. Concept mapping is a visual representation of patient problems and interventions that show their relationships to one another.

28. Case study:
    a. The nurse needs to recognize that many assumptions (beliefs) could interfere with the patient eating; such as, the food presented is not culturally appropriate. These assumptions must be clarified. The aim of critical thinking is the ability to focus on the important issues at hand (not eating his food) and make decisions that produce desired outcomes.
    b. Knowing the patient is central to individualizing nursing care so a patient feels cared for and cared about. Specific questions to ask: Why is this patient not eating the food that is given to him? What do I really know about this patient's dietary habits? What options do I have?

29. 4. Involves recognizing an issue exists, analyzing information, evaluating information, and making conclusions

30. 4. The five steps are assessment, diagnosis, planning, interventions, and evaluation.

CHAPTER 16

1. a. Collection of information from primary (patient) and secondary (family, caregiver) sources
   b. Interpretation and validation of data to determine if more data are needed or if the database is complete
2. The patient-centered interview during the history, periodic assessments during rounding or administering care and physical examination
3. a. Health perception–health management pattern
   b. Nutritional–metabolic pattern
   c. Elimination pattern
   d. Activity–exercise pattern
   e. Sleep–rest pattern
   f. Cognitive–perceptual pattern
   g. Self-perception–self-concept pattern
   h. Role–relationship pattern
   i. Sexuality–reproductive pattern
   j. Coping–stress tolerance pattern
   k. Value–belief pattern
4. a. Subjective data include patients' verbal descriptions of their health problems (feeling, perceptions, and self-reported symptoms).
   b. Objective data include observations or measurements of a patient's health status (see, hear, and touch).
5. a. Patient is the best source.
   b. Family caregivers and significant others
   c. Health care team
   d. Medical records
   e. Other records and scientific literature
6. is relationship based on an organized conversation focused on learning about a patient's concerns and needs.
7. a. Courtesy
   b. Comfort
   c. Connection
   d. Confirmation
8. a. Orientation and setting an agenda
   b. Working phase: Collecting assessment
   c. Terminating an interview
9. a. Observation: Nonverbal communication
   b. Open-ended: Prompts patients to describe a situation (tell their story) in more than one or two words
   c. Leading question: Risky, limits information
   d. Back channeling: Active listening prompts
   e. Probing: Encourages a full description without trying to control the direction of the story
   f. Closed-ended: Limit the patient's answers to one or two words
10. f
11. g
12. e
13. h
14. i
15. c
16. j
17. b
18. a
19. d
20. Diagnostic and laboratory data provide further explanation of alterations or problems identified during the history and physical examination.
21. Data validation is the comparison of data with another source to determine data accuracy.
22. A concept map is a visual representation that allows you to graphically show the connections between a patient's many health problems.
23. a. Specific considerations—as with all patients, it is critical to adapt each assessment to the uniqueness of each patients. The history taking requires cultural competence of the nurse. Collection of the information should come from the patient (primary source). Ask the patient her perceptions of the impending surgery. An older patient requires more time for assessment, especially if there are sensory alterations. Use effective communication skills when interviewing patient.
   b. Biological information, reason for seeking health care, previous health concerns, PMH, family history, spiritual health, review of systems. Assess the patient's functional health patterns to learn more about what the patient knows about recovery from surgery and restrictions.
   c. Other than the patient and caregiver; medical records which will contain medical history, lab and diagnostic test results, current physical findings
24. 4. Prompts patients to describe a situation in more than one or two words
25. 1. Some may be focused, and others may be comprehensive.
26. 3. Takes information provided in the patient's story and then more fully describes and identifies specific problem areas
27. 2. Asking questions about the normal functioning of each system; the changes are usually subjective data perceived by the patient.

CHAPTER 17

1. c
2. d
3. b
4. e
5. a
6. f
7. critically organizing all data elements about a patient into meaningful patterns
8. involves placing a label on your data pattern or cluster to clearly identify a patient's response to health problems
9. A diagnostic label is the name of the diagnosis; it describes the essence of the patient's response to health conditions.
10. A related factor is a patient's response to a health problem, which is related to a set of conditions that caused or influenced the response.
11. a. pathophysiological (biological or psychological)
   b. treatment – related
   c. situational (environmental or personal)
   d. maturational
12. a. diagnostic validity – standard diagnostic terminology must be used at the agency to ensure accuracy of the diagnostic statement.
   b. prioritization – ranking their hypothesis about patients, prioritizing their concerns and patient patients nursing diagnosis.

13. Avoid inaccurate or missing data, be thorough in your collection of data
14. Insufficient cluster of cues, premature or early closure, incorrect clustering
15. Inaccurate interpretation, failure to consider conflicting cues, insufficient number of cues, invalid cues, failure to consider cultural influences
16. Wrong label, evidence exists for another diagnosis, collaborative problem, failure to validate with the patient, failure to seek guidance
17. a. Identify the patient's response, not the medical diagnosis
    b. Identify diagnostic statement rather than the symptom
    c. Identify a related factor or risk factor treatable through nursing intervention
    d. Identify the problem caused by the treatment or diagnostic study rather than the treatment or study itself
    e. Identify the patient's response to the equipment rather than the equipment itself
    f. Identify the patient's problems rather than your problems with nursing care
    g. Identify the patient's problem rather than the nursing intervention
    h. Identify the patient's need rather than the goal of care
    i. Make professional rather than prejudicial judgments
    j. Avoid legally inadvisable statements
    k. Identify the problem and etiology to avoid a circular statement
    l. Identify only one patient problem in the diagnostic statement
18. Identify a patients nursing diagnosis, enter into the HER of the agency, , the computer system directs the nurse to select outcome and intervention options to individualized the care.
19. a. A collaborative problem is indicated when both medical and nursing interventions are needed to prevent or treat the problem—nurses cannot prevent seizures or bleeding, thus this is a collaborative problem.
20. 4. Provide the basis for the selection of nursing interventions to achieve outcomes for which the nurse is responsible
21. 4. It is the diagnostic label that describes the essence of a patient's response to health conditions.
22. 4. It is associated with the patient's actual or potential response to the health problem.
23. 2. It is the patient's actual or potential response to the health problem.

CHAPTER 18

1. Involves clinical judgement, reviewing a patient's diagnoses, prioritizing diagnoses and problems, setting outcomes to guide the plan of care, and choosing relevant interventions for patient care.

2. a. If untreated, result in harm to the patient or others
   b. Involve nonemergent, non-life-threatening needs of the patient
   c. Are not always directly related to a specific illness or prognosis but affect a patient's well-being
3. a. Workflow routine of a nursing unit
   b. Staffing levels
   c. Interruptions from other care providers
   d. Available material resources
4. a   7. a
5. b   8. b
6. b   9. a
10. Specific, Measurable, Attainable, Realistic, Timed
11. Addresses only one behavior or response
12. Terms describing quality, quantity, frequency, length, or weight allow the nurse to evaluate outcomes precisely.
13. For a patient's health to improve, he or she must be able to attain the outcomes of care that are set; mutually set attainable goals and outcomes.
14. A realistic goal or outcome is one that a patient is able to achieve.
15. A time-limited outcome is written so that it indicates when the nurse expects the response to occur.
16. Independent nursing interventions are nurse-initiated interventions that do not require direction or an order from another health care professional.
17. Dependent nursing interventions are physician-initiated interventions that require an order from a physician or other health care professional.
18. Collaborative interventions are interdependent nursing interventions that require the combined knowledge, skill, and expertise of multiple care professionals.
19. a. Desired patient outcomes
    b. Characteristics of the nursing diagnosis
    c. Research base knowledge for the intervention
    d. Feasibility for doing the intervention
    e. Acceptability to the patient
    f. Your own competency
20. The nursing care plan includes nursing diagnoses, expected outcomes, individualized nursing interventions, and evaluation findings. The plan promotes continuity of care and better communication for all health care providers.
21. The interprofessional care plan focuses on patient priorities and improves the coordination of all patient therapies and communication among all disciplines.
22. In a "nursing handoff," nurses collaborate and share information that ensures the continuity of care for a patient and prevents errors or delays in providing nursing interventions.
23. Consultation is a process in which the nurse seeks the expertise of a specialist to identify ways to handle problems in patient management or the planning and implementation of therapies.
24. a. Identify the general problem area
    b. Direct the consultation to the right professional
    c. Provide the consultant with relevant information about the problem area

d. Do not prejudice against or influence the consultants

e. Be available to discuss the findings and recommendations

f. Incorporate the recommendations into the plan of care

25. a. High-priority diagnosis that drive the priorities of safety, adequate oxygenation, and adequate circulation

b. Patient's lungs will be clear to auscultation.

26. 2. An objective behavior or response that you expect a patient to achieve in a short time, usually less than 1 week

27. 4. The measurable change in a patient's condition that you expect to occur in response to the nursing care

28. 3. The nurse sets patient-centered goals and expected outcomes and plans nursing interventions.

CHAPTER 19

1. Implementation begins after the nurse develops a plan of care. The interventions are designed to achieve the goals and expected outcomes needed to support or improve the patient's health status.

2. a. Direct care are treatments performed through interactions with patients.

b. Indirect care are treatments performed away from the patient but on behalf of the patient.

3. a. Helping role

b. Teaching–coaching function

c. Diagnostic and patient-monitoring function

d. Effective management of rapidly changing situations

e. Administering and monitoring therapeutic interventions and regimens

f. Monitoring and ensuring the quality of health care practices

g. Organizational and work role competencies

4. Are statements that include recommendations, intended to optimize patient care, that are informed by a systematic review of evidence and an assessment of the benefits and harms of alternative care options.

5. A standing order is a preprinted document containing orders for the conduct of routine therapies, monitoring guidelines, or diagnostic procedures for patients with identified clinical problems.

6. Nursing Interventions Classification (NIC) interventions offer a level of standardization to enhance communication of nursing care across settings and to compare outcomes.

7. a. Review the set of all possible nursing interventions for a patient's problem

b. Review all possible consequences associated with each possible nursing action

c. Determine the probability of all possible consequences

d. Judge the value of the consequence to the patient

8. reassess the patient before a procedure

9. review the nursing care plan and consider if revision to interventions is necessary based on patient's current condition

10. organize necessary resources and your delivery of care

11. anticipate and prevent complications based on what you know about the patient

12. Implement the interventions correctly

13. Activities of daily living are activities usually performed in the course of a normal day, such as ambulation, eating, dressing, bathing, and grooming.

14. Instrumental activities of daily living that support daily life include skills such as shopping, preparing meals, writing checks, and taking medications.

15. Physical care techniques involve the safe and competent administration of nursing procedures.

16. Lifesaving measures are physical care techniques that are used when a patient's physiological or psychological state is threatened.

17. Counseling is a direct care method that helps the patient use a problem-solving process to recognize and manage stress and to facilitate interpersonal relationships.

18. Teaching involves good interpersonal skills to create a change in a patient's knowledge and behavior.

19. An adverse reaction is a harmful or unintended effect of a medication, diagnostic test, or therapeutic intervention.

20. Preventive nursing actions promote health and prevent illness to avoid the need for acute or rehabilitative health care.

21. Are nursing treatments or procedures performed from a patient but on behalf of a patient.

22. Is when patents and families invest time in carrying out required treatments to achieve patient goals.

23. You would reassess the patient; compare assessment findings to validate existing nursing diagnosis; review the care plan; and decide whether the nursing interventions remain appropriate for your patient

24. 4. The nurse needs to exercise good judgment and decision making before actually delivering any interventions.

25. 2. Certain nursing situations require you to obtain assistance by seeking additional personnel, knowledge, or nursing skills. You will need assistance with this patient to help turn and position the patient safely.

26. 1. Guides decisions and interventions for specific health care problems or conditions

27. 1. An acquisition of new knowledge or psychomotor skills

CHAPTER 20

1. Whether a patient's condition or well-being improved after nursing interventions were delivered

2. a. Examine the results of care according to clinical data collected

    b. Compare achieved effects or outcomes with goals and expected outcomes

    c. Recognize errors or omissions

    d. Understand a patient situation, reflect on the situation, and correct the errors

3. a. assessing the patient
    b. knowing the patient
    c. education

4. a. being systematic and using criterion-based evaluation
    b. collaborating with patients and healthcare professionals
    c. using ongoing assessment data to revise a plan
    d. communicating results to patients and families

5. They include the expected outcomes established during planning. These outcomes are based upon a specific nursing diagnosis and the assessment findings used to form the diagnosis.

6. comparison before and after an intervention, a comparison after an intervention

7. similar to and often the same assessment skills and techniques you perform during a patient assessment.

8. a. provide a means for nurses and other health care providers to evaluate the status of patients, families, community
    b. provide an outcome measurement system using SNL for all health care settings, specialties, and patients across the life span
    c. offer a means to quantify the change in patient status after nursing interventions and to monitor patient progress

9. a. examine the outcome criteria to identify the exact desired patient behavior or response.
    b. evaluate a patient's actual behavior or response
    c. compare the established outcome criteria with the actual behavior or response
    d. judge the degree of agreement between outcome criteria and the actual behavior or response
    e. if there is not agreement (or only partial agreement) between the outcome criteria and the actual behavior or response, what is the reason?

10. The nurse's ability to recognize how a patient is responding and then adjusting interventions as a result. The nurse may change the frequency of an intervention, change how the intervention is delivered, or select a new intervention based on the patient's response.

11. Each time the nurse evaluates a patient, he or she determines if the plan of care should continue, discontinue, or be revised.

12. If the nurse and the patient agree that the expected outcomes and goals have been met, then that portion of the care plan is discontinued.

13. After reassessment, determine which nursing diagnosis is accurate for the situation and if the related factor or risk factor is accurate

14. Is each goal and expected outcome realistic for the problem, etiology, and time frame?

15. Examine the appropriateness of the intervention and the correct application of the intervention

16. The nurse is responsible for consistent, thorough documentation of the patient's progress toward the expected outcomes and use of nursing diagnostic language. When documenting a patient's response to the interventions, the nurse should describe the intervention, the evaluative measures used, the outcomes achieved, and the continued plan of care.

17. increase patient pain and suffering, prolong hospital stays, increase health care costs

18. (See Box 20.2)
    a. catheter association urinary tract infection
    b. central line blood stream infections
    c. patient falls
    d. patient falls with injury.
    e. pressure injury rate
    f. pain assessment/intervention/reassessment cycles completed
    g. peripheral IV infiltration rate
    h. physical restraint prevalence
    i. ventilator-associated pneumonia
    j. psychiatric patient assault rates

19. Inspect color, condition, and location of pressure injury; measure diameter of ulcer daily; note odor and color of drainage from ulcer

20. 2. Determines whether the patient's condition or well-being has improved after the application of the nursing process

21. 2. They are the expected favorable and measurable results of nursing care.

22. 3. If the goals have not been met, you may need to adjust the plan of care by the use of interventions, modify or add nursing diagnoses with appropriate goals and expected outcomes, and redefine priorities.

23. 1,3,4

CHAPTER 21

1. team building and training, trust, communication and a workplace that facilitates collaboration

2. a. Focus on change and innovation through team development
    b. Serve as a mentor for staff
    c. Develop and support moral agency of nurses

3. a. Develop interpersonal trust and ensure effective communication
    b. Have awareness of personal strengths and weaknesses
    c. Take initiative and sustain motivation
    d. Seek multiple perspectives and opinions to generate options and solutions
    e. Rebound from setbacks with positivity
    f. Understand what they can and cannot change
    g. Schedule time and space to regularly reflect, recharge, and reframe
    h. Take responsibility for decisions
    i. Display caring, understanding, an empathy for others
    j. Motivate and empower others
    k. Identify need to change and support
    l. Use different leadership styles appropriately

4. d
5. e
6. b
7. j
8. c
9. f
10. h
11. i
12. g
13. a

14. a. Collaborate with staff in establishing annual goals for the unit and systems needed
    b. Monitor professional nursing standards of practice
    c. Develop an ongoing staff development plan
    d. Recruit new employees
    e. Conduct routine staff evaluations
    f. Establish self as a role model
    g. Submit staff schedules
    h. Advocate for staff
    i. Conduct regular patient rounds and problem solve
    j. Establish, monitor, and implement a performance/quality improvement plan
    k. Review and recommend new equipment
    l. Conduct regular staff meetings
    m. Make rounds with health care providers
    n. Establish and support staff and interprofessional committees

15. a. Establishment of nursing practice or problem-solving committees or professional shared governance councils
    b. Interprofessional collaboration among nurses and health care providers
    c. Interprofessional rounding
    d. Staff communication
    e. Staff education

16. A focused and complete assessment of the patient's condition allows for accurate clinical judgement as to the patient's health problems and required nursing therapies.

17. The nurse forms a picture of the patient's total needs and sets priorities by deciding on what patient needs or problems need to be cared for first.

18. Implementing a plan of care requires you to be effective and efficient. Whereas effective use of time means doing the right things, efficient use of time means doing things right.

19. Administration of patient care occurs more smoothly when staff members work together.

20. Learn how, where, and when to use your time. Establish personal goals and time frames. Anticipate interruptions.

21. Evaluation is an ongoing process that compares actual patient outcomes with expected outcomes.

22. A professional environment is one in which staff members respect one another's ideas, share information, and keep one another informed.

23. a. Goal setting
    b. Time analysis
    c. Priority setting
    d. Interruption control
    e. Evaluation

24. a. Right task
    b. Right circumstances
    c. Right person
    d. Right direction or communication
    e. Right supervision

25. a. Assess the knowledge and skills of the delegate
    b. Match tasks to the delegate's skills
    c. Communicate clearly
    d. Listen attentively
    e. Provide feedback

26. You can delegate to an assistant to give the patient a bath, take his vital sign and take the patient for a walk

27. 4. As a student nurse, you have a responsibility for the care given to your patients, and you assume accountability for that care.

CHAPTER 22

1. d
2. b
3. e
4. c
5. a

6. a. Responsibility – the willingness to respect one's professional obligations and follow through
    b. Accountability – answering for one's own actions
    c. Confidentiality – respecting patient privacy
    d. Advocacy – application of one's skills and knowledge for the benefit of another person

7. A value is a personal belief about the worth of a given idea, attitude, custom, or object.

8. Values clarification is the need to distinguish among values, facts, and opinions.

9. Deontology is a system of ethics that defines actions as right or wrong based on their "right-making characteristics such as fidelity to promises, truthfulness, and justice." It does not look at the consequences of actions.

10. Utilitarianism is when the value of something is determined by its usefulness; the main emphasis is on the outcome or consequence of actions.

11. Feminist ethics focus on inequalities between people; they look to the nature of relationships for guidance.

12. An ethic of care focuses on understanding relationships, especially personal narratives.

13. Case-based reasoning turns away from conventional principles of ethics as a way to determine best actions and focuses instead on an intimate understanding of particular situations.

14. a. Ask the question: is this an ethical problem?
    b. Gather information relevant to the case
    c. Identify the ethical elements in the situation by clarifying values and recognizing the principles involved
    d. Name the problem
    e. Identify possible causes of action
    f. Create and implement an action plan
    g. Evaluate the action plan

15. a. Provide clinical ethical consultation
    b. Develop and/or revise policies pertaining to clinical ethics and hospital policy
    c. Facilitate education about issues
16. Posting information or pictures about patients, even without specific identifiers, is a violation of confidentiality.
17. Quality-of-life measures the value and benefits of certain medical interventions, which is central to discussions in futile care, cancer therapy, and do not resuscitate (DNR).
18. Antidiscrimination laws enhance the economic security of people with physical, mental, or emotional challenges.
19. End-of-life care: Almost any intervention beyond symptom management and comfort measures is seen as futile.
20. a. Respect for the patient's autonomy is a fundamental ethical commitment and needs to be taken into consideration when making clinical decisions with a patient.
    b. The nurse will remain committed to advocacy for this patient, speaking for the patient's point of view even though it conflicts with her own beliefs. Her commitment reflects a professional commitment to fidelity.
    c. The nurse's concern about managing difficult side effects represents the practice of nonmaleficence.
21. 2. Ethical problems come from controversy and conflict.
22. 4. The ethics committee is an additional resource for patients and health care professionals.
23. 4. Incorporate as much information as possible from a variety of sources such as laboratory and test results; the clinical state of the patient; current literature about the condition; and the patient's religious, cultural, and family situation.
24. 3. Privacy is a patient's right to avoid disclosure of their personal health information. Posting information or pictures about patients, even without specific identifiers, is a violation of confidentiality.

CHAPTER 23

1. e
2. h
3. f
4. b
5. c
6. g
7. d
8. a
9. a. defines nursing and reflects the values of the nursing profession
   b. reflect the knowledge and skill ordinarily possessed and used by nurses to perform within the scope of practice
10. a. health care laws
    b. best practice guidelines
    c. professional organization white papers
    d. evidence-based nursing knowledge
    e. citizen advocacy groups

11. Consumer rights and protection, affordable health care coverage, increased access to care, quality of care that meets the needs of patients
12. a. providing tax credits
    b. increasing insurance accountability for premiums and rate increases
    c. increases the number of choices available to patents to select insurers
13. It protects the rights of people with disabilities. It also is the most extensive law on how employers must treat health care workers and patients infected with HIV.
14. nurses must ensure that patient PHI is not inadvertently conveyed on social media and that protected data are not disclosed other than permitted by patients. Best practice , regardless of patient consent, is to never post patient information on social media.
15. Requires health insurances companies to provide coverage for mental health and substance use disorder treatment, just as they do for medical coverage.
16. The Patient Self-Determination Act requires health care institutions to provide written information to patients concerning their rights under state law to make decisions, including the right to refuse treatment and formulate advance directives.
17. An individual older than the age of 18 years has the right to make an organ donation; the person needs to make the gift in writing with his or her signature.
18. In conjunction with HIPPA and in response to new technology and social media
19. On patient rights, quality of life, quality of care, and the physical environment in which patients lived
20. a. Restraints should be used only to ensure the physical safety of the resident or other residents.
    b. Restraints should be used only when less restrictive interventions are not successful.
    c. Restraints should be used only on the written order of a physician, which includes a specific episode with start and end times.
21. The Board of Nursing licenses all RNs in the state in which they practice and can suspend or revoke a license if a nurse's conduct violates provisions in the licensing statute based on administrative law rules that implement and enforce the statute.
22. See Box 23.2
23. See Box 23.2
24. See Box 23.2
25. a. Explanation of the procedure or treatment
    b. Names and qualifications of people performing and assisting in the procedure
    c. A description of the serious harm that may occur
    d. Explanation of alternative therapies
    e. Has the right to refuse the treatment
    f. May refuse the treatment after it has begun
26. Good Samaritan laws encourage health care professionals to assist in emergencies, limit liability, and offer legal immunity for nurses who help at the scene of an accident.

27. Public health laws provide protection of the public's health, advocating for the rights of people, regulating health care and health care financing, and ensuring professional accountability for the care provided.

28. Determination of death requires irreversible cessation of circulatory and respiratory functions or that there is irreversible cessation of all functions of the entire brain, including the brainstem.

29. d   34. c
30. g   35. f
31. e   36. j
32. h   37. b
33. i   38. a

39. a. the nurse (dependent) owed a duty of care to the patient (plaintiff)
    b. the nurse did not carry out or breached the duty of care
    c. the patient was injured due to the breach in duty
    d. damages or remedies are allowed under state law

40. a. 1973 Roe versus Wade; state laws vary as to viability tests in the termination of pregnancy
    b. sometimes called physician–assisted suicide; a statue for a competent individual with a terminal illness who can make a request to end their life in a dignified manner governed by state laws

41. a. if a student harms a patient as a direct result of their actions or lack of actions, the student, instructor, agency, and university share the liability for the incorrect action.
    b. adequate staffing is required to assure patient safety and satisfaction with care. Nurse–to–patient ratios are determined in different ways (state laws, staffing committees, and patient needs).

42. a. Lacks the knowledge or skill needed
    b. Care exceeding the Nurse Practice Act is expected.
    c. Health of the nurse or her unborn child is directly threatened.
    d. Orientation to the unit has not been completed.
    e. Clearly states and documents a conscientious objection based on moral, ethical, or religious grounds
    f. Clinical judgment is impaired due to fatigue.

43. Identifying possible risks, analyzing them, acting to reduce risks, and evaluating the steps to taken to reduce them

44. The occurrence (incident) report provides a database for further investigation in an attempt to determine deviations from standards of care; corrective measures are needed to prevent recurrence and to alert risk management to a potential claim situation.

45. Call the nursing supervisor about your concerns and take the assignment only if your concerns are documented in writing

46. 1. Determines the legal boundaries within each state

47. 3. Need to perform only those tasks that appear in the job description for a nurse's aide or assistant

48. 4. Conduct that falls below the standards of care

49. 1. Unintentional touching without consent

50. 4. Need to follow the institution's policies and procedures on how to handle these situations and use the chain of command

CHAPTER 24

1. Communication is a lifelong learning process that is an essential part of patient-centered nursing care.

2. a. Take the initiative in establishing and maintaining communication
   b. Be authentic (one's self)
   c. Respond appropriately to the other person

3. perceptual biases, stereotypes

4. c   14. m
5. d   15. a
6. e   16. h
7. a   17. b
8. b   18. i
9. g   19. k
10. c   20. n
11. f   21. e
12. j   22. d
13. l

23. a. Voice tone
    b. Eye contact
    c. Body positioning

24. a. Intimate distance (0–18 inches)
    b. Personal distance (18 inches–4 feet)
    c. Social distance (9–12 feet)
    d. Public distance (12 feet and greater)

25. (Box 24.4)
    a. Preinteraction phase
    b. Orientation phase
    c. Working phase
    d. Termination phase

26. A technique for encouraging patients to share their thoughts, beliefs, fears, and concerns with the aim of changing their behaviors

27. Many nursing situations, especially those in community and home care settings, require the nurse to form helping relationships with entire families.

28. Communication with other members of the health care team affects patient safety and the work environment. The SBAR technique is a popular communication tool that standardizes communication.

29. Behaviors such as withholding information, backbiting, making snide remarks, nonverbal expressions of disapproval

30. a. Address the behavior when it occurs in a calm manner
    b. Describe how the behavior affects your functioning
    c. Ask for the abuse to stop
    d. Notify the manager to get support for the situation
    e. Avoid gossiping about the situation or the person with other staff
    f. Make a plan for taking action in the future
    g. Document the incidence in detail in your personal notes, not patient records

31. a. Courtesy
    b. Use of names
    c. Trustworthiness
    d. Autonomy and responsibility
    e. Assertiveness
32. a. Autonomy is being self-directed and independent in accomplishing goals and advocating for others.
    b. Assertiveness is expressing feelings and ideas without judging or hurting others.
33. (Box 24.6)
    a. Physiological status, emotional status, growth and development, unmet needs, attitudes and values, perceptions and personality, self-concept, self-esteem
    b. Social and working relationship, level of trust, level of caring, level of self-disclosure, shared history, balance of power and control
    c. Information exchange, goal achievement, problem resolution, expression of feelings
    d. Privacy level, noise level, comfort and safety level, distraction level
    e. Educational level, language and self-expression, customs and expectations
34. (Box 24.7)
    a. Make sure the patient knows that you are talking
    b. Face the patient with your face/mouth visible and don't chew gum
    c. Speak clearly, do not shout
    d. Speak slowly
    e. Check for hearing aids, etc.
    f. Quiet, well-lit environment with minimal distraction
    g. Allow time for the patient to respond
    h. Give the patient a chance to ask questions
    i. Keep communication short and to the point
35. a. Men tend to use less verbal communication but are more likely to initiate communication and address issues more directly.
    b. Women disclose more personal information and use more active listening.
36. Impaired verbal communication (state in which the individual's experiences are decreased, delayed, or absent or the person has an inability to receive, process, transmit, and use symbols)
37. Defining characteristics are the inability to articulate words, inappropriate verbalization, difficulty forming words, and difficulty in comprehending.
38. Related factors can be physiological, mechanical, anatomical, psychological, cultural, or developmental in nature.
39. a. Patient initiates conversation about the diagnosis.
    b. Patient is able to attend to appropriate stimuli.
    c. Patient conveys clear and understandable messages with health team.
    d. Patient will express increased satisfaction with the communication process.
40. e
41. g
42. m
43. o
44. f
45. a

46. p
47. n
48. l
49. k
50. b
51. j
52. i
53. c
54. d
55. h
56. g
57. k
58. j
59. f
60. h
61. c
62. e
63. d
64. a
65. i
66. b
67. Listen attentively, do not interrupt, ask simple questions, allow time, use visual cues, use communication aids
68. Use simple sentences, ask one question at a time, allow time for patient to respond, be an attentive listener, include family and friends
69. Check for hearing aids, reduce environmental noise, get patient's attention, face the patient, do not chew gum, speak in a normal voice, rephrase, provide sign language
70. Check for glasses, identify yourself, speak in a normal tone, do not rely on gestures or nonverbal communication, use indirect lighting, use 14-point print
71. Call the patient by name, verbally and by touch; speak to patient as though the patient can hear; explain all procedures; provide orientation
72. Speak to the patient in normal tone, establish a method to signal the desire to communicate, provide an interpreter, avoid using family members, develop communication aids
73. a. Determine whether he encourages openness and allow the patient to "tell his story" expressing both thoughts and feelings
    b. Identify any missed verbal or nonverbal cues or conversational themes
    c. Examine whether nursing responses blocked or facilitated the patient's efforts to communicate
    d. Determine whether nursing responses were positive and supportive or superficial and judgmental
    e. Examine the type and number of questions asked
    f. Determine the type and number of therapeutic communication techniques used
    g. Discover any missed opportunities to use humor, silence, or touch
74. "I am sorry we did not notify you more quickly. It sounds like you have been really worried about your husband."
75. 4. Means of conveying and receiving messages through visual, auditory, and tactile senses
76. 1. Awareness of the tone of verbal response and the nonverbal behavior results in further exploration
77. 3. The connotative meaning of a word is influenced by the thoughts, feelings, or ideas people have about the word.
78. 3. Motivates one person to communicate with the other
79. 4. Personal zone when taking a patient's history

CHAPTER 25

1. The nurse is a visible, competent resource for patients who want to improve their physical and psychological well-being. In the school, home, clinic, or workplace, nurses provide information and skills that allow patients to assume healthier behaviors.
2. As a nurse, you learn to identify patients' willingness to learn and motivate interest in learning. Injured or ill patients need information and skills to help them regain or maintain their levels of health.
3. New knowledge and skills are often necessary for patients to continue ADLs and learn to cope with permanent health alterations.
4. c
5. h
6. f
7. i
8. g
9. e
10. a
11. d
12. b
13. a. Assessment
    b. Communication
    c. Cultural
    d. Establishment
    e. Sensitivity
    f. Safety
14. a. Loss of health (grieving process)
    b. Health status
    c. Attentional set
15. Need to know a patient's level of knowledge and intellectual skills before beginning a teaching plan
16. Learning in children depends on the child's maturation; intellectual growth moves from the concrete to the abstract as the child matures. Information presented to children needs to be understandable and based on the child's developmental stage.
17. Adults tend to be self-directed learners; they often become dependent in new learning situations. The amount of information provided and the amount of time varies depending on the patient's personal situation and readiness to learn.
18. To learn psychomotor skills, the following physical characteristics are necessary: size, strength, coordination, and sensory acuity.
19. a. The nursing process requires assessment of all sources to date to determine a patient's total health care needs.
    b. The teaching process focuses on the patient's learning needs and willingness and capability to learn.
20. a. Information or skills needed by the patient to perform self-care and to understand the implications of a health problem
    b. Patient's experiences that influence the willingness and the need to learn
    c. Information that the family members require to support the patient's needs
21. a. Behavior
    b. Health beliefs and sociocultural background
    c. Perception of severity and susceptibility of a health problem and the benefits and barriers to treatment

d. perception of the severity and susceptibility of a health problem and the benefits and barriers in treatment
    e. Perceived ability to perform behaviors
    f. Desire to learn
    g. Attitudes about health care providers
    h. Learning style preference
22. a. cognitive function, memory, knowledge, association, and judgment
    b. cognitive domain of learning
    c. psychomotor domain of earning- physical strength, endurance, movement, dexterity, and coordination
    d. sensory deficits -visual or hearing loss
    e. patients reading level
    f. developmental level
    g. pain, fatigue, anxiety or depression
23. a. Distractions or persistent noise
    b. Comfort of the room, ventilation, temperature, lighting
    c. Room facilities and available equipment
24. a. Willingness to have family caregivers and others involved in the teaching plan
    b. Family caregiver's perceptions and understanding of the illness and its implications
    c. Caregiver's willingness and ability to participate in care
    d. Financial or material resources
    e. Teaching tools
25. a. decisional conflict
    b. lack of knowledge (affective, cognitive, psychomotor)
    c. impaired health maintenance
    d. impaired ability to manage diet/exercise regime
    e. self-care deficit
26. Identify what a patient needs to achieve to gain a better understanding of the information provided and better manage their illness
27. Priorities should be based on the patient's immediate needs (perception of what is most important, anxiety level, and amount of time available), nursing diagnoses, and the goals and outcomes established for the patient.
28. Time the teaching for when a patient is most attentive, receptive, and alert and organize the activities to provide time for rest and teaching–learning interactions
29. Organize teaching material into a logical sequence progressing from simple to complex ideas
30. c
31. e
32. i
33. j
34. h
35. a
36. g
37. d
38. f
39. b
40. The nurse is legally responsible for providing accurate, timely patient information that promotes continuity of care. Documentation of patient teaching supports quality improvement efforts and promotes third-party reimbursement.

41. Short sessions during which the nurse provides the most important information at the beginning and end of the education session
42. 2. An internal impulse is a force acting on or within a person that causes the person to behave in a particular way.
43. 4. Psychomotor learning involves acquiring skills that integrate mental and muscular activity.
44. 4. Mr. Jones. A mild level of anxiety motivates learning, but a high level of anxiety prevents learning from occurring.
45. 3. Complicated skills, such as learning to use a syringe, require considerable practice but are developmentally appropriate for school-age children.
46. 4. The objective describes an appropriate and achievable skill that the patient can be expected to master within a realistic time frame.

CHAPTER 26

1. Produces a written account of pertinent patient data, nursing clinical decision and interventions, and patient responses in a health care record
2. c
3. e
4. f
5. b
6. d
7. a
8. a patient's record within an integrated health care information system for an individual visit to a healthcare providers' office, or for an individual admission to an acute care facility that allows for seamless documentation of the progression of care
9. Favored term for an individuals' lifetime, computerized record, and means both the displayed or printed record
10. a. Improved quality, safety, and efficacy of health care
    b. Increases health care consumers' active involvement in their care
    c. Increases coordination of health care delivery
    d. Advances public health
    e. Safeguards the privacy and security of personal health records
11. a. Providers are required to notify patients of their privacy policy and make a reasonable effort to get written acknowledgment of this notification.
    b. HIPAA requires that disclosure or requests regarding health information are limited to the minimum necessary.
12. Is a combination of hardware and software that protects private networks from outside hackers, network damage, and theft or misuse of information.
13. Physical, psychosocial, environmental, self-care, spiritual, cultural, knowledge level, and discharge planning needs
14. A factual record contains descriptive, objective information about what a nurse sees, hears, feels, and smells.
15. An accurate record uses exact measurements, contains concise data, contains only approved abbreviations, uses correct spelling, and identifies the date and caregiver.

16. A complete record contains all appropriate and essential information.
17. Current records contain timely entries with immediate documentation of information as it is collected from the patient.
18. Organized records communicate information in a logical order.
19. d
20. b
21. c
22. a
23. d
24. c
25. e
26. b
27. f
28. a
29. With telephone reports, the nurse includes when the call was made, who made it, who was called, to whom information was given, what information was given, and what information was received.
30. a. Clearly determine the patient's name, room number, and diagnosis
    b. use clarification questions to avoid misunderstandings
    c. Write TO or VO, including the date and time, name of the patient, and the complete order, and sign the physician name and the nurse
    d. read back all orders
    e. Follow agency policies
    f. health care provider co signs orders within 24 hours
31. An incident or occurrence is any event that is not consistent with the routine operation of a health care unit or routine care of a patient. Examples include patient falls, needle-stick injuries, a visitor with an illness, medication errors, accidental omission of therapies, and any circumstances that lead to patient injury.
32. Model incorporates an interprofessional approach to delivery and documentation of patient care.
33. Are interprofessional care plans that identify patient problems, key interventions, and expected outcomes within an established time frame
34. When the activities on the pathway are not completed as predicted or a patient does not meet the expected outcomes
35. The use of information systems (HIS, CIS) and other technology to record, monitor, and deliver patient care and to perform managerial and organizational functions in health care
36. a. Nursing process, NANDA, NIC, and NOC
    b. Protocol or critical pathway
37. a. Better access to information
    b. Enhanced quality of documentation
    c. Reduced errors of omission
    d. Reduced hospital costs
    e. Increased nurse job satisfaction
    f. Compliance with requirements of accrediting agencies
    g. Development of a common clinical database
    h. Enhanced ability to track records
38. Is the specialty that integrates nursing science, computer science and information science to manage and communicate data, information, knowledge, and wisdom in nursing

39. Confirm that the fax number you have for the acute rehabilitation facility is correct before sending the fax. Use a cover sheet that indicates the specific person at the acute rehabilitation facility to whom you are directing the patient information. Utilize the encryption feature on the fax machine to encode the information making it impossible for staff at the acute rehabilitation facility to read the information you fax unless they have the encryption key. Place the information you printed out to fax in a secure canister marked for shredding.

40. 4. The patient's medical record should be the most current and accurate continuous source of information about the patient's health care status.

41. 4. When recording subjective data, document the patient's exact words within quotation marks whenever possible

42. 2. An effective change-of-shift report describes each patient's health status and lets staff on the next shift know what care the patients will require.

43. 3. An incident is any event that is not consistent with the routine operation of a health care unit or routine care of a patient.

44. 1,2,4

CHAPTER 27

1. a. Identify patients correctly
   b. Improve staff communication
   c. Use medicines safely
   d. Use alarms safely
   e. Prevent infection
   f. Identify patient safety risks
   g. Prevent mistakes in surgery
2. a. Oxygen
   b. Nutrition
   c. Optimum temperature
3. a. MVAs (leading cause)
   b. Poison
   c. Falls
   d. Fire
   e. Disasters
4. Any microorganism capable of producing an illness with the most common means of transmission by the hands
5. Reduces and in some cases prevents the transmission of disease from person to person
6. A harmful chemical or waste material discharged into the water, soil, or air
7. a. Patient's developmental level
   b. Mobility, sensory, and cognitive status
   c. Lifestyle choices
   d. Knowledge of common safety precautions
8. a. Lifestyle
   b. Impaired mobility
   c. Sensory or communication impairment
   d. Lack of sensory awareness
9. a. Falls
   b. Patient-inherent accidents (seizures, burns, inflicted cuts)

c. Procedure-related accidents (medication administrations, improper procedures)
d. Equipment-related accidents (rapid IV infusions, electrical hazards)

10. a. Activity and exercise
    b. Medication history
    c. History of falls
    d. Home maintenance
11. a. Risk for injury
    b. Impaired Cognition: Confusion
    c. Risk for poisoning
    d. Lack of Knowledge
12. a. Demonstrate effective use of technology and standardized practices that support safety and quality
    b. Demonstrate effective use of strategies to reduce the risk of harm to self or others
    c. Use of appropriate strategies to reduce reliance on memory
    d. Communicate observations or concerns related to hazards and errors to patients, families and the health care team
13. See Table 27.2.
14. See Table 27.2.
15. See Table 27.2.
16. See Table 27.2.
17. Assist them in making lifestyle modifications by referring them to resources
18. See Box 27.8.
19. a. Basic needs related to oxygen, nutrition, and temperature
    b. Modifications in home environment
    c. General preventive measures
20. a. On admission
    b. Routinely until discharge
21. A physical restraint is any manual method, physical or mechanical device, material, or equipment that immobilizes or reduces the ability of a patient to move his or her arms, legs, body, or head freely.
22. Medications used to manage a patient's behavior that are not a standard treatment or dosage for the patient's condition
23. a. Reduce the risk of patient injury from falls
    b. Prevent interruption of therapy
    c. Prevent a confused or combative patient from removing life support equipment
    d. Reduce the risk of injury to others by the patient
24. a. R—Rescue and remove all patients in immediate danger
    b. A—Activate the alarm
    c. C—Confine the fire by closing doors and windows and turning off oxygen and electrical equipment
    d. E—Extinguish the fire using an extinguisher
25. Seizure precautions are nursing interventions to protect patients from traumatic injury, positioning for adequate ventilation and drainage of oral secretions, and providing privacy and support after the event.
26. a. The identification of possible emergency situations and their probable impact

321

Answer Key

Copyright © 2023 Elsevier, Inc. All rights reserved.

b. The maintenance of an adequate amount of supplies

c. A formal response plan for staff and hospital operations to restore essential services and resume normal operations

27. Provide scheduled toileting rounds every 2 to 3 hours; keep the bed in low position with the side rails down; keep the pathway from the bed to the bathroom clear

28. 3. An individual's safety is most threatened when physiological needs are not met, including the need for water, oxygen, basic nutrition, and optimum temperature.

29. 4. Older-adulthood is the developmental stage that carries the highest risk of an injury from a fall because of the physiological changes that occur during the aging process, which increase the patient's risk for falls.

30. 3. The nurse should use the RACE to set priorities in case of fire. Rescue and remove all patients in immediate danger first.

31. 3,1,5,2,4

32. a. Ms. Cohen states, "I bump into things, and I'm afraid I'm going to fall." Cabinets in her kitchen are disorganized and full of breakable items that could fall out. Throw rugs are on the floors, bathroom lighting is poor (40-watt bulbs), her bathtub lacks safety strips or grab bars; and her home is cluttered with furniture and small objects. Ms. Cohen has kyphosis and has a hesitant, uncoordinated gait. She frequently holds walls for support. Ms. Cohen's left arm and leg are weaker than those on the right. Ms. Cohen has trouble reading and seeing familiar objects at a distance while wearing current glasses.

b. Basic human needs, potential risks to patient, developmental stage, influence of medication or illness

c. In the case of safety, the nurse integrates knowledge from previous experiences in caring for patients who had an injury or were at risk.

d. The American Nurses Association's standards for nursing practice address the nurse's responsibility in maintaining patient safety, agency practice standards, and The Joint Commission's patient safety goals.

e. Critical thinking attitudes such as perseverance and creativity, collection of unbiased accurate data regarding threats to the patient's safety, and a thorough review of the patient's home environment would be applicable in this case.

33.

Patient	Potential Nursing Teaching
6-month-old infant weighing 9.5kg (21 pounds)	Use a three point harness, forward-facing safety seat.
	The infant should remain rear-facing for as long as possible.
	A convertible seat is the only option for your infant.
8-year-old child who is 4 feet 4 inches tall	This child can sit in the front seat with a lap and shoulder restraint.
	Be sure to use a booster seat for your child.
	A forward-facing harness restraint is the safest option.
4-year-old who weighs 20.8 kg (46 pounds)	Use a rear-facing convertible safety seat.
	A booster seat with a lap and shoulder restraint is the best option.
	A forward-facing, car safety seat with a three point harness is recommended.

It is very important that infants and children ride in child safety seats that are appropriate for their age and weight.

- A 6-month-old infant weighing 20 pounds should remain rear-facing for as long as possible, until they reach the highest weight or height associated with the given safety seat. While a three point harness is appropriate, this infant is too young to ride forward-facing. A convertible seat can be used for an infant and a toddler, however, this is not the only option for this child.
- A 8-year-old child who is 4 feet 4 inches tall should use a booster seat with a lap and shoulder restraint. This child should not ride in the front seat as all children 12 years of age and under should be restrained in the back seat of the vehicle. A forward-facing, harness restraint is not required due to both age and height. A belt-positioning booster seat should be used until the vehicle's lap and shoulder seat belt fits properly. This is often when they have reached at least 4 feet, 9 inches in height and are 9 to 12 years of age.
- A 4-year-old who weighs 46 pounds should ride forward facing in a car safety seat with a three point harness. The child is too big to ride rear-facing but not yet old enough to ride in a booster seat.

CHAPTER 28

1.	d	9.	a
2.	m	10.	f
3.	o	11.	j
4.	l	12.	b
5.	g	13.	e
6.	n	14.	h
7.	k	15.	c
8.	p	16.	i

17. a. An infectious agent or pathogen
    b. A reservoir or source
    c. A portal of exit from the reservoir
    d. A mode of transmission
    e. A portal of entry to a host
    f. A susceptible host
18. a. Person-to-person or physical source and susceptible host
    b. Personal contact of a susceptible host with a contaminated inanimate object
    c. Large particles that travel up to 3 feet and come in contact with the host
    d. Droplets that suspended in the air during coughing or sneezing
    e. Contaminated items
    f. Internal and external transmissions
19. (Box 28.2)
    a. Incubation period: Interval between entrance of the pathogen into the body and appearance of the first symptoms
    b. Prodromal stage: Onset of nonspecific signs and symptoms to more specific symptoms
    c. Illness stage: Manifests signs and symptoms to type of infection
    d. Convalescence: Acute symptoms of infection disappear
20. a. Patient experiences localized symptoms such as pain, tenderness, warmth, and redness at the wound site.
    b. An infection that affects the entire body instead of just a single organ and can become fatal if undetected
21. a. The body contains microorganisms that reside on the surface and deep layers of the skin, in saliva and oral mucosa, and in the intestinal walls and genitourinary tract that maintain health.
    b. The skin, mouth, eyes, respiratory tract, urinary tract, genitourinary tract, and vagina have unique defenses against infection.
    c. Inflammation is the body's response to injury, infection, or irritation. It is a protective vascular reaction that delivers fluid, blood products, and nutrients to an area of injury.
22. a. Acute inflammation: Rapid vasodilatation that causes redness at the site and localized warmth, allowing more blood near the location of the injury (phagocytosis)
    b. Inflammatory exudate is the accumulation of fluid and dead tissue cells; WBCs form at the site. Exudate may be serous (clear, like plasma), sanguineous (containing RBCs), or purulent (containing WBCs and bacteria).
    c. Healing involves the defensive, reconstructive, and maturative stages.
23. a. Invasive procedures
    b. Antibiotic administration
    c. Presence of multidrug organisms
    d. Breaks in the infection protection and control activities

24. a. Urinary tract
    b. Surgical or traumatic wounds
    c. Respiratory tract
    d. Bloodstream
25. a. Exogenous infection comes from microorganisms outside the individual that do not exist in normal floras.
    b. Endogenous infection occurs when part of the patient's flora becomes altered and an overgrowth results.
    c. Are a type of HAI by an invasive diagnostic or therapeutic procedure
26. a. Infants have immature defenses, breastfed babies have greater immunity, viruses are common in middle-aged adults, older-adult cell-mediated immunity declines.
    b. A reduction in the intake of protein, carbohydrates, and fats reduces the body's defenses and impairs wound healing.
    c. Basal metabolic rate increases; increase serum glucose levels and decrease antiinflammatory responses with elevated cortisone levels
    d. People with diseases of the immune system (leukemia, AIDS) and chronic diseases (AODM) have weakened defenses against infection.
    e. Estrogens promote (but androgens suppress) immune responses during infections and after vaccination.
27. (Box 28-5)
28. See Table 28.4.
29. a. Risk for Infection
    b. Impaired Oral Mucous Membrane
    c. Social Isolation
    d. Impaired Tissue Integrity
    e. impaired nutritional status: deficient food intake
30. a. the patient demonstrates proper hand-hygiene prior to discharge
    b. the patient identifies the signs and symptoms of wound infection
    c. the patient is afebrile upon discharge
    d. the patients wound edges are approximated at time of discharge
31. a. Nutrition – a proper diet helps the immune system function and consists of a variety of foods from all food groups
    b. Hygiene – personal measures reduce organisms on the skin and maintain the integrity of mucous membranes
    c. Immunizations – adhere to the current CDC recommendations
    d. Adequate rest and regular exercise – increases lung capacity, circulation, energy, and endurance, which decreases stress and improves appetite, sleep, and elimination
32. a. Clean technique: hand-hygiene, barrier techniques, cleaning the environment routinely
33. a. Disinfection is a process that eliminates many or all microorganisms with the exception of bacterial spores from inanimate objects.
    b. Sterilization is the complete elimination or destruction of all microorganisms, including spores.

323

34. a. concentration of solution and duration of contact
    b. Type and number of pathogens
    c. Surface areas to treat
    d. Temperature of environment
    e. Presence of soap
    f. Presence of organic materials
35. a. When bathing, use soap and water to remove drainage, dried secretions, and excess perspiration
    b. Change dressings when they are wet or soiled
    c. Place tissues, soiled dressings, or soiled linen in fluid-resistant bags
    d. Place all needles, safety needles, and needleless systems into puncture-proof containers
    e. Keep surfaces clean and dry
    f. Do not leave bottle solutions open; date and discard them in 24 hours
    g. Keep drainage tubes and collection bags patent
    h. Wear gloves and protective eyewear and empty all drainage systems at the end of the shift
36. a. Education of health care facility staff and visitors
    b. Posters and written material for agency and visitors
    c. Education on how to cover your nose and mouth when you cough, using a tissue, and the prompt disposal of the contaminated tissue
    d. Placing a surgical mask on the patient if it will not compromise respiratory function or is applicable
    e. Hand-hygiene after contact with contaminated respiratory secretions
    f. Spatial separation greater than 3 feet from persons with respiratory infections
37. a. handwashing
    b. antiseptic hand wash
    c. antiseptic hand rub
    d. surgical hand antisepsis
38. a. Standard precautions are designed for all patients in all settings regardless of the diagnosis; they apply to contact with blood, body fluid, nonintact skin, and mucous membranes.
    b. Isolation precautions are based on the mode of transmission of disease. They are termed airborne; droplet; contact; and a new category, protective environment.
39. Direct – the care and handling of contaminated body fluids; they require a gown and gloves
40. Large droplets expelled into the air and by being 3 feet away; require surgical mask, proper hand hygiene, and dedicated-care equipment
41. Focus on smaller droplets; require a specially equipped room with a negative air flow and all personnel wear an N95 respirator every time when entering the room
42. Gowns prevent soiling clothing during contact with patients.
43. A full-face protection when you anticipate splashing or spraying of blood or bloody fluid into your face and a mask to satisfy droplet or airborne precautions
44. Glasses or goggles should be worn for procedures that generate splashes or splatters.
45. Need to wear when touching blood, body fluid, secretions, excretions, moist mucous membranes, nonintact skin, and contaminated items or surfaces

46. a. Collection and analysis of infection data
    b. Evaluation of products and procedures
    c. Development and review of policies and procedures
    d. Consultation on infection risk assessment, prevention and control strategies
    e. Education efforts directed at interventions to reduce infection risks
    f. Education of patients and families
    g. Implementation of changes mandated by regulatory, accrediting, and licensing agencies
    h. Application of epidemiological principles
    i. Antimicrobial management
    j. Participation in research projects
    k. monitoring antibiotic-resistant organisms in the institution
47. a. During procedures that require intentional perforation of the patient's skin (IV lines)
    b. When the skin's integrity is broken (trauma, surgical incision or burns)
    c. During procedures that involve procedures (insertion of catheters or surgical instruments)
48. a. A sterile object remains sterile only when touched by another sterile object.
    b. Place only sterile objects on a sterile field
    c. A sterile object or field out of the range of vision or an object held below a person's waist is contaminated.
    d. A sterile object or field becomes contaminated by prolonged exposure to air.
    e. When a sterile surface comes in contact with a wet, contaminated surface, the sterile object or field becomes contaminated by capillary action.
    f. Because fluid flows in the direction of gravity, a sterile object becomes contaminated if gravity causes a contaminated liquid to flow over the object's surface.
    g. The edges of a sterile field or container are considered to be contaminated.
49. a. Assemble all equipment
    b. Don caps, masks, and eyewear
    c. Open sterile packages
    d. Open sterile items on a flat surface
    e. Open a sterile item while holding it
    f. Prepare a sterile field
    g. Pour sterile solutions
    h. Surgical scrub
    i. Apply sterile gloves
    j. Don a sterile gown
50. a. Monitor patients postoperatively, including surgical sites, invasive sites, the respiratory tract, and the urinary tract
    b. Examine all invasive and surgical sites for swelling, erythema, or purulent drainage
    c. Monitor breath sounds
    d. Review laboratory results
51. Tell him that he must remain in the room most of the time to control for transmission of the infection but with proper precautions can leave the room for procedures.
52. 1. The incubation period is the interval between the entrance of the pathogen into the body and appearance of first symptoms.

53. 1. Iatrogenic infections are a type of health care–associated infection (HAI) caused by an invasive diagnostic or therapeutic procedure.

54. 1. If moisture leaks through a sterile package's protective covering, organisms can travel to the sterile object.

55. 1. Patients who are transported outside of their rooms need to wear surgical masks to protect other patients and personnel.

56. 2,5,4,1,3

57. The nurse is caring for a 76-year-old patient who is admitted to rule out sepsis. The patient's vital signs are: Temperature 102.3°F (39°C); blood pressure 110/62 mmHg; heart rate 88 beats/min; respiratory rate 20 breaths/min; oxygen saturation 96% on room air. Current laboratory results are shown in the table. **Highlight the assessment data that would be anticipated with sepsis.**

Laboratory Results	Parameter	Result	Reference Range
	WBC	18,000	5,000–10,000/mm^3
	Neutrophils	45%	55% – 70%
	Lymphocytes	12%	20% – 40%
	Basophils	1%	0.5% – 1.5%

The patient's temperature is elevated at 102.3°F (39°C). With systemic infection, fever is caused by the phagocytic release of pyrogens from bacterial cells. In addition, the patient's white blood cells are significantly elevated. Leukocytosis, or an increase in the number of circulating white blood cells, is the response of the body to white blood cells leaving the blood vessels. The white blood cell count is increased in infection. Neutrophils are part of the differential count and can be decreased in the older-adult with significant infection. Lymphocytes are also decreased in sepsis. Older-adults are less able to produce lymphocytes to combat an immune system challenge.

CHAPTER 29

1. a. The nurse may delegate the measurement of vital signs but is responsible for analyzing and interpreting their significance and selecting appropriate interventions.
   b. clean all devices used to measure vital signs between patients, decreasing the risk of infection.
   c. Assess ensure that is working correctly to provide accurate findings.
   d. Select equipment needs on the basis of the patient's condition and characteristics.
   e. Know the patient's usual range of vital signs
   f. Know the patient's health history, therapies, and medications
   g. Control or minimize environmental factors that affect vital signs
   h. Use an organized and systematic approach
   i. Collaborate with health care providers to decide on the frequency of vital sign assessment
   j. Use measurements to determine the indications for medication administration
   k. Analyze the results of the measurements on the basis of the patient's condition
   l. Verify and communicate significant changes with the patient's health care provider
   m. Educate the family or caregiver in the assessment and the significance of findings

2. h
3. j
4. f
5. e
6. a
7. g
8. b
9. i
10. c
11. d

12. Visible perspiration primarily occurring on forehead and upper thorax

13. a. Insulation of the body
    b. Vasoconstriction
    c. Temperature sensation

14. a. The degree of temperature extreme
    b. The person's ability to sense feeling comfortable or uncomfortable
    c. Thought processes or emotions
    d. Person's mobility or ability to remove or add clothes

15. a. Age
    b. Exercise
    c. Hormone level
    d. Circadian rhythm
    e. Stress
    f. Environment
    g. Temperature alterations (fever, hyperthermia, heatstroke, heat exhaustion, hypothermia)

16. e
17. h
18. b
19. f
20. c
21. g
22. d
23. a

24. Examples of answers can be found in Table 29-2.

25. a. Subtract 32 from the Fahrenheit reading and multiply the result by 5/9
    b. Multiply the Celsius reading by 9/5 and add 32 to the product

26. a. Risk for Impaired Thermoregulation
    b. Hyperthermia
    c. Hypothermia
    d. Fever
    e. chronic fever

27. a. increasing ventilation in the home
    b. Obtaining appropriate clothing to wear in cold weather

28. Those at risk include the very young and very old; persons debilitated by trauma, stroke, or diabetes; those who are intoxicated by drugs or alcohol; patients with sepsis; and those who have inadequate home heating and shelter. Fatigue, dark skin color, malnutrition, and hypoxemia also increase the risk.

29. a. Children have immature temperature-control mechanisms, so their temperatures can rise rapidly, and they are at risk for fluid-volume deficit.
    b. Drug fevers are often accompanied by other allergy symptoms such as rash or pruritus.

30. a. Pharmacologic therapy includes antipyretics and corticosteroids.
    b. Nonpharmacologic therapy includes tepid sponge baths, bathing with alcohol water solutions, applying ice packs to the axillae and groin areas, and cooling fans.

31. Move the patient to a cooler environment; remove excess body clothing; place cool, wet towels over the skin; and use fans

32. Remove wet clothes; wrap the patient in blankets

33. Body temperature will return to an acceptable range, other vital signs will stabilize, and the patient will report a sense of comfort.

34. a. Radial
    b. Apical

35. See Table 29.3.

36. a. When assessing the radial pulse, consider rate, rhythm, strength, and equality
    b. When assessing the apical pulse, consider rate and rhythm only

37. a. 120 to 160
    b. 90 to 140
    c. 80 to 110
    d. 75 to 100
    e. 60 to 90
    f. 60 to 100

38. See answers in Table 29.5.

39. Tachycardia is an abnormal elevated heart rate (> 100 beats/min in adults).

40. Bradycardia is a slow rate (< 60 beats/min in adults).

41. Pulse deficit is an inefficient contraction of the heart that fails to transmit a pulse wave to the peripheral site; it is the difference between the apical and the radial pulse rates.

42. A dysrhythmia is an abnormal rhythm, including early, late, or missed beats.

43. a. activity intolerance
    b. dehydration
    c. hypervolemia
    d. impaired cardiac function
    e. impaired peripheral tissue perfusion

44. Ventilation is the movement of gases in and out of the lungs.

45. Diffusion is the movement of oxygen and carbon dioxide between the alveoli and the red blood cells.

46. Perfusion is the distribution of red blood cells to and from the pulmonary capillaries.

47. Hypoxemia is low levels of arterial O_2.

48. a. Active
    b. Passive

49. See Box 29.6.

50. a. 30 to 60
    b. 30 to 50
    c. 25 to 32
    d. 20 to 30
    e. 16 to 20
    f. 12 to 20

51. Rate of breathing is regular but slow; < 12 breaths/min.

52. Rate of breathing is regular but rapid; > 20 breaths/min.

53. Respirations are labored and increased in depth, and the rate is > 20 breaths/min.

54. Respirations cease for several seconds.

55. Rate and depth of respirations increase.

56. Respiratory rate is abnormally low, and depth of ventilation is depressed.

57. Respiratory rate and depth are irregular; alternating periods of apnea and hyperventilation.

58. Kussmaul respirations are abnormally deep, regular, and increased in rate.

59. Biot respirations are abnormally shallow for two or three breaths followed by an irregular period of apnea.

60. SaO_2 is the percentage of hemoglobin that is bound with oxygen in the arteries and is the percent of saturation of hemoglobin; normal range is usually between 95% and 100%.

61. Measurement of exhaled carbon dioxide throughout exhalation; normally the range is 35-45 mm Hg

62. a. Activity intolerance
    b. Impaired airway clearance
    c. Impaired breathing
    d. Impaired gas exchange

63. Blood pressure is the force exerted on the walls of an artery by the pulsing blood under pressure from the heart.

64. Systolic pressure is the peak of maximum pressure when ejection occurs.

65. Diastolic pressure occurs when the ventricles relax; the blood remaining in the arteries exerts a minimum pressure.

66. Pulse pressure is the difference between systolic and diastolic pressure.

67. Cardiac output increases as a result of an increase in heart rate, greater heart muscle contractility, or an increase in blood volume.

68. Peripheral resistance is the resistance to blood flow determined by the tone of vascular musculature and diameter of blood vessels.

69. The volume of blood circulating within the vascular system affects blood pressure, which normally remains constant.

70. Viscosity is the thickness that affects the ease with which blood flows through blood vessels, determined by the hematocrit.

71. With reduced elasticity, there is greater resistance to blood flow, and the systemic pressure rises (systolic pressure).

72. a. Age
    b. Stress

c. Ethnicity and genetics
d. Gender
e. Daily variations
f. Medications
g. Activity and weight
h. Smoking
73. Table 29.8
  a. 40 (mean) mm Hg
  b. 85/54 mm Hg
  c. 95/65 mm Hg
  d. 105/65 mm Hg
  e. 110/65 mm Hg
  f. 119/75 mm Hg
  g. <120/80 mm Hg
74. Family history, obesity, cigarette smoking, heavy alcohol consumption, high sodium, sedentary lifestyle, exposure to continuous stress, diabetics, older, African Americans
75. Dehydrated, anemic, experienced prolonged bed rest, recent blood loss, medications
76. First: Clear, rhythmic tapping corresponding to the pulse rate that gradually increases in intensity (systolic pressure)
Second: Blowing or swishing sound as the cuff deflates

Third: A crisper and more intense tapping
Fourth: Muffled and low-pitched as the cuff is further deflated (diastolic pressure in infants and children)
Fifth: The disappearance of sound (diastolic pressure in adolescents and adults)
77. a. Activity intolerance
  b. Anxiety
  c. Impaired cardiac output
  d. Fluid imbalance
  e. Acute pain
78. See Box 29.11.
79. Respiratory rate of 22 and oxygen saturation of 94%
80. 4. The skin regulates the temperature through insulation of the body, vasoconstriction, and temperature sensation.
81. 3. The transfer of heat from one object to another with direct contact (solids, liquids, and gases)
82. 3. Victims of heat stroke do not sweat.
83. 2. 156 is the onset of the first Korotkoff sound (systolic pressure), and 88 is the fifth sound that corresponds with the diastolic pressure.
84. 5,2,4,1,3,6

85.

Apply ice packs to the axillae	Pyrexia	Temperature
Administer oxygen at 2 L/min via nasal cannula	Hypothermia	Pain level
Obtain cultures of body fluids (urine, sputum, blood)	Hypoxemia	Capnography
Remove all clothing	Hypotension	Blood glucose
Request an order for acetaminophen	Malignant hyperthermia	Pulse oximetry

This patient has a fever, or pyrexia, as evidenced by a body temperature of 102.4°F (39°C). For healthy young adults, the average oral temperature is 37°C (98.6°F). Pyrogens such as bacteria and viruses can elevate the body temperature by acting as antigens to trigger the immune system. In this case, the fever could have multiple causes and further assessment is required to determine the cause. Obtaining cultures of body fluids is an appropriate action to help isolate the cause of the pyrexia. An antipyretic, such as acetaminophen can be used to decrease the body temperature. The nurse will need to monitor the patient's temperature and pain level.

The patient does not have hypothermia (low temperature), hypoxemia (low oxygen saturation), hypotension (low blood pressure), or malignant hyperthermia. While the patient does have pyrexia, malignant hyperthermia (or an elevation in temperature) is associated with general anesthesia in certain susceptible people.

While it used to be acceptable to apply ice packs to the axillae and groin area to decrease the body temperature, it is now avoided as this can induce shivering. Shivering causes the body temperature to increase. Oxygen is not necessary for this patient as they have clear lung sounds with an oxygen saturation of 96% on room air. It is also not necessary to remove all patient clothing. This will likely make the patient uncomfortable and could also induce shivering which can increase body temperature. It is unnecessary to monitor capnography which is the measurement of exhaled carbon dioxide. The patient is oxygenating well with clear lung sounds. The patient has no history of diabetes and does not require continual assessment of blood sugar. Continual assessment of pulse oximetry is unnecessary as the patient is oxygenating well with clear lung sounds.

CHAPTER 30

1. a. Gather baseline data about the patient's health status
  b. Support, confirm, or refute subjective data obtained
  c. Identify and confirm nursing diagnoses
  d. Make clinical decisions about a patient's changing health status and management
  e. Evaluate the outcomes of care
2. a. Consider the patient's health beliefs, use of alternative therapies, nutrition habits, relationships with family, and comfort with physical closeness of exam
  b. Learn to recognize common characteristics and disorders among ethnic populations

c. Recognize variation in physical characteristics among ethnic populations

d. Recognize your own knowledge deficits

3. a. Infection control

b. Environment – requires privacy

c. Equipment – arrange any necessary equipment so it is readily available

d. Physical preparation of the patient – with proper dress and draping

e. Positioning – refer to Table 30-2 for preferred positions for exams

f. Psychological preparation of the patient – explain the purpose and steps of the exam

4. a. Gather all or part of the histories of infants and children from parents or guardians

b. Gain a child's trust before doing any type of examination, perform the exam in a nonthreatening area, talk and play first, and do the visual parts of the exam first

c. Offer support to the parents during the examination and do not pass judgment

d. Call children by their first names and address the parents as Mr. and Mrs

e. Treat adolescents as adults, provide confidentiality for adolescents; speak alone with them

5. a. Do not stereotype about aging patients' level of cognition

b. Be sensitive to sensory or physical limitations (more time)

c. Adequate space is needed

d. Use patience, allow for pauses, and observe for details

e. Certain types of information may be stressful to give

f. Perform the examination near bathroom facilities

g. Be alert for signs of increasing fatigue

6. a. Compare both sides for symmetry

b. If a patient is ill, first assess the systems of the body part most at risk

c. Offer rest periods if the patient becomes fatigued

d. Perform painful procedures near the end of the examination

e. Record assessments in specific terms in the record

f. Use common and accepted medical terms and abbreviations

g. Record quick notes during the examination to avoid delays

7. Inspection is looking, listening, and smelling to distinguish normal from abnormal findings.

8. a. Adequate lighting is available

b. Use a direct light source

c. Inspect each area for size, shape, color, symmetry, position, and abnormality

d. Position and expose body parts as needed, maintaining privacy

e. Check for side-to-side symmetry

f. Validate findings with the patient

9. Palpation involves using the hands to touch body parts.

10. a. Light palpation involves pressing inward 1 cm (superficial).

b. Deep palpation involves depressing the area 4 cm to assess the conditions of organs.

11. Tapping the skin with the fingertips to vibrate underlying tissues and organs

12. Auscultation is listening to the internal sounds the body makes.

13. a. Frequency indicates the number of sound wave cycles generated per second by a vibrating object.

b. Amplitude describes the loudness, soft to loud.

c. Quality describes sounds of similar frequency and loudness.

d. Duration describes length of time that sound vibrations last.

14. a. Gender and race

b. Age

c. Signs of distress

d. Body type

e. Posture

f. Gait

g. Body movements

h. Hygiene and grooming

i. Dress

j. Body odor

k. Affect and mood

l. Speech

m. Signs of patient-abuse

n. Substance-abuse

15. Physical injury or neglect are signs of possible abuse (evidence of malnutrition or presence of bruising). Also watch for fear of the spouse or partner, caregiver, or parent.

16. C: Have you ever felt the need to cut down on your use?
A. Have people annoyed you by criticizing your use?
G. Have you ever felt bad or guilty about your use?
E. Have you ever used or had a drink first thing in the morning as an "eye opener" to steady your nerves or feel normal?

17. a. Weigh patients at the same time of day

b. Weigh patients on the same scale

c. Weigh patients in the same clothes

18. a. Oxygenation

b. Circulation

c. Nutrition

d. Local tissue damage

e. Hydration

19. Pigmentation is skin color. It is usually uniform over the body.

20. Answers can be found in Table 30.8.

21. a. Diaphoresis (sedative hypnotic, alcohol)

b. Spider angiomas (alcohol, stimulants)

c. Burns (especially on fingers) (alcohol)

d. Needle marks (opioids)

e. Contusions, abrasions, cuts, scars (alcohol, hypnotics, IV opioids)

f. "Homemade" tattoos (cocaine, IV opioids)

g. Vasculitis (cocaine)

h. Red, dry skin (PCP)

22. *Indurated* means hardened.

23. *Turgor* is the skin's elasticity.

24. Occurs in localized pressure areas when patients remain in one position

25. Edema means areas of the skin that are swollen or edematous from a buildup of fluid in the tissues.

26. Unusual findings in the skin—skin tags, senile keratosis, cherry angiomas

27-35. Answers can be found in Box 30-6

36-38. Answers can be found in Box 30-7

39. Asymmetry, Border irregularity, Color, Diameter, Evolution

40. a. *Pediculus humanus capitis* (head lice)
    b. *Pediculus humanus corporis* (body lice)
    c. *Pediculus pubis* (crab lice)

41. Clubbing is a change in the angle between the nail and nail base, including softening, flattening, and enlargement of the fingertips.

42. Beau's lines are transverse depressions in the nails.

43. Koilonychia (spoon nails) are concave curves.

44. Splinter hemorrhages are red or brown linear streaks in nail beds.

45. Paronychia is inflammation of the skin at the base of the nail.

46. Hydrocephalus is the buildup of cerebrospinal fluid in the ventricles.

47. Hyperopia is a refractive error causing farsightedness.

48. Myopia is a refractive error causing nearsightedness.

49. Presbyopia is impaired near vision in middle-age and older-adults caused by loss of elasticity of the lens.

50. Retinopathy is a noninflammatory eye disorder resulting from changes in retinal blood vessels.

51. Strabismus is a congenital condition in which both eyes do not focus on an object simultaneously.

52. A cataract is an increased opacity of the lens that blocks light rays from entering the eye.

53. Glaucoma is intraocular structural damage resulting from increased intraocular pressure.

54. Macular degeneration is blurred central vision, often occurring suddenly, caused by progressive degeneration of the center of the retina.

55. a. Visual acuity that tests central vision with a Snellen chart
    b. Visual fields – objects seen in the periphery
    c. Extraocular movements – test the six muscles that guide the eye
    d. External eye structures
    e. Internal eye structures

56. a. Position and alignment
    b. Eyebrows
    c. Eyelids
    d. Lacrimal apparatus
    e. Conjunctivae and sclera
    f. Corneas
    g. Pupils and irises

57. Exophthalmos is a bulging of the eye.

58. An ectropion is an eyelid margin that turns out.

59. An entropion is an eyelid margin that turns in.

60. Conjunctivitis is the presence of redness, which indicates an allergy or an infection.

61. A ptosis is an abnormal drooping of the eyelid over the pupil.

62. Pupils equal, round, and reactive to light and accommodation

63. a. Retina
    b. Choroids
    c. Optic nerve disc
    d. Macula
    e. Fovea centralis
    f. Retinal vessels

64. a. External ear (auricle, outer ear canal, and tympanic membrane)
    b. Middle ear (three bony ossicles)
    c. Inner ear (cochlea, vestibule, and semicircular canals)

65. The normal tympanic membrane appears translucent, shiny, and pearly gray.

66. a. Conduction – interrupts sound waves as they travel from the outer ear to the cochlea of the inner ear (no sound transmitted from outer and middle ear structures)
    b. Sensorineural – sound is transmitted through the outer and middle ear structures but the sound becomes interrupted beyond the bony ossicles
    c. Mixed – combination of the conduction and sensorineural loss

67. Injury to the auditory nerve resulting from high-maintenance doses of antibiotics

68. Excoriation is skin breakdown characterized by redness and skin sloughing.

69. Polyps are tumor-like growths.

70. Leukoplakia are thick white patches that are often precancerous lesions seen in heavy smokers and people with alcoholism.

71. Varicosities are swollen, tortuous veins that are common in older-adults.

72. Exostosis is extra bony growth between the two palates.

73. a. Neck muscles
    b. Lymph nodes of the head and neck
    c. Carotid arteries
    d. Jugular veins
    e. Thyroid gland
    f. Trachea

74. 1. Occipital nodes at the base of the skull
    2. Postauricular nodes over the mastoid
    3. Preauricular nodes just in front of the ear
    4. Retropharyngeal nodes at the angle of the mandible
    5. Submandibular nodes
    6. Submental nodes in the midline behind the mandibular tip

75. Systemic disease or neoplasm

76. a. Patient's nipples
    b. Angle of Louis

c. Suprasternal notch
d. Costal angle
e. Clavicles
f. Vertebrae

77. Symmetrical, separating thumbs 3 to 5 cm; reduced chest excursion may be caused by pain, postural deformity, or fatigue.
78. Vocal or tactile fremitus are vibrations that you can palpate externally caused by sound waves.
79. Vesicular sounds are soft, breezy, and low-pitched sounds that are created by air moving through smaller airways.
80. Bronchovesicular sounds are blowing sounds that are medium pitched and of medium intensity that are created by air moving through large airways.
81. Bronchial sounds are loud and high pitched with a hollow quality that are created by air moving through the trachea close to the chest wall.
82. Answers can be found in Table 30.21
83. The point of maximal impulse is where the apex of the heart is touching the anterior chest wall at approximately the fourth to fifth intercostal space just medial to the left midclavicular line.
84. Mitral and tricuspid valve closure causes the first heart sound (S1), the "lub."
85. Aortic and pulmonic valve closure causes the second heart sound (S2), the "dub."
86. When the heart attempts to fill an already distended ventricle, a third heart sound (S3) can be heard; abnormal in adults.
87. When the atria contract to enhance ventricular filling, a fourth sound is heard (S4); normal in healthy older-adults and athletes; not normal in adults.
88. Lies between the sternal body and manubrium and feels the ridge in the sternum approximately 5 cm below the sternal notch
89. Second intercostal space on the right
90. Left second intercostal space
91. Left third intercostal space
92. Fourth or fifth intercostal space along the sternum
93. Fifth intercostal space just to the left of the sternum; left midclavicular line
94. Tip of the sternum
95. A murmur is a sustained swishing or blowing sound heard at the beginning, middle, or end of the systolic or diastolic phase.
96. a. Auscultate all valve areas for placement in the cardiac cycle (timing), where best heard (location), radiation, loudness, pitch, and quality
    b. Determine if they occur between S_1 and S_2 (systolic), and S_2 and S_1 (diastolic)
    c. The location is not necessarily over the valves.
    d. Listen over areas besides where the murmur is heard best to assess for radiation (neck and back)
    e. Feel for a thrust or intermittent palpable sensation at the auscultation site in serious murmurs and rate the intensity (a thrill)
97. Grade 1 = barely audible in a quiet room
    Grad. 2 = clearly audible but quiet
    Grad. 3 = moderately loud
    Grad. 4 = loud with associated thrill
    Grad. 5 = very loud thrill easily palpable
    Grad. 6 = louder; heard without stethoscope
98. Syncope is caused by a drop in heart rate and blood pressure.
99. An absent pulse wave (blockage)
100. Narrowing
101. A bruit is the blowing sound caused by turbulence in a narrowed section of a blood vessel.
102. 1. Place the patient in a supine position, avoid neck hyperextension or flexion, observe for engorgement
     2. raise the HOB until pulsations become evident between the angle of the jaw and the clavicle
     3. inspect jugular vein at 45 degree angle
103. See Table 30.25
104. Inspect the calves for localized redness, tenderness, and swelling over vein sites
105. a. Ages 40–44 should have the choice to start annual breast cancer screening with mammograms
     b. Ages 45–54 should get a mammogram every year
     c. Ages 55 and over should have mammograms every 2 years
     d. Early and more extensive screening for personal history of breast cancer, family history, genetic mutation, previous radiation therapy to the chest before 30-years-old
106. a. Clockwise or counterclockwise forming small concentric circles
     b. Vertical technique – up and down each quadrant
     c. Center of the breast in a radial fashion
107. a. Location in relation to the quadrant
     b. Diameter
     c. Shape (round or discoid)
     d. Consistency (soft, firm or hard)
     e. Tenderness
     f. Mobility
     g. Discreteness (clear or unclear boundaries)
108. Benign (fibrocystic) breast disease is characterized by bilateral lumpy, painful breast, sometimes with nipple discharge.
109. Striae are stretch marks (due to obesity or pregnancy).
110. A hernia is a protrusion of abdominal organs through the muscle wall.
111. Distention is swelling by intestinal gas, tumor, or fluid in the abdominal cavity.
112. Peristalsis is movement of contents through the intestines, which is a normal function of the small and large intestine.
113. Borborygmi are growling sounds, which are hyperactive bowel sounds.

114. Rebound tenderness is the pain a patient may experience when the nurse quickly lifts his or her hand away after pressing it deeply into the involved area.
115. An aneurysm is a localized dilation of a vessel wall.
116. Chancres are syphilitic lesions, which appear as small, open ulcers that drain serous material.
117. A Papanicolaou specimen is used to test for cervical and vaginal cancer.
118. Common symptoms include a painless enlargement of one testis and the appearance of a palpable, small, hard lump on the side of the testicle.
119. Digital examination is used to detect colorectal cancer in the early stages and prostatic tumors.
120. A kyphosis is a hunchback, an exaggeration of the posterior curvature of the thoracic spine.
121. Lordosis is a swayback, an increased lumbar curvature.
122. Scoliosis is a lateral spinal curvature.
123. Osteoporosis is a metabolic bone disease that causes a decrease in quality and quantity of bone.
124. A goniometer is an instrument that measures the precise degree of motion in a particular joint.
125. Flexion = movement decreasing angle between two adjoining bones
126. Extension = increasing angle between two adjoining bones
127. Hyperextension = beyond its normal resting extended position
128. Pronation = that the frontal or ventral surfaces face downward
129. Supination = front or ventral surface faces upward
130. Abduction = away from the midline
131. Adduction = toward the midline
132. Internal rotation = rotation of the joint inward
133. External rotation = rotation of the joint outward
134. Eversion = turning of the body part away from the midline
135. Inversion = turning the body part toward the midline
136. Dorsiflexion = flexion of toes and foot upward
137. Plantar flexion = bending of toes and foot downward
138. Hypertonicity is increased muscle tone.
139. Hypotonicity is a muscle with little tone.
140. Atrophied muscles are reduced in size; they feel soft and boggy.
141. The Mini-Mental State Examination measures orientation and cognitive function.
142. Delirium (acute mental disorder) is characterized by confusion, disorientation, and restlessness.
143. a. There is reduced clarity of awareness of the environment.
    b. Ability to focus, sustain, or shift attention is impaired.
    c. Irrelevant stimuli easily distract the person.
    d. Accompanying change in cognition.
    e. Recent memory commonly is affected.
    f. Disorientation usually occurs.
    g. Language disturbances
    h. Perceptual disturbances
144. The Glasgow Coma Scale provides an objective measurement of consciousness on a numerical scale over time.
145. a. A person cannot understand written or verbal speech.
    b. A person understands written and verbal speech but cannot write or speak appropriately when attempting to communicate.
146. I. Olfactory – sense of smell
    II. Optic – visual acuity
    III. Oculomotor – extraocular eye movements, pupil constriction
    IV. Trochlear – downward, inward eye movements
    V. Trigeminal – sensory nerve to skin of face, motor nerve to muscles of jaw
    VI. Abducens – lateral movement of eyeballs
    VII. Facial – facial expression, taste
    VIII. Auditory – hearing
    IX. Glossopharyngeal – taste, ability to swallow
    X. Vagus – sensation of pharynx, movement of vocal cords, parasympathetic innervation to glands and organs
    XI. Spinal accessory – movement of head and shoulders
    XII. Hypoglossal – position of tongue
147. a. Pain
    b. Temperature
    c. Position
    d. Vibration
    e. Crude and finely localized touch
148. The cerebellum controls muscular activity, maintains balance and equilibrium, and helps to control posture.
149. a. Deep tendon reflexes (biceps, triceps, patellar, Achilles)
    b. Cutaneous reflexes (plantar, gluteal, abdominal)
150. Moist crackles in the base of bilateral lungs
151. 4. A thorough explanation of the purpose and steps of each assessment lets patients know what to expect and what to do so they can cooperate.
152. 3. Normally, the skin lifts easily and snaps back immediately to its resting position; the back of the hand is not the best place to test for turgor.
153. 3. Circumscribed elevation of skin filled with serous fluid, smaller than 1 cm
154. 2. Use a systematic pattern when comparing the right and left sides. You need to compare lung sounds in one region on one side of the body with sounds in the same region on the opposite side of the body.
155. 4. After the ventricles empty, ventricular pressure falls below that in the aorta and pulmonary artery, allowing the valves to close and causing the second heart sound.
156. 2,3,5
157. Correct answers are shown in yellow highlight.

Nurses' Notes:	72-year-old female presents alert and oriented to person, place, and time. Senile keratosis noted on the face near the eyes. The patient is missing two back teeth, oral mucosa is glistening and moist with leukoplakia. The ventral surface of the tongue is pink and smooth with large veins between the frenulum fold. Patient reports no pain when chewing food. Scant amount of yellow exudate along the posterior pharynx. The trachea is midline. Right carotid bruit with auscultation of S_1S_2. Stomach is soft with positive bowels sounds in four quadrants. Skin shows tenting when pinched. Patient reports no difficulty with urination. The patient is able to ambulate with even gate. Vital signs: 98.8°F (37°C), 120/64 mmHg, 88 beats/min, 18 breaths/min, oxygen saturation 98% on room air. The patient reports a history of smoking.

Senile keratosis is a thickening of the skin that normally occurs in older-adults. Loose or missing teeth are common in older-adults because bone resorption increases. The patient reports no pain with chewing food so there is no indication that the missing teeth are a new issue or concern. Oral mucosa should be glistening and moist. However, leukoplakia are thick white patches that are often seen in heavy smokers. Yellow exudate along the posterior pharynx is likely from infection and requires follow-up. The trachea should be midline. When auscultating the carotid arteries, a bruit is not a normal finding and requires follow-up. A bruit can indicate a narrowing in the artery. Auscultation of S1S2 is a normal finding as is the presence of bowel sounds in four abdominal quadrants. Skin tenting when pinched indicates increased skin turgor. This can be a sign of dehydration and requires follow-up. Vital signs are within normal limits. Follow-up regarding smoking cessation is an important part of health promotion.

CHAPTER 31

1. a. The federal government protects the health of the people by ensuring that medications are safe and effective. Currently, the Food and Drug Administration ensures that all medications undergo vigorous testing before they are sold.
   b. The state governments conform to federal legislation but also have additional controls such as alcohol and tobacco.
   c. Health care institutions have individual policies to meet federal and state regulations.
   d. The Nurse Practice Act defines the scope of a nurse's professional functions and responsibilities.
2. A chemical name provides an exact description of the medication's composition and molecular structure.
3. A generic name is created by the manufacturer who first develops the medication; this becomes the official name.
4. The trade name is one that the manufacturer has trademarked to identify the particular version they manufacture.
5. A medication classification indicates the effect of the medication on a body system, the symptoms the medication relieves, or the medication's desired effect.

6. The form of the medication determines its route of administration.
7. Pharmacokinetics is the study of how medications enter the body, reach their site of action, metabolize, and exit the body.
8. Absorption refers to the passage of medication molecules into the blood from the site of administration.
9. a. Route of administration
   b. Ability of the medication to dissolve
   c. Blood flow to the site of administration
   d. Body surface area (BSA)
   e. Lipid solubility
10. a. Circulation – vascularity of the various tissues and organs
    b. Membrane permeability – must be able to pass through all the tissues and biological membranes of the organ
    c. Protein binding – most medications partially bind with albumin, reducing the ability of the drug to exert activity
    d. Metabolism – biotransformation
    e. Excretion – chemical makeup of the drug determines the organ for excretion
11. After a medication reaches its site of action, it becomes metabolized into a less active or inactive form that is easier to excrete.
12. The kidneys are the primary organ for drug excretion. When renal function declines, a patient is at risk for medication toxicity.
13. Therapeutic effects are the expected or predictable physiological response to a medication.
14. Side effects are predictable and often unavoidable secondary effects a medication predictably will cause.
15. Adverse effects are unintended, undesirable, and often unpredictable severe responses to medication.
16. Toxic effects develop after prolonged intake of a medication or when a medication accumulates in the blood because of impaired metabolism or excretion.
17. Idiosyncratic reactions are unpredictable effects in which a patient overreacts or underreacts to a medication or has a reaction that is different from normal.
18. Allergic reactions are unpredictable responses to a medication. Examples include hives or itching.
19. Anaphylactic reactions are allergic reactions that are life threatening and characterized by sudden

constriction of bronchiolar muscles, edema of the pharynx and larynx, and severe wheezing and shortness of breath.

20. Medication interaction occurs when one medication modifies the action of another medication; it may alter the way another medication is absorbed, metabolized, or eliminated from the body.

21. A synergistic effect is when the combined effect of the two medications is greater than the effect of the medications when given separately.

22. Occurs over time; usually noted when patients receive higher doses of medication to achieve the same therapeutic effect

23. Addiction is physical and psychological.

24. The MEC is the plasma level of a medication below which the medication's effect will not occur.

25. The peak concentration is the highest serum level concentration.

26. The trough concentration is the lowest serum level concentration.

27. The biological half-life is the time it takes for excretion processes to lower the serum medication concentration by half.

28. a. Oral – easiest and most common
    b. Buccal – in the mouth against the mucous membranes
    c. Sublingual – under the tongue

29. a. Intradermal – into the dermis just under the epidermis
    b. Subcutaneous – into tissues just below the dermis of the skin
    c. Intramuscular – injection into a muscle
    d. Intravenous – into a vein

30. Epidural injections are administered in the epidural space via a catheter, usually used for postoperative analgesia.

31. Intrathecal administration is via a catheter that is in the subarachnoid space or one of the ventricles of the brain.

32. Intraosseous infusion of medication is administered directly into the bone marrow; it is commonly used in infants and toddlers.

33. Intraperitoneal medications, such as chemotherapeutic agents, insulin, and antibiotics, are administered into the peritoneal cavity.

34. Intrapleural medications, commonly chemotherapeutics, are administered directly into the pleural space.

35. Intraarterial medications are administered directly into the arteries.

36. Intracardiac medications are injected directly into the cardiac tissue.

37. Intraarticular medications are injected into a joint.

38. a. Directly applying a liquid or ointment
    b. Inserting a medication into a body cavity
    c. Instilling fluid into a body cavity
    d. Irrigating a body cavity
    e. Spraying a medication into a body cavity

39. Inhaled medications are readily absorbed and work rapidly because of the rich vascular alveolar capillary network present in the pulmonary tissue.

40. a. Metric – each basic unit of measurement is organized into units of 10
    b. Household – convenient but inaccurate

41. A solution is a given mass of solid substance dissolved in a known volume of fluid or a given volume of liquid dissolved in a known volume of another fluid.

42. Dose ordered/Dose on hand × Amount on hand = Amount to administer

43. a. Use only metric system on prescriptions, labels, and dosing
    b. Never administer medications using household spoons
    c. Round all dosing instructions to the nearest 0.1, 0.5 or 1 mL
    d. Medication needs to be tailored based on age, weight, and body mass index
    e. Provide education using hands-on demonstration
    f. Consider using picture-based education for low literacy

44. a. Weigh the patient in kilograms before administering medications
    b. Doses are usually smaller than adults – TB or 1 mL syringes.
    c. IM doses are very small and should not exceed 1mL (children) 0.5 mL (infants).
    d. Most medications are not round off to the nearest tenth, but rather to the nearest thousandth.
    e. Measure doses that are less than 1 mL in syringes
    f. Estimate the dose before beginning the calculation
    g. Compare and evaluate the amount of medication ordered over 24 hours with the recommended dosage (safe dose)

45. If the order is given verbally to the nurse by the provider, it is a verbal order.

46. A standing or routine order is carried out until the prescriber cancels it by another order or until a prescribed number of days elapse.

47. A prn order is a medication that is given only when a patient requires it.

48. A single or one-time dose is given only once at a specified time.

49. A STAT order describes a single dose of a medication to be given immediately and only once.

50. Now is used when a patient needs a medication quickly but not right away; the nurse has up to 90 minutes to administer.

51. a. Unit dose
    b. Automated medication dispensing systems (AMDS)

52. a. Inaccurate prescribing
    b. Administration of the wrong medicine
    c. Giving the medication using the wrong route or time interval
    d. Administering extra doses
    e. Failing to administer a medication

333

Answer Key

53. a. Obtain, verify, document
    b. Consider and compare
    c. Reconcile
    d. Communicate
54. a. The right medication
    b. The right dose
    c. The right patient
    d. The right route
    e. The right time
    f. The right documentation
    g. The right indication
55. a. Be informed of the medication's name, purpose, action, and potential undesired effects
    b. Refuse a medication regardless of the consequences
    c. Have qualified nurses or physicians assess a medication history
    d. Be properly advised of the experimental nature of medication therapy and give written consent
    e. Receive labeled medications safely without discomfort
    f. Receive appropriate supportive therapy
    g. Not receive unnecessary medications
    h. Be informed if medications are a part of a research study
56. a. History
    b. History of allergies
    c. Medication data
    d. Diet history
    e. Patient's perceptual or coordination problems
    f. Patient's current condition
    g. Patient's attitude about medication use
    h. Factors affecting adherence to medication therapy
    i. Patient's learning needs
57. a. Impaired health maintenance
    b. Lack of knowledge (medication)
    c. Nonadherence (medication regimen)
    d. Adverse medication interaction
    e. Complex medication regimen (polypharmacy)
58. a. Will verbalize understanding of desired effects and adverse effects of medications
    b. Will state signs, symptoms, and treatment of hypoglycemia
    c. Will monitor blood sugar to determine if medication is appropriate to take
    d. Will prepare a dose of ordered medication
    e. Will describe a daily routine that will integrate timing of medication with daily activities
59. a. Health beliefs
    b. Personal motivations
    c. Socioeconomic factors
    d. Habits
60. a. Patient's full name
    b. Date and time that the order is written
    c. Medication name
    d. Dosage
    e. Route of administration
    f. Time and frequency of administration
    g. Signature of provider

61. a. The name of the medication
    b. Dose
    c. Route
    d. Exact time of administration
    e. Site
62. When patients need to take several medications to treat their illnesses, take two or more medications from the same chemical class, use two or more medications with the same or similar actions or mix nutritional supplements or herbal products with medications, polypharmacy happens.
63. a. Patient responds to therapy.
    b. Patient has the ability to assume responsibility for self-care.
64. See Box 31.13.
65. a. Medication history and reconciling medications
    b. Assess if patient has an existing patch before application
    c. Wear disposable gloves when applying and removing patches
    d. Apply a noticeable label to the patch
    e. Document removal of medication on the MAR
    f. Document the location of the patient's body where the medication was placed on the medication administration record (MAR)
66. Decongestant spray or drops
67. a. Avoid instilling any eye medication directly onto the cornea
    b. Avoid touching the eyelids or other eye structures with eye droppers or ointment tubes
    c. Use medication only for the patient's affected eye
    d. Never allow a patient to use another patient's eye medications
68. a. Vertigo
    b. Dizziness
    c. Nausea
69. a. Suppositories
    b. Foam
    c. Jellies
    d. Creams
70. Exerting local effects (promoting defecation) or systemic effects (reducing nausea)
71. a. Delivers a measured dose of medication with each push of a canister; often used with a spacer
    b. Releases medication when a patient raises a level and then inhales
    c. Hold dry, powdered medication and create an aerosol when the patient inhales through a reservoir that contains the medication
72. a. Draw medication from ampule quickly; do not allow it to stand open
    b. Avoid letting the needle touch contaminated surface
    c. Avoid touching the length of the plunger or inner part of the barrel
    d. Prepare the skin, use friction and a circular motion while cleaning with an antiseptic swab, and start from the center and move outward

334

73. a. The patient's size and weight
   b. Type of tissue into which the medication is to be injected
74. a. Contain single doses of medications in a liquid
   b. A single-dose or multidose container with a rubber seal at the top (closed system)
75. a. Do not contaminate one medication with another
   b. Ensure that the final dose is accurate
   c. Maintain aseptic technique
76. Rate of action (rapid, short, intermediate, and long acting); each has a different onset, peak, and duration of action.
77. a. Need to maintain their individual routine when preparing and administering their insulin
   b. Do not mix insulin with any other medication or diluents
   c. Never mix insulin glargine or insulin detemir with other types of insulin
   d. Inject rapid-acting insulin mixed with NPH within 15 minutes before a meal
   e. Verify insulin dosages with another nurse while preparing them
78. a. Use a sharp beveled needle in the smallest suitable length and gauge
   b. Position the patient as comfortably as possible to reduce muscle tension
   c. Select the proper injection site using anatomical landmarks
   d. Apply a vapocoolant spray or topical anesthetic to the site if possible
   e. Divert the patient's attention from the injection through conversation
   f. Insert the needle quickly and smoothly
   g. Hold the syringe while the needle remains in tissues
   h. Inject the medication slowly and steadily
79. a. The outer posterior aspect of the upper arms
   b. The abdomen (below the costal margins to the iliac crests)
   c. The anterior aspects of the thighs
80. 0.5 to 1.5 mL; smaller volumes to children
81. a. 25-gauge, 5/8-inch needle inserted at a 45-degree angle
   b. 1/2-inch needle inserted at a 90-degree angle
82. 90 degrees
83. a. 2 to 5 mL into a large muscle
   b. 2 mL
   c. 1 mL
84. Deep site away from nerves and blood vessels; preferred site for medications for adults; children and infants for large volumes and viscous and irritating solutions
85. For adults and children, muscle is thick and well developed; anterior lateral aspect of the thigh
86. Easily accessible, but muscle not well developed; use small amounts (< 2 ml); not used in infants or children; potential for injury to radial and ulnar nerves; immunizations for children; recommended site for hepatitis B and rabies injections

87. Minimizes local skin irritation by sealing the medication in muscle tissue
88. Skin testing; injected into the dermis where medication is absorbed slowly
89. a. Infusion of large volumes of IV fluids (may contain medications)
   b. Injection of a bolus or small volume of medication
   c. Piggyback infusion
90. a. Fast-acting medications must be delivered quickly.
   b. It provides constant therapeutic blood levels.
   c. It can be used when medications are highly alkaline and irritating to the muscle and subcutaneous tissue.
91. a. They reduce risk of rapid infusion by IV push.
   b. They allow for administration of medications that are stable for a limited time in solution.
   c. They allow for control of IV fluid intake.
92. A small (25- to 250-mL) IV bag connected to short tubing lines that connect to the upper Y port of a primary infusion line
93. A small (50- to 150-mL) container that attaches below the primary infusion bag
94. A battery-operated machine that allows medications to be given in very small amounts of fluid (5 to 60 mL)
95. a. Cost saving
   b. Effectiveness of nurse's time by eliminating constant monitoring of flow rates
   c. Increased mobility, safety, and comfort for the patient
96. Assess the patient for cough or change in voice tone or quality after swallowing. Assess patient's gag reflex by offering 50 mL of water in 5-mL allotments. Give medication either as a liquid or as a solid based on patient's swallowing ability.
97. 3. Definition of pharmacokinetics
98. 1. Absorption refers to the passage of medication molecules into the blood from the site of administration.
99. 1. Definition of onset
100. 1. An oral route
101. 2. If mixing rapid- or short-acting insulin with intermediate-acting insulin, take the insulin syringe and aspirate a volume of air equivalent to the dose of insulin to be withdrawn from the intermediate-acting insulin first.
102. 2,3,5
103. To administer the medication as ordered, the nurse will first Roll the NPH insulin between the palms. Then the nurse will Inject 5 units of air into the intermediate (NPH) insulin using a U-100 syringe.

Patients with diabetes mellitus often require more than one type of insulin. This allows for longer and tighter control of the blood sugar. Insulin can only be mixed if compatible. In this case, the patient has regular insulin which is short acting and NPH insulin that is intermediate acting ordered. To administer this medication, the nurse

335

Answer Key

will first roll the cloudy insulin between the palms to re-suspend the insulin preparation. NPH insulin is cloudy. Regular insulin is clear. Insulin should not be shaken as this can create air bubbles that can affect dosing. After rolling the NPH insulin vial between the palms, the nurse will use a U-100 syringe to inject 5 units of air into the NPH insulin. The nurse will not touch the tip of the syringe to the insulin and will remove the syringe from the vial without aspirating. With the same syringe, the nurse will draw up the regular insulin first (6 units) followed by the 5 units of NPH, with accuracy checks in between the steps.

CHAPTER 32

1. Complementary therapies are therapies used in addition to conventional treatment recommended by the patient's health care provider.
2. Alternative therapies include the same interventions as complementary but frequently become the primary treatment that replaces allopathic medical care.
3. See Table 32.1.
4. See Table 32.1.
5. See Table 32.1.
6. See Table 32.1.
7. See Table 32.1.
8. a. Emphasizes the importance of the relationship between the practitioner and patient
   b. Focuses on the whole person
   c. Is informed by evidence
   d. Makes use of appropriate therapeutic approaches, health care professionals, and disciplines
9. muscle tension, gastrointestinal discomfort, pain or sleep disturbances.
10. Reduces generalized decreased cognitive, physiological, and/or behavioral arousal; decreased heart and respiratory rates, blood pressure, and oxygen consumption and increased alpha brain activity and peripheral skin temperature
11. Relaxation training helps to teach the individual how to effectively rest and reduce tension in the body.
12. The goal of passive relaxation is to still the mind and body intentionally without the need to tighten and relax any particular body part.
13. The outcome of relaxation therapy is lowered heart rate and blood pressure, decreased muscle tension, improved sense of well-being, and reduced symptoms of distress.
14. During the first few months when the person is learning to focus on body sensations and tensions, there is increased sensitivity in detecting muscle tension. Occasionally, intensification of symptoms or the development of new symptoms can occur.
15. Meditation is any activity that limits stimulus input by directing attention to a single unchanging or repetitive stimulus.
16. Meditation has been used to successfully reduce hypertensive risks; reduce relapses in alcohol treatment programs; reduce depression, anxiety, and distress

in cancer patients; and benefit people with posttraumatic stress disorders and chronic pain.
17. Meditation is contraindicated for people who have a strong fear of losing control or who are hypersensitive; medication use.
18. Imagery is a group of visualization techniques that uses the conscious mind to create mental images to stimulate physical changes in the body, improve perceived well-being, or enhance self-awareness.
19. Creative visualization is one form of self-directed imagery that is based on the principle of mind–body connectivity.
20. Imagery can be helpful in controlling or relieving pain, decreasing nightmares and improving sleep, and treating chronic diseases.
21. Biofeedback is a mind–body technique that uses instruments to teach self-regulation and voluntary self-control over specific physiological responses.
22. Biofeedback can be useful in treating headaches, smoking cessation, strokes, attention deficit hyperactivity, epilepsy, and a variety of gastrointestinal and urinary tract disorders.
23. Repressed emotions or feelings are sometimes uncovered during biofeedback, and the patient may have difficulty coping.
24. The most important concept is yin and yang, which represent opposing yet complementary phenomena that exist in a state of dynamic equilibrium.
25. a. Burning moxa, a cone or stick of dried herbs that have healing properties on or near the skin
   b. Placing a heated cup on the skin to create a slight suction
   c. Martial art—moving meditation
   d. Choreographed movements or gestures
26. Acupuncture, herbal therapies, tai chi
27. Limitations include: concern about the safety of Chinese herbal treatments, they are not FDA regulated, and interactions with traditional medications, such as Aspirin and Clopidogrel.
28. a. *Qi* is the vital energy of the body.
   b. Meridians are channels of energy that run in regular patterns through the body and over its surface.
   c. Acupoints are holes through which qi can be influenced by the insertion of needles.
29. a. Centering
   b. Assessment
   c. Unruffling
   d. Treatment
   e. Evaluation
30. Therapeutic touch is used in the treatment of pain in adults and children, dementia, trauma, and anxiety.
31. Therapeutic touch is contraindicated in persons who are sensitive to human interaction and touch.
32. When the spine is misaligned, energy flow is impeded, and the innate healing abilities of the body are impaired; improves acute pain and disability.
33. Acute myelopathy, fractures, dislocations, rheumatoid arthritis, and osteoporosis

34. menopausal depression, antiinflammatory effects, lowers blood sugar
35. Problems with herbal therapies include contamination with other chemicals or herbs, toxic agents, a variety of standards used from one company to another.
36. The integrative medicine approach is a multiple-practitioner treatment group; a pluralistic, complementary health care system; it is consistent with the holistic approach nurses learn to practice.
37. Ability to focus attention for an extended time. Stopping a focus on unnecessary goal-directed activity. Being able to tolerate experiences that are uncertain.
38. 2. The perception that the treatments offered by the medical profession do not provide relief for a variety of common illnesses
39. 3. They have not received approval for use as drugs and are not regulated by the FDA; therefore, they can be sold as food or food supplements only.
40. 2. It is important for the nurse to know the current research being done in this area to provide accurate information not only to patients but also to other health care professionals.

CHAPTER 33

1. Self-concept is an individual's view of him- or herself. It is a complex mixture of unconscious and conscious thoughts, attitudes, and perceptions.
2. a. Sense of competency
   b. Perceived reactions of others to one's body
   c. Ongoing perceptions and interpretations of the thoughts and feelings of others
   d. Personal and professional relationships
   e. Academic and employment-related identity
   f. Personality characteristics that affect self-expectations
   g. Perceptions of events that have an impact on life
   h. Mastery of prior and new experiences
   i. Cultural identity
3. d   5. b
4. a   6. c
7. A self-concept stressor is any real or perceived change that threatens identity, body image, or role performance.
8. g   12. h
9. d   13. b
10. f   14. e
11. c   15. a
16. a. Thoughts and feelings about lifestyle, health, and illness
   b. Awareness of how one's own nonverbal communication affects patients and families
   c. Personal values and expectations and how they affect patients
   d. Ability to accept differences in self-concept and self-esteem
   e. Ability to convey a nonjudgmental attitude toward patients
   f. Preconceived attitudes toward cultural differences

17. The focus is on identity, body image, and role performance; perceptions of these factors to reveal his or her level of self-esteem, and the number and intensity of stressors.
18. See Box 33-5.
19. a. Disturbed body image
   b. Disturbed personal identity
   c. Impaired role performance
   d. Situational low self-esteem
20. The patient will discuss a minimum of three areas of her life in which she is functioning well. The patient will be able to voice the recognition that losing her job is not reflective of her worth as a person. The patient will attend a support group for out-of-work professionals.
21. Healthy lifestyle measures include proper nutrition, regular exercise within the patient's capabilities, adequate sleep and rest, and stress-reducing practices.
22. Expected outcomes include nonverbal behaviors indicating positive self-concept, statements of self-acceptance, and acceptance of change in appearance or function.
23. Smoking, hazardous alcohol consumption, unprotected sexual activity
24. 3. Adolescence is a particularly critical time when many variables affect self-concept and self-esteem.
25. 4. Involves attitudes related to the body, including physical appearance, structure, or function, which is affected by cognitive and physical development as well as cultural and societal attitudes
26. 4. Certain behaviors become common depending on whether they are approved and reinforced.
27. 2. Attitudes toward body image can occur as a result of situational events such as the loss of or change in a body part.
28. a. Observe Mrs. Johnson's behaviors that suggest an alteration in self-concept. Assess Mrs. Johnson's cultural background. Assess Mrs. Johnson's coping skills and resources. Converse with Mrs. Johnson to determine her feelings, perceptions about changes in body image, self-esteem, or role. Assess the quality of Mrs. Johnson's relationships.
   b. Self-awareness is critical; nurses derive their self-concepts and professional identify from their public image, work environment, and education as well as their professional, social, and cultural values.
   c. Humanities, sciences, nursing research, and clinical practice; components of self-concept (identity, body image, self-esteem, role performance); self-concept stressors related to identity, body image, self-esteem, and role; therapeutic communication principles and nonverbal indicators of distress; cultural and societal issues that influence body image; pharmacologic effects of medicine (pain medication); Erikson's psychosocial theory of development
   d. Support Mrs. Johnson's autonomy to make choices and express values that support positive self-concept. Apply intellectual standards of relevance and plausibility for care to be acceptable to

337

Mrs. Johnson. Susan needs to safeguard Mrs. Johnson's right to privacy by judiciously protecting information of a confidential nature.

   e. Looking for the range of behaviors suggestive of an altered self-concept; cultural differences, role performance, perception of the stressors and of change; previous coping behaviors

29. The patient is demonstrating <u>body image</u>, <u>self-concept</u>, and <u>self-esteem</u> issues.

The patient has a healthy body weight yet believes that she is fat. This is a distortion of body image which can lead to eating disorders in young adults. Body image involves attitudes related to the body, including physical appearance, structure, or function. The self-harm behaviors that are observed and reported (cutting of skin) indicate issues with self-concept and self-esteem. Self-esteems is an individual's overall feeling of self-worth. To engage in behaviors of self-harm, there are underlying issues that require intervention specific to self-esteem. When self-esteem is low, a person is more likely to engage in risky behavior. Self-concept is how one feels about oneself. This patient feels they are fat and demonstrates behavior that lacks self-worth.

Role performance is the way in which individual's carry out their perceived roles such as parent or supervisor. This patient does not demonstrate an issue with role performance. Identity confusion exists when people do not maintain a clear, consistent, and continuous consciousness of personal identity. This patient does not demonstrate identity confusion. Role strain is a combination of role conflict and role ambiguity. It is generally associated as a feeling of frustration when a person feels inadequate or unsuited to a role such as providing care for a disabled child. This patient does not demonstrate role strain.

CHAPTER 34

1. f	7. j
2. h	8. k
3. g	9. l
4. i	10. b
5. e	11. c
6. d	12. a

13. a. Peer, family, and social support are often lacking.
   b. Barriers to health care that include fear of discrimination, insensitivity, and lack of knowledge about their specific health needs
   c. High risk for STIs, depression, and victimization
14. Desire, arousal, or orgasm
15. a. Diabetes, kidney disease, alcohol dependence, depression, neurological disorders, vascular insufficiency, and diseases of the prostate
   b. Statins, antihypertensives, antidepressants, antipsychotics, and benzodiazepines
16. a. Reduced sex drive
   b. Decreased sexual interest
   c. Mood changes
17. a. Impact of pregnancy and menstruation on sexuality
   b. Discussing sexual issues
   c. Decisional issues

18. a. Contraception
   b. Abortion
   c. STI prevention
19. a. Syphilis
   b. Gonorrhea
   c. Chlamydia
   d. Trichomoniasis
   e. HPV
   f. HSV type II
20. a. Infertility
   b. Sexual abuse
   c. Personal and emotional conflicts
   d. Sexual dysfunction
21. a. Physical
   b. Functional
   c. Relationship
   d. Lifestyle
   e. Developmental factors
   f. Self-esteem factors
22. Permission, limited information, specific suggestions, intensive therapy
23. a. Problematic sexual behavior
   b. Difficulty coping
   c. Lack of knowledge of contraception
   d. Impaired sexual functioning
   e. Risk for impaired reproductive function
24. a. Discuss stressors that contribute to sexual dysfunction with partner within 2 weeks
   b. Identify alternative, satisfying, and acceptable sexual practices for oneself and one's partner within 4 weeks
25. a. Contraception
   b. Safe-sex practices
   c. Prevention of STIs
   d. Women: Regular breast self-examinations, mammograms, Pap test
   e. Men: Testicular examinations
26. a. Avoid alcohol (in excess) and tobacco
   b. Eat well-balanced meals
   c. Plan sexual activity for times when the couple feels rested
   d. Take pain medication if needed before sexual intercourse
   e. Use pillows and alternate positioning to enhance comfort
   f. Encourage touch, kissing, hugging, and other tactile stimulation
   g. Communicate your concerns and fears to your partner and health care provider
27. Individuals experience major physical changes, the effects of drugs and treatments, emotional stress of a prognosis, concern about future functioning, and separation from others.
28. a. Ask patients questions about risk factors, sexual concerns, and their level of satisfaction
   b. Note behavioral cues
29. Tell me how you would describe your sexual health?
30. 4. The child identifies with the parent of the same sex and develops a complementary relationship with the parent of the opposite sex.

31. 4. Normal sexual changes occur as people age.
32. 1. Methods that are effective for contraception do not always reduce the risk of STIs.
33. a. Assess Mr. Clements' developmental stage in regard to sexuality. Consider self-concept as a factor that will influence sexual satisfaction and functioning. Provide physical assessment of urogenital area. Determine Mr. Clements' sexual concerns. Assess safe-sex practices and the use of contraception. Assess the medical conditions and medications that may be affecting his sexual functioning. Assess the impact of high-risk behaviors on sexual health.
     b. A basic understanding of sexual development, sexual orientation, sociocultural dimensions, the impact of self-concept, STIs, and safe-sex practices; ways to phrase questions regarding sexuality and functioning; disease conditions that affect sexual functioning; how interpersonal relationship factors may affect sexual functioning
     c. Explore discomfort by discussing topics related to sexuality and develop a plan for addressing these discomforts. Reflect on personal sexual experiences and how he has responded.
     d. Apply intellectual standards of relevance and plausibility for care to be acceptable to Mr. Clements. Safeguard Mr. Clements' right to privacy by judiciously protecting information of a confidential nature. Apply the principles of ethic of care.
     e. Display curiosity; consider why Mr. Clements might behave or respond in a particular manner. Display integrity; his beliefs and values may differ from Mr. Clements'. Admit to inconsistencies in his and Mr. Clements' values. Risk taking: be willing to explore both personal and Mr. Clements' sexual issues and concerns.
34.

Patient	Developmental Assessment Data
3-year-old natal male	Knows there are boys and girls
	Waits to see what peers do in a situation
	Identifies with his male caregiver
6-year-old natal female	Prefers to be in group with other females
	Seems anxious and worried if she fits in with others
	Asks her mom about how to make friends
12-year-old natal female	Reports anxiety and asks, "Do you think I am normal?"
	Identifies sexual intimacy as a basic need
	Reports breast development and body changes

Sexuality changes as a person grows and ages. Each stage of development brings changes in sexual functioning and the role of sexuality in relationships. In early childhood (3-years-old), the child becomes aware of the differences between sexes and they begin to interpret behaviors with the binary categories of male and female. A 3-year-old will also identify with a parent or caregiver of the same sex while developing a complimentary relationship with the parent or caregiver of the opposite sex. A 3-year-old is not yet interested in peers and peer behavior does not influence behavior. A school-age child (6-years-old) will prefer being with groups of the same sex. A 6-year-old will look to parents, educators, and peers for advice and direction on how to relate to others, such as asking a parent how to make friends. A 6-year-old is less likely to be anxious about fitting in as this occurs later in preadolescence. A 12-year-old is entering puberty and adolescence and is experiencing emotional and body changes. Anxiety and an intense desire to fit in and be "normal" is common. Breast development would be anticipated. However, sexual intimacy as a basic need occurs later in life during young adulthood.

CHAPTER 35

1. Spirituality is an awareness of one's inner self and a sense of connection to a higher being, nature, or to some purpose other than oneself.
2. e
3. f
4. d
5. b
6. g
7. c
8. h
9. a
10. i
11. a. The strength of a patient's spirituality influences how he or she copes with sudden illness and how quickly he or she moves to recovery.
    b. Dependence on others for routine self-care needs often creates feelings of powerlessness; this, along with the loss of a sense of purpose in life, impairs the ability to cope with alterations in functioning.
    c. Terminal illness creates an uncertainty about what death means and thus makes patients susceptible to spiritual distress.
    d. A near-death experience is a psychological phenomenon of people who either have been close to clinical death or have recovered after being declared dead.

339

12. Individuals have some source of authority (a supreme being; a code of conduct; a specific religious leader, family or friends, oneself, or a combination) and guidance in their lives that lead them to choose and act on their beliefs.

13. Individuals who accept change in life, make decisions about their lives, and are able to forgive others in times of difficulty have higher levels of spiritual well-being.

14. People who are connected to themselves, others, nature, and God or another supreme being cope with the stress brought on by crisis and chronic illness.

15. When people are satisfied with life, more energy is available to deal with new difficulties and to resolve problems.

16. Remaining connected with their cultural heritage often helps patients define their place in the world and to express their spirituality.

17. Fellowship is a type of relationship that an individual has with other persons.

18. Rituals include participation in worship, prayer, sacraments, fasting, singing, meditating, scripture reading, and making offerings or sacrifices.

19. Expression of spirituality is highly individual and includes showing an appreciation for life in the variety of things that people do, living in the moment and not worrying about tomorrow, appreciating nature, expressing love toward others, and being productive.

20. a. Impaired spiritual distress
    b. Decreased spiritual distress
    c. Hopelessness
    d. Powerlessness
    e. Spiritual distress

21. a. the patient expresses feelings of peacefulness
    b. the patient reports a feeling connected with family and others
    c. The patient initiates social interactions with family and friends.
    d. the patient participates in spiritual rites and practices

22. Giving attention, answering questions, listening, and having a positive and encouraging (but realistic) attitude, being with rather than doing for

23. a. Mobilizing hope for the nurse as well as the patient
    b. Finding an interpretation or understanding of the illness, pain, anxiety, or other stressful emotion that is acceptable to the patient
    c. Assisting the patient in using social, emotional, and spiritual resources

24. Support systems serve as a human link connecting the patient, the nurse, and the patient's lifestyle before an illness. The support system is a source of faith and hope and often is an important resource in conducting meaningful religious rituals.

25. Food and rituals are sometimes important to a person's spirituality.

26. Plan care to allow time for religious readings, spiritual visitations, or attendance at religious services

27. Prayer offers an opportunity to renew personal faith and belief in a higher being in a specific, focused way that is either highly ritualized and formal or spontaneous and informal.

28. Meditation creates a relaxation that reduces daily stress, lowers blood pressure, slows the aging process, reduces pain, and enhances the function of the immune system.

29. The nurse's ability to enter into a therapeutic and spiritual relationship with the patient will support a patient during times of grief.

30. Reveal the patient's developing an increased or restored sense of connectedness with family; maintaining, renewing, or reforming a sense of purpose in life and for some confidence and trust in a supreme being or power

31. Ask the patient if she would like to pray with the nurse; ask the patient if she would like pastoral care to visit; provide the patient privacy while she is praying the rosary

32. 3. Must be able to practice the five pillars of Islam; health and spirituality are connected

33. 2. Their belief is not to kill any living creature.

34. 3. Muslims wash the body of the dead family member and wrap it in white cloth with the head turned to the right shoulder.

35. 2. The defining characteristics reveal patterns that reflect a person's actual or potential dispiritedness.

36. 3. When patients use meditation in conjunction with their spiritual beliefs, they often report an increased spirituality that they commonly describe as experiencing the presence of power, force or energy, or what was perceived as God.

37. a. Constructs that define spirituality: Self-transcendence, connectedness, faith, and hope
    b. Using the nurse's past experience in selecting interventions that support the patient's well-being, the nurse will exhibit confidence in her skills and develop a trusting relationship with Lisa. Be open to any possible conflict between the patient's opinion and the nurse's; decide how to reach mutually beneficial outcomes.
    c. The concepts of faith, hope, spiritual well-being, and religion; caring practices in the individual approach to a patient; available services in the community (health care providers and agencies)
    d. Standards of autonomy and self-determination to support Lisa's decisions about the plan; ANA Code of Ethics; nurses who are comfortable with their own spirituality often are more likely to care for their patients' spiritual needs
    e. Lisa will express her will to live with family members; Lisa will describe a feeling of peacefulness to her family; Lisa will express a personal sense of spiritual well-being.

CHAPTER 36

1. l
2. n
3. m
4. o
5. f
6. k
7. b
8. j
9. i
10. d
11. h
12. c
13. g
14. e
15. a

16. a. Human development
    b. Personal relationships
    c. Nature of the loss
    d. Coping strategies
    e. Socioeconomic status
    f. Culture
    g. Spiritual and religious beliefs
    h. Hope

17. It is important to assess the patient's coping style, the nature of the family relationships, personal goals, cultural and spiritual beliefs, sources of hope, and availability of support systems.

18. Box 36.4

19. a. Impaired Family Coping
    b. Death Anxiety
    c. Pain (acute or chronic)
    d. Dysfunctional Grief
    e. Anticipatory Grief

20. a. patient expresses spiritual beliefs about death
    b. patient verbalizes acceptance of the loss
    c. patient participates in planning the funeral service

21. Palliative care is the prevention, relief, reduction, or soothing of symptoms of disease or disorders throughout the entire course of an illness, including care of a dying individual and bereavement follow-up for the family.

22. a. Provides relief from pain and other distressing symptoms
    b. Supports life and regards dying as a normal process
    c. Neither hastens nor postpones health
    d. Integrates psychological and spiritual aspects of patient care
    e. Offers support system to help patients actively live
    f. Offers a support system to help family cope
    g. Enhances the quality of life and positively influences the course of the illness
    h. Uses a team approach to address the needs
    i. Is applicable early in the course of illness, in conjunction with other therapies

23. a. Patient and family are the unit.
    b. Coordinated home care with access to inpatient and nursing home beds when needed
    c. Symptom management
    d. Physician-directed services
    e. Provision of an interdisciplinary care team
    f. Medical and nursing services available at all times
    g. Bereavement follow-up

    h. Trained volunteers for visitation and respite support

24. a. Use therapeutic communication
    b. Provide psychosocial care
    c. Manage symptoms
    d. Promote dignity and self-esteem
    e. Maintain a comfortable and peaceful environment
    f. Promote spiritual comfort and hope
    g. Protect against abandonment and isolation
    h. Support the grieving family
    i. Assist with end-of-life decision making

25. a. Help the survivor accept that the loss is real
    b. Support efforts to adjust to the loss using a problem-solving approach
    c. Encourage establishment of new relationships
    d. Allow time to grieve
    e. Describe behaviors and feelings that survivors frequently experience
    f. Provide continuing support
    g. Be alert for signs of ineffective, harmful coping mechanisms

26. Organ and tissue donation provides information about who can legally give consent, which organs or tissues can be donated, associated costs, and how donation will affect burial or cremation.

27. Autopsy is the surgical dissection of a body after death to determine the cause and circumstances of death or discover the pathway of a disease.

28. Postmortem care is the care of the body after death, maintaining the integrity of rituals and mourning practices.

29. Short-term goals include talking about the loss without feeling overwhelmed, improved energy level, normalized sleep and dietary patterns, reorganization of life patterns, improved ability to make decisions, and finding it easier to be around people.

30. Long-term goals include the return of a sense of humor and normal life patterns, renewed or new personal relationships, and decrease of inner pain.

31. Complicated grief occurs when a person has difficulty progressing through the loss experience; grief is the emotional response to loss; people grieve based on their experiences, cultural expectations, and spiritual values.

32. 1. Life changes are natural and often positive, which are learned as change always involves necessary losses.

33. 3. Care of the terminally ill patient and his or her family

34. 2. Cushions and postpones awareness of the loss by trying to prevent it from happening

35. 3. To help patients and families achieve the best possible quality of life, determine the goals of care, and select the appropriate interventions

36. 2,3,5

37. a. Knowledge related to the characteristics of grief resolution; the clinical symptoms of an improved level of comfort
    b. Previous patient responses to planned nursing interventions for symptom management or loss of a significant other

c. Used established expected outcomes to evaluate the patient response to care; evaluated the patient's role in the grieving process

d. Persevere in seeking successful comfort measures for the grieving patient

e. Evaluate signs and symptoms of Mrs. Allison's grief; evaluate family members' ability to provide supportive care; evaluate the patient's level of comfort; ask if the patient's/family's expectations are being met

38.

Assessment Finding	Stages of Dying	Attachment Theory	Both Grief Theories
States, "I don't believe he is gone."	X		
States, "I just don't want to talk about the loss right now. We don't have to think about it all the time."			X
States, "I don't want to eat or drink, I have pain in my chest, and I feel sick at my stomach."		X	
States, "If God would just take me instead of my husband, it would be better."	X		
The patient is openly sobbing at times and demonstrates acute physical distress.		X	

Knowledge of grief theories and normal responses to loss and bereavement helps you to better understand these complex experiences and how to help a grieving person. When the patient states, "I don't believe he is gone" this is a form of denial which is the first stage in the Stages of Dying. When the patient states, "I just don't want to talk about the loss right now, We don't have to think about it all the time" that could be denial associated with the stages of dying or a form of numbing which is associated with the attachment theory. Numbing protects the person from the full impact of the loss. When the patient states, "I don't want to eat or drink, I have pain in my chest, and I feel sick at my stomach" the patient is demonstrating yearning and searching associated with the attachment theory where physical reports often accompany the intensity of grief. When the patient states, "If God would just take me instead of my husband, it would be better" this reflects the process of bargaining which is identified as one of the stages of dying. Openly sobbing with acute physical distress reflects yearning and searching within the attachment theory.

CHAPTER 37

1. j
2. c
3. k
4. m
5. g
6. f
7. n
8. o
9. r
10. p
11. d
12. q
13. s
14. i
15. a
16. e
17. h
18. b
19. l
20. t

21. a. Uses a systems approach and helps you understand your patients' individual responses to stressors as well as families' and communities' responses; views a patient, family, or community as constantly changing in response to the environment and stressors

b. Focuses on promoting health and managing stress. People want to live in ways that enable them to be as healthy as possible and capable of assessing their own abilities and assets.

22. Adjusting to chronic illness. The physical limitations posed by a disease state and the uncertainty associated with treatment and illness.

23. Maturational factors vary with life stage: Children (relate to physical appearance), preadolescent (self-esteem issues), adolescent (identity), adults (major changes in life circumstances), and older-adults (loss of autonomy)

24. Sociocultural factors include poverty and physical disabilities, loss of parents and caregivers (children), violence, and homelessness.

25. Is a condition that can overwhelm health care providers and cause physical, mental, and emotional health issues. It is a state of burnout and secondary traumatic stress.

26. Occurs when a medical error occurs that inflicts significant harm on a patient and their families

27. (Box 37.4)
a. Patient safety
b. Perception of the stressor
c. Available coping resources
d. Maladaptive coping used
e. Adherence to healthy practices

28. a. Grooming and hygiene
b. Gait
c. Characteristics of the handshake
d. Actions while sitting
e. Quality of speech
f. Eye contact
g. The attitude of the patient

29.
  a. Anxiety
  b. Despair
  c. Difficulty Coping
  d. Risk for Posttrauma Response
  e. Stress Overload

30.
  a. You direct nursing activities to identify individuals and populations who are possibly at risk for stress
  b. Include actions directed at symptoms such as protecting the patient from self-harm
  c. Assist the patient in readapting and can include relaxation training and time management

31.
  a. You direct nursing activities to identify individuals and populations who may be at risk for stress
  b. Increase resistance to stress
  c. Learn skills that reduce physiological response to stress

32.
  a. Improves muscle tone and posture, controls weight, reduces tension, and promotes relaxation
  b. Family, friends, and colleagues listen, offer advise, and provide emotional support that benefits a patient experiencing stress
  c. Developing lists of prioritized tasks – tasks that require immediate attention, those that are important and those that can be delayed
  d. In a relaxed state, a person uses imagination in a way that allows visualization of a soothing, peaceful setting.
  e. Diminishes physiological tension through a systematic approach to releasing tension in major muscle groups
  f. Helps individuals communicate effectively regarding their needs and desires, which is important for reducing stress
  g. Provides a therapeutic outlet for stress. Patients can express a full range of emotion and vent their feelings without hurting anyone else's feelings.
  h. Moment-to-moment present awareness with an attitude on nonjudgment, acceptance, and openness

33. Crisis intervention is a specific type of brief psychotherapy with prescribed steps. First is patient safety an the second is anxiety using techniques.

34. Reports of feeling better when the stressor is gone; improved sleep patterns and appetite; improved ability to concentrate

35. Who can you talk to on a routine basis? What do you do when you feel lonely? Tell me about any changes you have experienced in lifestyle habits, such as sleeping, eating, smoking, and drinking.

36. 1. Stress is an experience a person is exposed to through a stimulus or stressor.

37. 1. Alarm reaction, resistance stage, and the exhaustion stage

38. 3. The nurse helps the patient make the mental connection between the stressful event and the patient's reaction to it.

39. 1,3,4,5

40.
  a. General adaptation syndrome (GAS), communication principles that contribute to assessing a patient's behaviors, factors influencing stress, and coping and sociocultural factors
  b. Experience with previous patients; personal experiences with stress and coping increase your ability to empathize
  c. Practice standards for psychiatric mental health nursing, nursing theories, interprofessional approaches
  d. Maintain ongoing communication with Sandra and John because coping with stress takes time; need to actively involve the patient and his wife in the process of problem identification, prioritizing, and goal setting
  e. Ask Sandra if her fatigue and stress levels have decreased; ask Sandra and John to describe modifications they have made in their daily routine; any revision in the plan of care includes steps to address patient expectations.

41. The employee health nurse determines that the nurse working in the COVID unit is most likely experiencing <u>compassion fatigue.</u> The employee health nurse suggests the most important thing is to <u>recognize the concern.</u> The employee health nurse presents several strategies to help the nurse including <u>practicing self-care.</u>

The nurse working in the COVID unit is exhibiting clear signs of compassion fatigue. This term is used to describe a state of burnout and secondary traumatic stress. Over time, giving of oneself in often intense caring environments can result in emotional exhaustion, leaving a nurse feeling irritable, restless, and unable to focus and engage with patients. The nurse is not exhibiting signs of anxiety, PTSD, second-victim syndrome, or dissociation.

Early recognition of compassion fatigue is the priority nursing action. Recognizing that this is temporary and will get better is not accurate as caring for COVID patients is continuing and this does not address the immediate concern of compassion fatigue that the nurse is experiencing now. It is not realistic to take time off of work and while seeing a mental health provider or attending a support group may be an option, the priority is to recognize the concern of compassion fatigue. If this goes unrecognized, it can progress to the use of negative coping mechanisms.

After recognizing the compassion fatigue the employee health nurse will equip the patient (in this case the health care provider) with resources and tools to address the compassion fatigue. This includes making self-care a priority, talking with those who can relate about the stress, as well as using multiple relaxation strategies such as deep breathing and relaxation exercises. Taking PRN benzodiazepines is not recommended and can progress to a negative coping strategy. Moving to a different unit is likely not an option nor is taking medical leave. Becoming more informed about COVID cases could actually be harmful as information overload can lead to additional worry. Limiting access to legitimate information as the pandemic evolves is advised.

CHAPTER 38

1. k
2. d
3. p
4. n
5. l
6. m
7. e
8. q
9. o
10. s
11. t
12. f
13. g
14. r
15. b
16. h
17. i
18. j
19. c
20. a

21. a. Widen your base of support by separating the feet to a comfortable distance
    b. The center of gravity closer to your base of support to increase balance
    c. Bend your knees and flex the hips until squatting, and maintain proper back alignment to keep the trunk erect

22. a. Congenital defects
    b. Disorders of bones, joints, and muscles
    c. Central nervous system damage
    d. Musculoskeletal trauma

23. a. Poor dietary habits
    b. Playing video games with excess screen time
    c. Lack of exercise

24. a. developmental changes
    b. behavioral aspects
    c. environmental issues
    d. lifestyle
    e. cultural and ethnic origin
    f. family and social support

25. The infant's spine is flexed and lacks the antero-posterior curves; as growth and stability increase, the thoracic spine straightens, and the lumbar spinal curve appears, allowing for sitting and standing.

26. Posture is awkward because of slight swayback and protruding abdomen; toward the end of toddlerhood, posture appears less awkward, curves in the cervical and lumbar vertebrae are accentuated, and foot eversion disappears.

27. Adolescents experience a tremendous growth spurt. In girls, the hips widen, and fat is deposited in upper arms, thighs, and buttocks. In boys, long bone growth and muscle mass are increased.

28. Healthy adults also have the necessary musculoskeletal development and coordination to carry out ADLs.

29. Older-adults experience a progressive loss of total bone mass because of physical inactivity, hormonal changes, and increased osteoclastic activity.

30. a. Precontemplation
    b. Contemplation
    c. Preparation
    d. Action
    e. Maintenance

31. a. Determine normal physiological changes in body alignment resulting from growth and development for each patient
    b. Identify deviations in body alignment caused by incorrect posture
    c. Provide opportunities for patients to observe their posture
    d. Identify learning needs of patients for maintaining correct body alignment
    e. Identify trauma, muscle damage or nerve dysfunction
    f. Obtain information concerning other factors that contribute

32. a. Sitting
    b. Standing
    c. Range of motion
    d. Gait
    e. Exercise

33. a. Observe the patient entering the room, and note speed, stride, and balance
    b. Ask the patient to walk across the room, turn, and come back
    c. Ask the patient to walk heel-to-toe in a straight line

34. See Box 38.5.

35. a. Activity Intolerance
    b. Risk for fall related to Injury
    c. Impaired Mobility
    d. Impaired Physical Mobility
    e. Acute or Chronic Pain

36. a. Participates in prescribed physical activity while maintaining appropriate heart rate, blood pressure, and breathing rate
    b. Verbalizes an understanding of the need to gradually increase activity based on tolerance and symptoms
    c. Expresses understanding of balancing rest and activity

37. Subtract the patient's current age from 220 and obtain the target heart rate by taking 60% to 90% of the maximum

38. a. Walking, running, bicycling, aerobic dance, jumping rope, and cross-country skiing
    b. Active ROM and stretching all muscle groups and joints
    c. Weight training, raking leaves, shoveling snow, and kneading bread

39. Active: The patient is able to move his or her joints independently. Passive: The nurse moves each joint.

40. Walking helps to prevent contractures by increasing joint mobility.

41. a. A single straight-legged cane is used to support and balance a patient with decreased leg strength.
    b. A quad cane provides more support and is used for partial or complete leg paralysis or some hemiplegia.

42. a. Four-point gait: Each leg is moved alternately with each opposing crutch so three points are on the floor at all times.
    b. Three-point gait: Bears weight on both crutches and then on the uninvolved leg, repeating the sequence.
    c. Two-point gait: There is at least partial weight bearing on each foot.
    d. Swing-through gait: Weight is placed on supportive legs; crutches are one stride in front and then swings through with the crutches, supporting the patient's weight.

43. a. Pulse
    b. Blood pressure
    c. Oxygen saturation
    d. Strength
    e. Fatigue
    f. Psychological well-being
44. 1. Identify the patient using at least two identifiers
    2. Perform hand hygiene
    3. Directly assess physical capacity of a patient to transfer
    4. Assess for weakness, dizziness, or risk for orthostatic (postural) hypotension
    5. Refer to medical record for most recent recorded weight and height for the patient
45. 4. Ligaments are white, shiny, flexible bands of fibrous tissue that bind joints and connect bones and cartilage.
46. 2. Exercise increases cardiac output.
47. 1,4,5,6. These all influence activity tolerance.
48. a. Consult and collaborate with members of the health team to increase Mrs. Smith's activity. Involve Mrs. Smith and her family in designing her activity and exercise plan. Consider Mrs. Smith's ability to increase her activity level and follow an exercise program.
    b. The role of physical therapist and exercise trainers in improving Mrs. Smith's activity and exercise program; determine Mrs. Smith's ability to increase her level of activity; impact of medication on Mrs. Smith's activity tolerance
    c. Consider previous patient and personal experiences to therapies designed to improve exercise and activity tolerance. Consider personal experience with exercise regimens.
    d. Therapies need to be individualized to Mrs. Smith's activity tolerance. Apply the goals of the American College of Sports Medicine in the application.
    e. Be responsible and creative in designing interventions to improve Mrs. Smith's activity tolerance
49. 1. To find the target heart rate, multiply your current age by 60%.
    2. Encourage regular stretching and limit periods of long sitting.
    3. It is expected to have some mild dizziness when walking briskly for endurance.
    4. Weight-bearing exercises, like hiking or climbing stairs are encouraged.
    5. High impact aerobics can help develop balance and muscle strength.
    6. Even exaggerating normal movements can help to build strength.
    7. Once muscle is lost, it is too late to build strength again.
    8. Remember to limit fluids to avoid potential fluid overload.
    Exercise to maintain mobility is very important for older-adults. After ensuring that each participant is cleared for regular exercise, the nurse will teach the following:

1. To find the target heart rate, the nurse will first teach the patient to subtract their current age in years from 220. This calculates maximum heart rate. Then the nurse will have the patient calculate his or her target heart rate by taking 60% to 90% of the maximum. The nurse will not teach the patient to multiply your current age by 60% as this is incorrect.
2. The nurse will encourage older-adult patients to stretch regularly and limit periods of sitting. This reduces the risk of joint contractures.
3. It is important to teach the patient to listen to their own body when exercising. The nurse will not teach that it is expected to have dizziness as it is not expected to have dizziness when walking briskly. Endurance activities should not cause dizziness, chest pain or pressure, or a feeling like heartburn.
4. Weight-bearing exercises, like hiking or climbing stairs are encouraged as this can help to strengthen bones.
5. High-impact exercises are avoided for older-adults as this can lead to bone fracture.
6. Even exaggerated normal movements can be helpful for the older-adult to increase circulation and improve joint mobility.
7. The nurse will teach that it is never too late to start an exercise program. Muscle strength can be regained.
8. It is important for the older-adult to drink fluids during any activity that makes them sweat. Avoiding fluids during exercise could lead to dehydration.

CHAPTER 39

1. d
2. c
3. a
4. b
5. Region where two or more bones are attached
6. Bands of fibrous tissue that bind joints together, connect bones and cartilages, and aid joint flexibility and support
7. Fibrous bands of tissue that connect muscle to bone
8. Nonvascular and support connective tissue
9. Contract and relax are the working elements of movement.
10. Regulates movement and posture
11. a. Can cause pain, impair alignment and mobility
    b. Weakness and wasting of muscles, which increase disability and deformity
    c. Impaired body alignment, balance, and mobility
    d. Results in bruises, contusions, tears, sprains, and fractures
12. A person's ability to move about freely
13. The inability to move freely
14. Cells and the tissue reduce in size and function in response to prolonged inactivity resulting from bed rest, trauma, casting, or local nerve damage.
15. Decreases the metabolic rate; alters the metabolism of CHO, fats, and proteins; causes fluid and electrolyte and calcium imbalances; and causes GI disturbances
16. a. Collapse of alveoli
    b. Inflammation of the lung from stasis or pooling of secretions

17. a. A drop in blood pressure greater than 20 mm Hg in systolic pressure or 10 mm Hg in diastolic pressure within 3 minutes of rising in an upright position
    b. Accumulation of platelets, fibrin, clotting factors, and cellular elements of the blood attached to the interior wall of a vein or artery that occludes the lumen of the vessel
18. a. Loss of endurance, decreased muscle mass and strength, and joint instability
    b. Impaired calcium metabolism and impaired joint mobility (bone tissue is less dense or atrophied)
    c. Osteoporosis
    d. Joint contractures (fixation of a joint)
    e. Footdrop (permanent plantar flexion)
19. a. Urinary stasis (renal pelvis fills before urine enters the ureters), which increases the risk of UTI
    b. Renal calculi (calcium stones that lodge in the renal pelvis), usually due to hypercalcemia
20. Pressure injury (impairment of the skin as a result of prolonged ischemia in tissues) characterized by inflammation and usually forms over a bony prominence
21. a. Emotional and behavioral responses
    b. Sensory alterations
    c. Changes in coping
22. Delays the child's gross motor skills, intellectual development, or musculoskeletal development
23. Social isolation
24. Physiological systems are at risk, loss of job
25. Weaker bones, increased risk of falls, increased physical dependence on others
26. a. The maximum amount of movement available at a joint in one of the three planes of the body: sagittal, frontal, or transverse; exercises are active, active assisted, and passive
    b. Manner or style of walking, including rhythm, cadence, length of stride, and speed
    c. Physical activity for conditioning the body, improving health, and maintaining fitness
    d. Includes assessing the patient standing, sitting, and lying
27. Height and weight, turgor of the skin (dehydration ad edema), review intake and output (fluid balance) and lab data (abnormalities), dietary and food pattern
28. Inspect chest wall movements (asymmetrical chest wall movement), auscultation (diminished breath sounds, crackles, or wheezes)
29. Monitor blood pressure (orthostatic hypotension) and heart rate (increased cardiac workload) and assess the arteriovenous system (capillary refill for tissue perfusion)
30. Assess for decreased muscle tone and strength, loss of muscle mass, reduced ROM and contractures
31. Inspection (break in skin integrity and color changes)
32. Patient's intake and output, adequacy of patient's dietary choices, bowel sounds, passing flatus, and frequency and consistency of bowel movements

33. Observe the patient's behavior (confusion or delirium; boredom, anxiety, and feelings of isolation, depression, and anger)
34. a. Hypercoagulability (clotting disorders, fever, dehydration)
    b. Venous wall abnormalities (orthopedic surgery, varicose veins)
    c. Blood flow stasis (immobility, obesity, and pregnancy)
35. a. Ineffective Airway Clearance
    b. Risk for Impaired Skin Integrity
    d. Risk for Constipation
    e. Social Isolation
36. a. Skin color and temperature return to normal baseline within 20 minutes of position change.
    b. Changes position at least every 2 hours
37. a. Prevention of work-related injury
    b. Exercise
    c. Bone health in patients with osteoporosis
38. a. A high-protein, high-caloric diet
    b. Vitamin B and C supplements
39. a. Deep breathe and cough every 1 or 2 hours
    b. Chest physiotherapy (CPT)
    c. Ensure intake of 1100–1400 mL/day of fluid
40. a. Reduce orthostatic hypotension; early mobilization
    b. Reduce cardiac workload; avoid Valsalva movements
    c. Prevent thrombus formation; prophylaxis (anticoagulant, mechanical prevention with graduated compression stockings, intermittent pneumatic compression devices and foot pumps)
41. a. Perform active, active assisted and passive ROM exercises
    b. Positioning techniques – use of trochanter roll (prevents external rotation of hips), hand rolls (thumb in slight adduction and in opposition to fingers), trapeze bar
42. a. Turning and positioning and skin care
    b. Use of therapeutic devices to relieve pressure (air loss mattresses, heel boots)
43. a. Well hydrated
    b. Prevent urinary stasis and calculi and infections
44. a. Anticipate change in the patient's status and provide routine and informal socialization
    b. Stimuli to maintain patient's orientation
45. a. Head of bed (HOB) elevated 45 to 60 degrees and the knees are slightly elevated [increased cervical flexion, sliding to the foot of the bed, deceased circulation to the feet, external rotation of the hips, unsupported feet and pressure on heels and sacrum and increased shearing]
    b. Rest on their backs; all body parts are in relation to each other [increased cervical flexion, shoulders internally rotated, thumb not in opposition to fingers, hips externally rotated, pressure points to occipital region of head, coccyx elbows and heels]
    c. Lies face or chest down [neck and lumbar spine hyperextension, plantar flexion of ankles, pressure points to chin, elbows, breasts, hips, knees, and toes]

d. The patient rests on the side with body weight on the dependent hip and shoulder [lateral flexion of neck, spinal curves out of alignment, shoulder and hip joints internally rotated, adducted, lack of foot support, pressure points on ear, shoulder, anterior iliac spine, trochanter, and ankles]

e. Weight is on anterior ileus, humerus, and clavicle [lateral flexion of the neck, internal rotation, adduction to shoulders and hips, lack of foot support, pressure points to ileum, shoulder, knees, and ankles]

46. Activities beyond ADLs that are necessary to be independent in society

47. Always stand on the patient's affected side and support the patient by using a gait belt

48. Increase in bruising, bleeding gums, guaiac-positive stools

49. 1. Footdrop. Allowing the foot to be dorsiflexed at the ankles prevents this.

50. 3. Immobility causing decreased lung elastic recoiling and secretions accumulating in portions of the lungs

51. 2,3,4. Homan's sign is no longer a reliable indicator in assessing for DVT.

52. 4. This technique produces a forceful, productive cough without excessive fatigue.

53. 1,3,4,5. Impaired mobility affects multiple body systems.

54. The nurse has begun assessment of an 81-year-old patient admitted to a medical-surgical floor with generalized weakness. During the assessment, the patient states, "I've been in bed for what seems like forever. I'm just too tired to get up and do anything at all." The nurse notes a reddish area at the base of the spine measuring 2 inches by 2 inches (5.08 cm x 5.08 cm). Crepitus, slight resistance, and hypotonia are noted when passive range of motion is performed on the lower extremities. Joint swelling in the fingers and wrists is observed. Vital signs include blood pressure of 100/70 mm Hg, temperature 97.8°F (36.6°C), respirations 12 per minute, and pulse 64 beats per minute.

Generalized weakness can be indicative of numerous health disorders. It is important for the nurse to recognize cues that may contribute to or be the cause of weakness. The patient's perception of "being in bed forever" warrants further assessment and reporting, as does the patient's statements of being "too tired to get up and do anything at all". These pieces of information illustrate that this is not a new condition, which can be important when determining next steps for care. The reddish area at the base of the spine could indicate the presence of a pressure injury; this must be well-documented and reported to the provider so that immediate interventions can be put in place to further prevent damage to tissue integrity. Hypotonia is a type of muscle tone abnormality; this condition can contribute to weakness as decreased muscle tone can culminate in diminished energy and difficulty ambulating. Joint swelling in the fingers and wrists should be reported, as these may be signs of osteoporosis which can also contribute to weakness if the patient avoids movement due to pain.

Crepitus and slight resistance are normal findings associated with immobility; these do not need to be reported to the health care provider. All vital signs are within expected parameters, and the urinalysis results are normal.

CHAPTER 40

1. a. The epidermis is the outer layer of the skin.
   b. The dermis is the thicker layer containing bundles of collagen and elastic fibers.
   c. The subcutaneous layer contains blood vessels, nerves, lymph, and loose connective tissue with fat cells.

2. a. Protection
   b. Sensation
   c. Temperature regulation
   d. Excretion and secretion

3. Dry mouth

4. Inflammation of the gums

5. Tooth decay produced by interaction of food and bacteria

6. a. Social practices
   b. Personal preferences
   c. Body image
   d. Socioeconomic status
   e. Health beliefs and motivation
   f. Cultural variables
   g. Developmental stage
   h. Physical condition

7. Assessment of the skin includes the color, texture, thickness, turgor, temperature, and hydration.

8. a. Dry skin: Bathe less frequently and rinse the body of all soap, because residue left on the skin can cause irritation and breakdown. Add moisture to the air through the use of a humidifier. Increase fluid intake when the skin is dry. Use moisturizing cream to aid healing. (Cream forms a protective barrier and helps maintain fluid within skin.) Use cream such as Eucerin. Use creams to clean skin that is dry or allergic to soaps and detergents.
   b. Acne: Wash hair and skin thoroughly each day with warm water and soap to remove oil. Use cosmetics sparingly because oily cosmetics or creams accumulate in pores and tend to make condition worse. Implement dietary restrictions if necessary. (Eliminate from the diet all foods that aggravate the condition.) Use prescribed topical antibiotics for severe forms of acne.
   c. Skin rashes: Wash the area thoroughly and apply antiseptic spray or lotion to prevent further itching and aid in the healing process. Apply warm or cold soaks to relieve inflammation if indicated.
   d. Contact dermatitis: Avoid causative agents (e.g., cleansers and soaps)
   e. Abrasion: Be careful not to scratch the patient with jewelry or fingernails. Wash abrasions with mild soap and water; dry thoroughly and gently. Observe dressings or bandages for retained moisture because it increases risk of infection.

347

9. a. Calluses: Thickened portion of epidermis consists of mass of horny, keratotic cells. Calluses are usually flat and painless and are found on undersurface of foot or on palm of hand.
   b. Corns: Friction and pressure from ill-fitting or loose shoes cause keratosis. Corns are seen mainly on or between toes over bony prominences. Corns are usually cone shaped, round, and raised. Soft corns are macerated.
   c. Plantar warts: Fungating lesion appears on sole of foot and is caused by the papilloma virus.
   d. Tinea pedis: Athlete's foot is a fungal infection of the foot; scaliness and cracking of skin occur between the toes and on the soles of the feet. Small blisters containing fluid appear.
   e. Ingrown nails: The toenail or fingernail grows inward into soft tissue around the nail. Ingrown nails often result from improper nail trimming.
   f. Paronychia: inflammation of tissue surrounding nail after hangnail or other injury.
   g. Foot odors: Foot odors are the result of excess perspiration that promotes microorganism growth.
10. Halitosis is bad breath.
11. Cracked lips
12. Inflamed tongue
13. Dandruff: Scaling of scalp is accompanied by itching. In severe cases, dandruff is on the eyebrows.
14. Ticks: Small, gray-brown parasites burrow into the skin and suck blood.
15. Pediculosis: Lice; tiny, grayish-white parasitic insects that infest mammals
16. Pediculosis capitis: Parasite is on scalp attached to hair strands. Eggs look like oval particles similar to dandruff. Bites or pustules may be observed behind the ears and at the hairline.
17. Pediculosis corporis: Parasites tend to cling to clothing, so they are not always easy to see. Body lice suck blood and lay eggs on clothing and furniture.
18. Pediculosis pubis: Parasites are in pubic hair. Crab lice are grayish white with red legs.
19. Alopecia: Alopecia occurs in all races. Balding patches are in the periphery of the hair line. Hair becomes brittle and broken.
20. a. Oral problems: Patients who are unable to use their upper extremities because of paralysis, weakness, or restriction (e.g., cast or dressing); dehydration; inability to take fluids or food by mouth (NPO); presence of nasogastric or oxygen tubes; mouth breathers; chemotherapeutic drugs; over-the-counter lozenges, cough drops, antacids, and chewable vitamins; radiation therapy to the head and neck; oral surgery, trauma to the mouth, or placement of oral airway; immunosuppression; altered blood clotting; diabetes mellitus
    b. Skin problems: Immobilization; reduced sensation because of stroke, spinal cord injury, diabetes, or local nerve damage; limited protein or caloric intake and reduced hydration (e.g., fever, burns, gastrointestinal alterations, poorly fitting

dentures); excessive secretions or excretions on the skin from perspiration, urine, watery fecal material, and wound drainage; presence of external devices (e.g., casts, restraints, bandage, dressing); vascular insufficiency
    c. Foot problems: Patients who are unable to bend over or have reduced visual acuity
    d. Eye care problems: Reduced dexterity and hand coordination
21. a. Activity Intolerance
    b. Impaired mobility
    c. Impaired Health Maintenance
    d. Impaired Skin Integrity
    e. low self-esteem
22. a. Will be able to bathe independently in front of sink
    b. Will use assist devices for bathing
    c. Will dress self, using dressing stick and sock aid
23. a. Make all instructions relevant after assessing knowledge, motivations, and health beliefs
    b. Adapt instruction to a patient's personal bathing facilities
    c. Teach the patient ways to avoid injury
    d. Reinforce infection-control practices
24. a. Complete bed bath (Skill 40.1): Bath administered to totally dependent patient in bed
    b. Partial bed bath (Skill 40.1): Bed bath that consists of bathing only body parts that would cause discomfort if left unbathed, such as the hands, face, axillae, and perineal area. Partial bath also includes washing back and providing a back rub. Dependent patients in need of partial hygiene or self-sufficient bedridden patients who are unable to reach all body parts receive a partial bath.
25. a. Provide privacy
    b. Maintain safety
    c. Maintain warmth
    d. Promote independence
    e. Anticipate needs
26. Urinary or fecal incontinence, rectal and perineal dressings, indwelling catheters, and morbid obesity
27. A back rub promotes relaxation, relieves muscular tension, and decreases perception of pain.
28. a. Inspect feet daily
    b. Wash feet daily in lukewarm water
    c. Wear well-fitting shoes and clean dry socks, never go barefoot
    d. Keep skin soft and smooth with emollient lotion
    e. Trim toenails straight across and square-file edges smooth
    f. Elevate feet and wiggle toes
    g. Protect feet from hot and cold
29. Brushing: cleans the teeth of food particles, plaque, and bacteria. Massages the gums and relieves discomforts.
30. Flossing removes plaque and tartar between the teeth.
31. Dentures need to be cleaned on a regular basis to avoid gingival infection and irritation.

32. Brushing and combing help keep the hair clean and distribute oil evenly along hair shafts; they also prevent hair from tangling.

33. Shampooing frequency depends on a person's daily routines and the condition of the hair.

34. Mustache and beard require daily grooming because of food particles and mucus that collect on the hair.

35. Shave facial hair after the bath or shampoo; to avoid causing discomfort, gently pull the skin taut and use short, firm razor strokes in the direction the hair grows.

36. Cleansing the eyes involves simply washing with a clean washcloth moistened in water (see Skill 40-1). Never apply direct pressure over the eyeball because it causes serious injury. When cleansing the patient's eyes, obtain a clean washcloth and cleanse from the inner canthus to the outer canthus. Use a different section of the washcloth for each eye.

37. Using a bulb irrigating syringe, gently wash the ear canal with warm solution (37°C or 98.6°F), being careful not to occlude the canal, which results in pressure on the tympanic membrane. Direct the fluid slowly and gently toward the superior aspect of the ear canal, maintaining the flow in a steady stream.

38. a. A CIC hearing aid is the newest, smallest, and least visible; it fits entirely in the ear canal.
    b. An ITE hearing aid fits into the external ear and allows for more fine tuning; it is powerful and easy to adjust.
    c. A BTE hearing aid hooks around and behind the ear and is connected to an ear mold; it allows for fine tuning and is useful for patients with progressive hearing loss.
    d. A digital hearing aid analyzes sounds to remove background noise; it is beneficial for those with mild to severe hearing loss.

39. a. Fowler's: Head of bed raised to angle of 45 degrees or more; semisitting position; the foot of the bed may also be raised at the knees
    b. Semi-Fowler's: Head of bed raised approximately 30 degrees; inclination less than Fowler position; the foot of the bed may also be raised at the knees
    c. Trendelenburg: Entire bedframe tilted with the head of the bed down
    d. Reverse Trendelenburg: Entire bedframe tilted with the foot of the bed down
    e. Flat: Entire bedframe horizontally parallel with the floor

40. Wash feet daily in warm water and then pat dry. Apply moisturizing lotion to the feet. File the nails straight across.

41. 2. A bath that is administered to a totally dependent patient in bed

42. 1. The condition of the skin depends on the exposure to environmental irritants; with frequent bathing or exposure to low humidity, the skin becomes very dry and flaky.

43. 3. Each patient has individual desires and preferences about when to bathe, shave, and perform hair care.

44. 3. Use a medicated shampoo for eliminating lice, which are easily able to spread to furniture and other people if not treated.

45. 1,2. CHG should not be used on the face only clear water and mild soap. The sticky feeling is the CHG protecting against infection.

46. 1,2,4. The focus on high risk for impaired skin integrity is prevention. The patient with an actual lesion will require wound care.

47. a. Understanding of anatomy and physiology of the skin, pathophysiology of disease states (diabetic, hypertension, body mass index [BMI] of 40), developmental stage
    b. Reflection on early clinical experiences
    c. Therapeutic communication skills; professional guidelines American Diabetic Association (ADA)
    d. Social practices, personal preferences, body image, socioeconomic status for modifications needed at home
    e. Current physical conditions, chronic illnesses, limited mobility

48. Offers to clip the patient's toenails that are long
    Places dentures on a napkin by the sink
    Encourages the patient to wash their face and perineum
    Provides commercial mouthwash for rinsing after oral care

A complete bed bath is a bath administered to a totally dependent patient in bed. The nurse has clarified to the AP that full assistance is needed. Patients with diabetes require a health care provider's order to trim toenails, as the risk for cutting skin around the nails and introducing a pathogen is high; the nurse will therefore intervene when the AP offers to perform this task. Placing dentures on a napkin increases the chance that the dentures could be thrown away accidentally. The nurse will intervene, and then re-teach that dentures should be placed in an enclosed cup labeled with the patient's name on the bedside stand while hygiene is performed. Because the patient is fully dependent and requires a complete bed bath, the nurse will intervene when the AP encourages the patient to wash their face and perineum. Even small activities like this can exhaust a patient who is to receive full care. Commercial mouthwash should be avoided, as it is strong and often contains alcohol which can compromise oral tissue integrity. The nurse will intervene and clarify that if any type of rinse is used (provided the patient is not at risk for aspiration), it should be normal saline.

Donning clean gloves before care is an appropriate action by the AP. Draping the unexposed parts of the body is appropriate, as this provides privacy during the complete bed bath. Testing water temperature prior to using it for bathing is appropriate, as this action can alert the AP to whether the water is too cool or too hot. Raising the bed to a comfortable position is appropriate, as this allows the AP to use proper body mechanics when completing the task.

CHAPTER 41

1. e
2. g
3. i
4. j
5. h
6. d
7. f
8. b
9. a
10. c
11. c
12. e
13. h
14. f
15. b
16. g
17. a
18. d

19. Conduction through both atria (atrial depolarization)
20. Impulse travel time from the SA node through the AV node (0.12 to 0.2 seconds)
21. The impulse traveled through the ventricles –ventricle depolarization (0.06 to 0.1 seconds)
22. Time needed for ventricular depolarization and repolarization (0.12 to 0.42 seconds)
23. a. Physiological
    b. Developmental
    c. Lifestyle
    d. Environmental
24. a. Pregnancy (inspiratory capacity declines)
    b. Obesity (reduced lung volumes)
    c. Musculoskeletal abnormalities (structural configurations, trauma, muscular disease, CNS)
    d. Trauma (flail chest, incisions)
    e. Neuromuscular diseases (decrease the ability to expand and contract the chest wall)
    f. CNS alterations (reduced inspiratory lung volumes)
    g. Chronic diseases (chronic hypoxemia)
25. Hyperventilation is the state of ventilation in which the lungs remove carbon dioxide faster than it is produced by cellular metabolism (anxiety, infection, acid–base imbalance).
26. Hypoventilation occurs when alveolar ventilation is inadequate to meet the body's oxygen demand (atelectasis and COPD).
27. Hypoxia is inadequate tissue oxygenation at the cellular level (decreased hemoglobin levels, high altitudes, poisoning, pneumonia, shock, chest trauma).
28. Cyanosis is blue discoloration of the skin and mucous membranes caused by the presence of desaturated hemoglobin in capillaries.
29. Dysrhythmias
30. a. greater than 100 beats/min (reduce cardiac output by decreasing diastolic filling time)
    b. Less than 60 beats/min (lower cardiac output because of the decreased heart rate)
    c. Electric impulse in the atria is chaotic and from multiple sites (decreases cardiac output by altering preload and contractility).
    d. is a sudden, rapid onset of tachycardia originating above the AV node
    e. impulse originates in the ventricle, QRS complex is wide and bizarre
31. a. Left-sided heart failure is characterized by decreased functioning of the left ventricle (fatigue, breathlessness, dizziness, and confusion as a result of tissue hypoxia form diminished cardiac output).
    b. Right-sided heart failure is characterized by impaired functioning of the right ventricle (weight gain, distended neck veins, hepatomegaly and splenomegaly, and dependent peripheral edema).
32. a. Hardening (flow of blood through the valves is obstructed)
    b. Impaired closure (backflow of blood through an adjacent chamber)
33. Myocardial ischemia results when the supply of blood to the myocardium from the coronary arteries is insufficient to meet the myocardial oxygen demand.
34. Angina pectoris is caused by a transient imbalance between myocardial oxygen supply and demand.
35. Myocardial infarction results from a sudden decrease in coronary blood flow or an increase in myocardial oxygen demand without adequate coronary perfusion.
36. Infants and toddlers are at risk for upper respiratory tract infections because of the teething process (develop nasal congestion that encourages bacterial growth), frequent exposures, and secondhand smoke.
37. School-age children and adolescents are at risk from exposure to respiratory infections, secondhand smoke, and smoking.
38. Young and middle-aged adults are at risk from unhealthy diet, lack of exercise, stress, OTC medications, illegal substances, and smoking.
39. Older-adults are at risk from aging changes and osteoporosis.
40. a. Smoking cessation
    b. nutrition
    c. hydration
    d. exercise
    e. avoidance of substance-abuse
    f. reduce stress
41. a. Asbestos
    b. Talcum powder
    c. Dust
    d. Airborne fibers
42. a. Instant feedback about the patient's level of oxygenation
    b. End-tidal CO_2 monitoring provides instant information about the patient's ventilation, perfusion, and cellular metabolism.
43. a. Cardiac function: Pain, dyspnea, fatigue, peripheral circulation, cardiac risk factors
    b. Respiratory function: Cough, shortness of breath, wheezing, pain, environmental exposure, frequency of infections, risk factors, medication use, smoking use
44. a. Cardiac pain does not occur with respiratory variations.
    b. Pleuritic chest pain is peripheral and radiates to the scapular regions.
    c. Musculoskeletal pain often presents after exercise, trauma, or prolonged coughing episodes.
45. Fatigue is often an early sign of a worsening of the chronic underlying process.
46. Dyspnea is a clinical sign of hypoxia that is usually associated with exercise or excitement associated with many medical and environmental factors.

47. Orthopnea is an abnormal condition in which the patient has shortness of breath when lying down. This may lead the patient to use multiple pillows when lying down.

48. Cough is a sudden, audible expulsion of air from the lungs. It is a protective reflex to clear the trachea, bronchi, and lungs of irritants and secretions.

49. Wheezing is a high-pitched musical sound caused by high-velocity movement of air through a narrowed airway.

50. Inspection: Reveals skin and mucous membrane color, general appearance, level of consciousness, adequacy of systemic circulation, breathing patterns, and chest wall movement

51. Palpation: Documents the type and amount of thoracic excursion; areas of tenderness; identifies tactile fremitus, thrills, heaves, and PMI

52. Percussion: Detects the presence of abnormal fluid or air in the lungs

53. Auscultation: Identifies normal and abnormal heart and lung sounds

54. a. Holter monitor: Portable ECG worn by the patient. The test produces a continuous ECG tracing over a period of time. Patients keep a diary of activity, noting when they experience rapid heartbeats or dizziness. Evaluation of the ECG recording along with the diary provides information about the heart's electrical activity during activities of daily living.

    b. Exercise stress test: ECG is monitored while the patient walks on a treadmill at a specified speed and duration of time. Used to evaluate the cardiac response to physical stress. The test is not a valuable tool for evaluation of cardiac response in women because of an increased false-positive finding.

    c. Thallium stress test: An ECG stress test with the addition of thallium-201 injected IV. Determines coronary blood flow changes with increased activity.

    d. EPS: Invasive measure of intracardiac electrical pathways. Provides more specific information about difficult-to-treat dysrhythmias. Assesses adequacy of antidysrhythmic medication.

    e. Echocardiography: Noninvasive measure of heart structure and heart wall motion. Graphically demonstrates overall cardiac performance.

    f. Scintigraphy: Radionuclide angiography. Used to evaluate cardiac structure, myocardial perfusion, and contractility.

    g. Cardiac catheterization and angiography: Used to visualize cardiac chambers, valves, the great vessels, and coronary arteries. Pressures and volumes within the four chambers of the heart are also measured.

55. a. Pulmonary function tests: Determine the ability of the lungs to efficiently exchange oxygen and carbon dioxide. Used to differentiate pulmonary obstructive disease from restrictive disease.

    b. PEFR: Reflects changes in large airway sizes and is an excellent predictor of overall airway resistance in patients with asthma. Daily measurement is for early detection of asthma exacerbations.

    c. Bronchoscopy: Visual examination of the tracheobronchial tree through a narrow, flexible fiberoptic bronchoscope. Performed to obtain fluid, sputum, or biopsy samples and to remove mucous plugs or foreign bodies.

    d. Lung scan: Used to identify abnormal masses by their size and location. Identification of masses is used in planning therapy and treatments.

    e. Thoracentesis: Specimen of pleural fluid is obtained for cytologic examination. The results may indicate an infection or neoplastic disease. Identification of infection or a type of cancer is important in determining a plan of care.

56. a. Activity intolerance
    b. Impaired cardiac output
    c. Fatigue
    d. Acute pain
    e. Impaired breathing

57. a. Respiratory rate is between 12 and 20 breaths/minute.
    b. Achieves bilateral lung expansion
    c. Breathes without the use of accessory muscles

58. a. vaccinations-seasonal flu, Pneumococcal, COVID-19
    b. healthy lifestyle – diet, exercise
    c. avoid exposure to secondhand smoke

59. a. Hydration
    b. Humidification
    c. Nebulization
    d. Coughing and deep breathing

60. a. While exhaling, the patient opens the glottis by saying "huff."
    b. For patients without abdominal muscle control
    c. diaphragm descends when breathing in and ascends when breathing out

61. a. Consists of drainage, positioning, and turning
    b. Chest percussion and vibration

62. a. Bleeding disorders
    b. Osteoporosis
    c. Fractured ribs

63. An airway clearance technique that can be used with and without oscillation. PEP allows air to be inhaled easily but forces the patient to exhale against resistance.

64. Consists of an inflatable vest that is attached to an air-pulse generator. This loosens and removes secretions from the airway by delivering high-frequency, small volume expiratory pulses to the patient's external chest wall.

65. a. Benefits include an increase in general strength and lung expansion.
    b. Frequent changes of position are effective for reducing stasis of pulmonary secretions and decreased chest wall expansion (semi-Fowler is the most effective position).
    c. Incentive spirometry encourages voluntary deep breathing and prevents atelectasis by using visual feedback.

66. a. the simplest type, prevents obstruction of the trachea by displacement of the tongue into the oropharynx
    b. tube is passed thru the patient's mouth, past the pharynx and into the trachea
    c. used for long-term assistance –a surgical incision is made into the inferior border of the cricoid cartilage of the trachea, and a tube is inserted.
67. a. open – using a sterile catheter for ach suction session
    b. closed – reusable suction catheter that is encased in a plastic sheath to protect it between suction sessions.
68. a. Reversing hypoxia and acute respiratory acidosis
    b. Relieving respiratory distress
    c. Preventing or reversing atelectasis and respiratory muscle fatigue
    d. Allowing for sedation and/or other neuromuscular blockage
    e. Decreasing oxygen consumption
    f. Stabilizing the chest wall
69. a. Continuous positive airway pressure (CPAP) – maintains a steady stream of pressure throughout a patient's breathing cycle
    b. Bilevel positive airway pressure (BiPAP) – provides assistance during inspiration and preventing alveolar closure during expiration
70. a. increased ability to communicate with caregivers and family
    b. better ability to cough and clear secretions
    c. allowance for eating and drinking
71. a. To remove air and fluids from the pleural space
    b. To prevent air or fluid from reentering the pleural space
    c. To reestablish normal intrapleural and intrapulmonic pressures
72. a. Hemothorax is an accumulation of blood and fluid in the pleural cavity between the parietal and visceral pleurae, usually caused by trauma.
    b. Pneumothorax is a collection of air in the pleural space, caused by loss of negative intrapleural pressure.
73. The goal of oxygen therapy is to prevent or relieve hypoxia by delivering the lowest amount of oxygen possible, which leads to adequate tissue oxygenation.
74. a. Nasal cannula: A nasal cannula is a simple, comfortable device used for oxygen delivery (Skill 41.4). The two cannulas, about 1.5 cm (0.5 inch) long, protrude from the center of a disposable tube, and are inserted into the nares.
    b. provides heated, humidified oxygen thru a nasal cannula at flow rates of as high as 60 L/minute while an air-oxygen blender allows for the titration of the FiO_2
    c. Face mask: An oxygen face mask is a device used to administer oxygen, humidity, or heated humidity. It fits snugly over the mouth and nose and is secured in place with a strap. It assists in providing humidified oxygen. Can deliver 6-12 L/min
    c. Venturi mask: The Venturi mask delivers oxygen concentrations of 24% to 60% with oxygen flow rates of 4 to 12 L/min, depending on the flow-control meter selected.

75. a basic emergency procedure of artificial respiration and manual external cardiac massage
76. Chest compression, early defibrillation, establishing an airway, and rescue breathing
77. a. Physical exercise
    b. Nutrition counseling
    c. Relaxation and stress management techniques
    d. Prescribed medications and oxygen
78. Pursed-lip breathing involves deep inspiration and prolonged expiration through pursed lips to prevent alveolar collapse.
79. Diaphragmatic breathing requires the patient to relax the intercostal and accessory respiratory muscles while taking deep inspirations; it improves efficiency of breathing by decreasing air trapping and reducing the work of breathing.
80. The airway has visible secretions, has excessive coughing, or the patient shows a decrease in pulse oximetry reading.
81. 1. These are the three steps in the process of oxygenation.
82. 1. The heart must work to overcome this resistance to fully eject blood from the left ventricle.
83. 2. Gases move into and out of the lungs through pressure changes (intrapleural and atmospheric).
84. 3. All other answers are related to the subjective sensation of dyspnea.
85. 2. CPT includes postural drainage, percussion, and vibration.
86. 1,2,3; she denies alcohol and drug use, and although she lives on the 3rd floor this does not cause COPD but may be a challenge for her due to decreased lung capacity.
87. a. Identify recurring and present signs and symptoms associated with Mr. Edwards' impaired oxygenation. Determine the presence of risk factors that apply to Mr. Edwards. Ask Mr. Edwards about the use of medication. Determine Mr. Edwards' activity status. Determine Mr. Edwards' tolerance to activity.
    b. Cardiac and respiratory anatomy and physiology; cardiopulmonary pathophysiology; clinical signs and symptoms of altered oxygenation; developmental factors affecting oxygenation; impact on lifestyle; environmental impact
    c. Caring for patients with impaired oxygenation, activity intolerance, and respiratory infections; observations of changes in patient respiratory patterns made during poor air quality days; personal experience with how a change in altitudes or physical conditioning affects respiratory patterns; personal experience with respiratory infections or cardiopulmonary alterations
    d. Apply intellectual standards of clarity, precision, specificity, and accuracy when obtaining a health history for a patient with cardiopulmonary alterations
    e. Carry out the responsibility of obtaining correct information about Mr. Edwards and explaining risk factors, health promotion and disease prevention activities, and therapies for disease or symptom management. Display confidence in assessing Mr. Edwards' management of illness.

1. a. Extracellular fluid is the fluid outside the cell (interstitial, intravascular, and transcellular fluid).
   b. Intracellular fluid comprises all fluid within the cells of the body (two-thirds of total body water).
2. Cations are positively charged electrolytes (sodium, potassium, calcium, and magnesium).
3. Anions are negatively charged electrolytes (chloride, and bicarbonate).
4. A fluid that has the same tonicity as normal blood
5. Is more dilute than the blood
6. Is more concentrated than normal blood
7. Requires energy in the form of ATP to move electrolytes across cell membranes against the concentration gradient
8. Osmosis is a process by which water moves through a membrane that separates fluids with different particle concentrations.
9. Osmotic pressure is the drawing power of water and depends on the number of molecules in solution.
10. Diffusion is the passive movement of a solute in a solution across a semipermeable membrane from an area of higher concentration to an area of lower concentration.
11. Filtration is the net effect of four forces, two that move fluid out of the capillaries and small venules and two that move fluid back into them.
12. Is the force of the fluid pressing outward against a surface
13. Osmotic pressure – Inward-pulling force caused by blood proteins that helps move fluid from the interstitial area back into the capillaries
14. a. Fluid intake
    b. Fluid distribution
    c. Fluid output
15. ADH regulates the osmolality of the body fluids by influencing how much water is excreted. The release of ADH decreases if body fluids become too dilute, which allows more water to be excreted in the urine.
16. Renin converts angiotensinogen to angiotensin I, which is then converted to angiotensin II (vasoconstriction). Aldosterone causes reabsorption of sodium and water in isotonic proportion in the distal renal tubules; it also increases urinary excretion of potassium and hydrogen ions.
17. Cells in the atria of the heart release ANP when they are stretched; helps regulate extracellular fluid volume by influencing how much sodium and water are excreted.
18. a. Extracellular fluid volume deficit is present when there is insufficient isotonic fluid in the extracellular compartment (hypovolemia).
    b. Extracellular fluid volume excess is too much fluid in the extracellular compartment.
19. a. Water deficit, a hypertonic condition; caused by loss of more water than salt or gain of more salt than water
    b. Water excess, hypotonic condition; caused by more water than salt or a loss of more salt than water
20. Table 42.4
21. Table 42.5

Imbalance	Laboratory Finding	Signs and Symptoms
Hypokalemia	Serum K^+ level < 3.5 mEq/L (< 3.5 mmol/L); ECG abnormalities may occur	Bilateral muscle weakness that begins in quadriceps and may ascend to respiratory muscles; abdominal distention; decreased bowel sounds; constipation; cardiac dysrhythmias; signs of digoxin toxicity at normal digoxin levels
Hyperkalemia	Serum K^+ level > 5.0 mEq/L (> 5.0 mmol/L); ECG abnormalities may occur	Bilateral muscle weakness in quadriceps, transient abdominal cramps and diarrhea, cardiac dysrhythmias, cardiac arrest
Hypocalcemia	Total serum $Ca^{++} < 8.4$ mg/dL (< 2.1 mmol/L) or serum ionized $Ca^{++} < 4.5$ mg/dL (< 1.1 mmol/L); ECG abnormalities may occur	Positive Chvostek sign (contraction of facial muscles when facial nerve is tapped), positive Trousseau sign (carpal spasm with hypoxia), numbness and tingling of fingers and circumoral (around mouth) region, hyperactive reflexes, muscle twitching and cramping, tetany, seizures, laryngospasm, cardiac dysrhythmias
Hypercalcemia	Total serum $Ca^{++} > 10.5$ mg/dL (> 2.6 mmol/L) or serum ionized $Ca^{++} > 5.3$ mg/dL (> 1.3 mmol/L); ECG abnormalities may occur	Anorexia, nausea and vomiting, constipation, fatigue, diminished reflexes, lethargy, decreased level of consciousness, confusion, personality change, cardiac dysrhythmias; possible flank pain from renal calculi; with hypercalcemia caused by shift of calcium from bone: pathological fractures; signs of digoxin toxicity at normal digoxin levels

Imbalance	Laboratory Finding	Signs and Symptoms
Hypomagnesemia	Serum Mg^{++} level < 1.5 mEq/L (< 0.75 mmol/L)	Positive Chvostek sign and Trousseau signs, hyperactive deep tendon reflexes, insomnia, muscle cramps and twitching, grimacing, dysphagia, tachycardia, hypertension, tetany, seizures, cardiac dysrhythmias; signs of digoxin toxicity at normal digoxin levels
Hypermagnesemia	Serum Mg^{++} level > 2.5 mEq/L (> 1.25 mmol/L); ECG abnormalities may occur	Lethargy, hypoactive deep tendon reflexes, bradycardia, hypotension; acute elevation in magnesium levels: flushing, sensation of warmth; severe hypermagnesemia: flaccid muscle paralysis, decreased rate and depth of respirations, cardiac dysrhythmias, cardiac arrest

22. a. Acid production—two types: carbonic acid (CO_2) and metabolic acids (lactic acid)
   b. Acid buffering—buffers that work together to maintain normal pH (HCO_3)
   c. Acid excretion—through the lungs (carbonic acid) and kidneys (metabolic acids)

23.

Acid–Base Imbalance	Laboratory Findings	Signs and Symptoms
Respiratory acidosis	pH < 7.35 $PaCO_2$ > 45 mm Hg (6.0 kPa) HCO_3^- level normal if uncompensated or > 26 mEq/L (> 26 mmol/L) if compensated	Headache, lightheadedness, decreased level of consciousness (confusion, lethargy, coma), cardiac dysrhythmias
Respiratory alkalosis	pH > 7.45 $PaCO_2$ < 35 mm Hg (< 4.7 kPa) HCO_3^- level normal if short lived or uncompensated or < 22 mEq/L (< 22 mmol/L) if compensated K^+ level may be decreased (< 3.5 mEq/L) Ionized Ca^{++} level may be decreased (< 4.5 mg/dL)	Increased rate and depth of respirations (hyperventilation), lightheadedness, numbness and tingling of extremities and circumoral region (paresthesias), excitement and confusion possibly followed by decreased level of consciousness, cardiac dysrhythmias
Metabolic acidosis	pH < 7.35 $PaCO_2$ normal if uncompensated or < 35 mm Hg (4.7 kPa) if compensated HCO_3 level < 22 mEq/L (< 22 mmol/L) Anion gap normal or high, depending on cause K^+ level may be elevated (> 5.0 mq/L), depending on cause	Decreased level of consciousness (lethargy, confusion, coma), abdominal pain, cardiac dysrhythmias, increased rate and depth of respirations (compensatory hyperventilation)
Metabolic alkalosis	pH > 7.45 $PaCO_2$ normal if uncompensated or > 45 mm Hg (> 6.0 kPa) if compensated HCO_3^- > 26 mEq/L (> 26 mmol/L) K + level often decreased (< 3.5 mEq/L) Ionized Ca^{++} level may be decreased (< 4.5 mg/dL)	Lightheadedness, numbness and tingling of fingers, toes, and circumoral region (paresthesias); possible excitement and confusion followed by decreased level of consciousness, cardiac dysrhythmias (may be attributable to hypokalemia)

24. Infants and children have greater water needs and are more vulnerable to fluid volume alterations; fever in children creates an increase in the rate of insensible water loss; adolescents have increased metabolic processes; older-adults have decreased thirst sensation that often causes electrolyte imbalances.

25. Respiratory diseases, burns, trauma, GI alterations, and acute oliguric renal disease

26. Second to fifth postoperative day; increased secretion of aldosterone, glucocorticoids, and antidiuretic hormone (ADH) causes increased extracellular fluid volume (ECF); decreased osmolality and increased potassium excretion

27. The greater the body surface burned, the greater the fluid loss.

28. Changes depend on the type and progression of the cancer and its treatment.

29. Decreased cardiac output, which reduces kidney perfusion and activates the RAAS
30. Vomiting and diarrhea can cause ECV deficit; hypernatremia, clinical dehydration and hypokalemia, and nasogastric suctioning can cause metabolic alkalosis.
31. Sweating in a hot environment can lead to ECV deficit, hypernatremia, or clinical dehydration.
32. Recent changes in appetite or the ability to chew and swallow (breakdown of glycogen and fat stores, metabolic acidosis, hypoalbuminemia, edema)
33. History of smoking or alcohol consumption can increase likelihood of respiratory acidosis.
34. a. Diuretics: metabolic alkalosis, hyperkalemia, and hypokalemia
    b. Corticosteroids: metabolic alkalosis, hypokalemia
    c. Hyperkalemia
    d. Hyponatremia
    e. Hypokalemia, hyperkalemia, metabolic alkalosis
    f. Hyperkalemia, mild metabolic alkalosis
    g. Hypermagnesemia
    h. Mild ECV excess, hyponatremia
35. See Table 42.10.
36. a. Fluid imbalance
    b. Dehydration
    c. Electrolyte Imbalance
    d. Acid–base imbalance
    e. Lack of knowledge of fluid regime
37. a. Patient will be free of complications associated with the IV device throughout the duration of IV therapy.
    b. Patient will demonstrate fluid balance as evidenced by moist mucous membranes, balanced I & O, and stable weights within 48 hours.
38. Enteral replacement of fluids may be appropriate when the patient's GI tract is healthy but the patient cannot ingest fluids.
39. Patients who retain fluids and have fluid volume excess require restriction of fluids; patients who have hyponatremia
40. includes total parenteral nutrition (TPN), crystalloids (IV fluids and electrolyte therapy), and colloids (blood and blood component)
41. Total parenteral nutrition (TPN) is a nutritionally adequate hypertonic solution consisting of nutrients and electrolytes administered centrally or peripherally; it is formulated to meet a patient's needs.
42. IV therapy is used to correct or prevent fluid and electrolyte imbalances.
43. a. Isotonic: dextrose 5% in water, 0.9% sodium chloride (normal saline), lactated Ringer's solution
    b. Hypotonic: 0.45% sodium chloride (1/2 normal saline), 0.33% sodium chloride (1/3 normal saline), 0.225% sodium chloride (1/4 normal saline)
    c. Hypertonic: dextrose 10% in water, 3% to 5% sodium chloride, dextrose 5% in 0.9% sodium chloride, dextrose 5% in 0.45% sodium chloride, dextrose 5% in lactated Ringer's solution
44. Vascular assist devices (VADs) are catheters, cannulas, or infusion ports designed for repeated access to the vascular system.
45. A venipuncture is a technique in which a vein is punctured through the skin by a rigid stylet (butterfly), a stylet covered with a plastic cannula (ONC), or a needle attached to a syringe.
46. a. Use the smallest-gauge catheter or needle possible
    b. Avoid the back of the hand
    c. Avoid placement of IV line in veins that are easily bumped (less subcutaneous support tissue)
    d. Avoid vigorous friction with cleaning site
    e. Use minimal or no tourniquet pressure
    f. If using a tourniquet, place over a sleeve
    g. Lower the insertion angle for venipuncture 10-15 degrees after penetrating the skin (veins superficial)
    h. Stabilize the vein (veins roll away)
    i. Secure IV site with a catheter device; avoid excessive use of tape
    j. Medications increase the likelihood of bruising and bleeding
47. Electronic infusion pumps deliver an accurate hourly rate.
48. a. Keeping the system sterile and intact
    b. Changing solutions, tubing, and contaminated site dressings
    c. Assisting the patient with self-care activities
    d. Monitoring for complications of IV therapy
49. See Table 42.12.
50. a. Increase circulating blood volume after surgery, trauma, or hemorrhage
    b. Increase the number of RBCs and to maintain hemoglobin levels in patients with severe anemia
    c. Provide selected cellular components as replacement therapy
51. A, B, O, and AB blood types
52. The universal blood donor is type O−.
53. The universal blood recipient is type AB+.
54. A transfusion reaction is an antigen–antibody reaction and can range from mild response to severe anaphylactic shock, which can be life threatening.
55. Autotransfusion is the collection and reinfusion of a patient's own blood.

355

56.

Reaction	Cause	Clinical Manifestations
Acute intravascular hemolytic	Infusion of ABO-incompatible whole blood, RBCs, or components containing ≥ 10 mL of RBCs Antibodies in recipient's plasma attach to antigens on transfused RBCs, causing RBC destruction	Chills, fever, low back pain, flushing, tachycardia, tachypnea, hypotension, hemoglobinuria, hemoglobinemia, sudden oliguria (acute kidney injury), circulatory shock, cardiac arrest, death
Febrile, nonhemolytic	Antibodies against donor white blood cells	Sudden shaking chills (rigors), fever (rise in temperature $\geq 1°C$ or more), headache, flushing, anxiety, muscle pain
Mild allergic	Antibodies against donor plasma proteins	Flushing, itching, urticaria (hives)
Anaphylactic	Antibodies to donor plasma, especially anti-IgA	Anxiety, urticaria, dyspnea, wheezing progressing to cyanosis, severe hypotension, circulatory shock, possible cardiac arrest
Circulatory overload	Blood administered faster than the circulation can accommodate	Dyspnea, cough, crackles, or rales in dependent portions of lungs, distended neck veins when upright
Sepsis	Bacterial contamination of transfused blood components	Rapid onset of chills, high fever, severe hypotension, and circulatory shock May occur: vomiting, diarrhea, sudden oliguria (acute kidney injury), DIC

57. a. Stop the transfusion immediately
   b. Keep the IV line open with 0.9% normal saline (NS) by replacing the IV tubing down to the catheter hub
   c. Notify the health care provider
   d. Remain with the patient, observing signs and symptoms; monitor vital signs (VS) every 5 minutes
   e. Prepare to administer emergency drugs per protocol
   f. Prepare to perform cardiopulmonary resuscitation
   g. Obtain a urine specimen and send to the laboratory (RBC hemolysis)
   h. Save the blood container, tubing, attached labels, and transfusion record and return them to the laboratory
58. Slow the IV infusion rate
59. 4. Extracellular fluid is all the fluid outside of the cell and has three compartments.
60. 3. A combination of increased $PaCO_2$, excess carbonic acid, and an increased hydrogen ion concentration

61. 1. Any condition that results in the loss of GI fluids predisposes the patient to the development of dehydration and a variety of electrolyte disturbances.
62. 3, 5, 6; deficient carbonic acid resulting in alveolar hyperventilation
63. 4,7,5,1,9,2,6,8,3
64. a. Knowledge of risk factors for fluid imbalances and physiology of aging; this age group has a high risk for fluid imbalances; specific clinical assessments for signs and symptoms of imbalances; skills and techniques of safe IV therapy
   b. An individualized approach is the foundation of care.
   c. Infusion Nurses Society (INS) standards of practice
   d. Accountability, discipline, and integrity assist you in identifying appropriate nursing diagnoses.
   e. VS return to normal, no postural hypotension, I & O measurements are balanced, daily weight is returned to normal; Mrs. Beck describes effective home management of fluid balance

1. f	6. k	11. m	15. p
2. i	7. a	12. l	16. o
3. h	8. n	13. c	17. e
4. j	9. b	14. q	
5. g	10. d		

18.

Developmental Stage	Sleep Patterns
Neonates	A neonate up to the age of 3 months averages about 16 hours of sleep a day, sleeping almost constantly during the first week. The sleep cycle is generally 40 to 50 minutes with wakening occurring after one to two sleep cycles. Approximately 50% of this sleep is REM sleep, which stimulates the higher brain centers. This is essential for development, because neonates are not awake long enough for significant external stimulation.
Infants	Infants usually develop a nighttime pattern of sleep by 3 months of age. Infants normally take several naps during the day but usually sleep an average of 8 to 10 hours during the night for a total daily sleep time of 15 hours. About 30% of sleep time is in the REM cycle. Awakening commonly occurs early in the morning, although it is not unusual for infants to awaken during the night.
Toddlers	By the age of 2 years, children usually sleep through the night and take daily naps. Total sleep averages 12 hours a day. After 3 years of age, children often give up daytime naps. It is common for toddlers to awaken during the night. The percentage of REM sleep continues to fall. During this period, toddlers may be unwilling to go to bed at night because of a need for autonomy or a fear of separation from their parents.
Preschoolers	On average, preschoolers sleep about 12 hours a night (about 20% is REM). By the age of 5 years, preschoolers rarely take daytime naps except in cultures where a siesta is the custom. Preschoolers usually have difficulty relaxing or quieting down after long, active days and have problems with bedtime fears, waking during the night, or nightmares. Partial wakening followed by normal return to sleep is frequent. In the waking period, children exhibit brief crying, walking around, unintelligible speech, sleepwalking, or bedwetting.
School-age children	The amount of sleep needed varies during the school years. Six-year-old children average 11 to 12 hours of sleep nightly, and 11-year-old children sleep about 9 to 10 hours. Children who are 6 or 7 years old usually go to bed with some encouragement or by doing quiet activities. Older children often resist sleeping because of an unawareness of fatigue or a need to be independent.
Adolescents	On average, teenagers get about 7 ½ hours of sleep per night. The typical adolescent is subject to a number of changes such as school demands, after-school social activities, and part-time jobs that reduce the time spent sleeping.
Young adults	Most young adults average 6 to 8 ½ hours of sleep a night. Approximately 20% of sleep time is REM sleep, which remains consistent throughout life. It is common for the stresses of jobs, family relationships, and social activities frequently to lead to insomnia and the use of medication for sleep. Daytime sleepiness contributes to an increased number of accidents, decreased productivity, and interpersonal problems in this age group. Pregnancy increases the need for sleep and rest. Insomnia, periodic limb movements, restless leg syndrome, and sleep-disordered breathing are common problems during the third trimester of pregnancy.
Middle adults	During middle adulthood, the total time spent sleeping at night begins to decline. The amount of stage 4 sleep begins to fall, a decline that continues with advancing age. Insomnia is particularly common, probably because of the changes and stresses of middle age. Anxiety, depression, and certain physical illnesses cause sleep disturbances. Women experiencing menopausal symptoms often experience insomnia.

Developmental Stage	Sleep Patterns
Older-adults	Complaints of sleeping difficulties increase with age. More than 50% of adults 65 years or older report problems with sleep. Episodes of REM sleep tend to shorten. There is a progressive decrease in stages 3 and 4 NREM sleep; some older-adults have almost no stage 4 sleep, or deep sleep. Older-adults awaken more often during the night, and it takes more time for them to fall asleep. The tendency to nap seems to increase progressively with age because of the frequent awakenings experienced at night.
	The presence of chronic illness often results in sleep disturbances for older-adults. For example, an older-adult with arthritis frequently has difficulty sleeping because of painful joints. Changes in sleep pattern are often attributable to changes in the CNS that affect the regulation of sleep. Sensory impairment reduces an older person's sensitivity to time cues that maintain circadian rhythms.

19. Sleepiness, insomnia, and fatigue often result as a direct effect of commonly prescribed medications including hypnotics, diuretics, alcohol, caffeine, beta-adrenergic blockers, benzodiazepines, narcotics, anticonvulsants, antidepressants, and stimulants.

20. Rotating shifts cause difficulty adjusting to the altered sleep schedule, performing unaccustomed heavy work, engaging in late-night social activities, and changing evening mealtimes.

21. Most persons are sleep deprived and experience excessive sleepiness during the day, which can become pathological when it occurs at times when individuals need or want to be awake.

22. Personal problems or certain situations (retirement, physical impairment, or the death of a loved one) frequently disrupt sleep.

23. Good ventilation is essential for a restful sleep, as are the size and firmness of the bed; light levels affect the ability to fall asleep.

24. Exercise 2 hours or more before bedtime allows the body to cool down and maintain a state of fatigue that promotes relaxation.

25. Eating a large, heavy, or spicy meal at night often results in indigestion that interferes with sleep; caffeine, alcohol, and nicotine produce insomnia.

26. Patients, bed partners, and parents of children

27. a. Description of sleeping problems
    b. Usual sleep pattern
    c. Physical and psychological illness
    d. Current life events
    e. Emotional and mental status
    f. Bedtime routines
    g. Bedtime environment
    h. Behaviors of sleep deprivation

28. a. Adequate sleep
    b. Fatigue
    c. Impaired sleep
    d. Impaired alertness
    e. Sleep deprivation

29. a. patient will express feeling rested after sleep
    b. patient reports fewer awakenings during the night
    c. patient fall asleep within 30 minutes of going to bed
    d. patient reports sleeping 8 hours each night

30. Eliminate distracting noises; promote comfortable room temperature, ventilation, bed, and mattress to provide support and firmness

31. Sleep when fatigued or sleepy, bedtime routines for children and adults need to avoid excessive mental stimulation before bedtime

32. Use a small night light and a bell at the bedside to alert family members

33. Clothing, extra blankets, void before retiring

34. Increasing daytime activity lessens problems with falling asleep.

35. Pursue a relaxing activity for adults; children need comforting and night lights

36. A dairy product that contains l-tryptophan is often helpful to promote sleep; do not drink caffeine, tea, colas, and alcohol before bedtime.

37. Melatonin 0.3 mg to 3 mg 2 hours before bedtime (nutritional supplement to aid in sleep), valerian, kava

38. Reduce lights, reduce noise (See Box 43.12)

39. Keep beds clean and dry and in a comfortable position; application of dry or moist heat; splints; and proper positioning

40. Plan care to avoid awakening patients for nonessential tasks; allow patients to determine the timing and methods of delivery of basic care

41. Reduce the risk of postoperative complications for patients with sleep apnea (airway); use of CPAP

42. Giving patients control over their health care minimizes uncertainty and anxiety; back rubs; cautious use of sedatives.

43. a. Patient falls asleep after reducing noise and darkening a room.
    b. Patient describes the number of awakenings during the previous night.
    c. Patient and family demonstrate understanding after receiving instructions on sleep habits.

44. Answers are c and e only
Limit fluids to 4 hours before sleep. Ensure room temperature is comfortably cool. Maintain a regular bedtime and wake-up schedule. Eliminate naps unless they are part of the schedule, and if so, limit to 20 minutes. Use warm bath and relaxation techniques. Avoid activities such as exercise or watching TV before bedtime.

45. 2. Another name is the diurnal rhythm

46. 3. A natural protein found in milk, cheeses, and meats
47. 4. See Box 43-3 for other symptoms of sleep deprivation; most physiological symptoms are decreased, not increased.
48. 4. The related factor of the sleep disturbance is physiological for this patient (leg pain).
49. 2. A sleep-promotion plan frequently requires many weeks to accomplish.
50. 2,4,5
51. a. Evaluate the signs and symptoms of Julie's sleep disturbance. Review Julie's sleep pattern. Have her sleep partner report Julie's response to therapies. The expected outcomes developed during the care plan serve as the standards to evaluate its success. Ask the patient if her expectations of care are being met.
    b. The characteristics of a desirable sleep pattern; basis for the expected outcomes in the plan of care
    c. Nursing Scope and Standards of Practice, clinical guidelines for the treatment of primary insomnia as guidelines
    d. Humility may apply if an intervention is unsuccessful; rethink the approach. In the case of chronic sleep problems, perseverance is needed in staying with the plan of care or in trying new approaches.
    e. Use of established expected outcomes to evaluate Julie's plan of care (improved duration of sleep, fewer awakenings, she feels more rested)

52.

Assessment Finding	Sleep apnea	Medication-induced side effect
Stops breathing for up to 1 minute	X	
Sleepwalks		X
Snores loudly	X	
Enlarged tonsils	X	
Excessive daytime sleepiness	X	
Decreased oxygen saturation	X	
Eats while asleep		X
Respiratory depression		X

Interruptions in sleep caused by sleep apnea can produce concerning symptoms, as can side effects of medication intended to facilitate sleep. It is important that the nurse differentiates these symptoms so that assessment findings and possible concerns can be accurately communicated to the health care provider. Symptoms associated with sleep apnea include breathing cessation for 10 seconds up to 2 minutes, loud snoring, enlarged tonsils, excessive daytime sleepiness (despite having slept the night prior), and a decrease in oxygen saturation. Medication-induced side effects include sleep walking (zolpidem), eating while sleeping (zolpidem), and respiratory depression (benzodiazepines).

CHAPTER 44

1. An unpleasant, subjective sensory and emotional experience associated with actual or potential tissue damage or described in terms of such damage
2. physical, psychosocial, social, and financial
3. a. Transduction: Converts energy produced by stimuli (thermal, chemical, or mechanical) into electrical energy
   b. Transmission: Excitatory neurotransmitters send electrical impulses across the synaptic cleft between the nerve fibers, enhancing the pain impulse.
   c. Perception: The point the person is aware of the pain; gives awareness and meaning to pain, resulting in a reaction
   d. Modulation: The inhibition of pain impulse is the last phase of the normal pain process, which occurs due to release of inhibitory neurotransmitters.
4. Pain has emotional and cognitive components in addition to physical sensations. Gating mechanisms located along the CNS regulate or block pain impulses. Pain impulses pass through when a gate is open and are blocked when a gate is closed.
5. Level of pain a person is willing to accept
6. e
7. l
8. f
9. a
10. c
11. j
12. i
13. b
14. k
15. d
16. g
17. h
18. m

19. a. Acute pain is protective, has a cause, is of short duration, and has limited tissue damage and emotional response.
    b. Chronic pain lasts longer than anticipated, does not always have a cause, and leads to great personal suffering.
20. a. Chronic episodic pain is pain that occurs sporadically over an extended duration of time.
    b. Idiopathic pain is chronic in the absence of an identifiable physical or psychological cause or pain perceived as excessive for the extent of an organic pathological condition.
21. a. Patients who abuse substances (drugs and alcohol) overreact to discomforts.
    b. Patients with minor illnesses have less pain than those with severe physical alteration.
    c. Administering analgesics regularly leads to drug addiction.
    d. The amount of tissue damage in an injury accurately indicates pain intensity.
    e. Health care personnel are the best authorities on the nature of a patient's pain.
    f. Psychogenic pain is not real.
    g. Chronic pain is psychological.
    h. Patients who are hospitalized will experience pain.
    i. Patients who cannot speak do not feel pain.
22. a. Age-children and aging
    b. Fatigue – heightens the perception of pain and deceased coping abilities
    c. Genes – can possibly increase or decrease a person's sensitivity to pain and determines pain threshold or tolerance
    d. Neurologic function – any factor that interrupts or influences normal pain reception or perception affects a patient's awareness of and response to pain
23. a. Previous experience – prior experience does not mean that a person accepts pain more easily in the future
    b. Family and social support – can make the experience less stressful; the presence of parents is especially important for children experiencing pain
    c. Spiritual factors – benefits for individuals' physical and emotional health
24. a. Attention – the degree to which the patient focuses on pain
    b. Anxiety and fear – perceive pain differently if it suggests a threat, loss, punishment, or challenge
    c. Coping styles – pain can be a lonely experience that often causes patients to feel a loss of control
25. Individuals learn what is expected and accepted by their culture; different meanings and attitudes are associated with pain across various cultural groups.
26. a. Quality of life
    b. Self-care
    c. Work
    d. Social support

27. a. Ask about pain regularly. Assess pain systematically.
    b. Believe the patient and family in their report of pain and what relieves it
    c. Choose pain-control options appropriate for the patient, family, and setting
    d. Deliver interventions in a timely, logical, and coordinated fashion
    e. Empower patients and their families. Enable them to control their course to the greatest extent possible.
28. a. Timing (onset, duration, and pattern)
    b. Location
    c. Severity
    d. Quality
    e. Aggravating and precipitating factors
    f. Relief measures
    g. Contributing symptoms
29. a. Difficulty Coping with pain
    b. Inadequate pain control
    c. Fatigue
    d. Impaired Mobility
    e. Impaired Sleep
    f. Social Interaction
30. a. Patient reports that pain is a 3 or less on a scale of 0 to 10.
    b. modifies activities that intensify pain
    c. Uses pain-relief measures safely
    d. Is able to complete ADLs independently
31. a. Change patient's perception of pain, and provide patient with a greater sense of control (distraction, prayer, relaxation, guided imagery, music, and biofeedback)
    b. Aim to provide pain relief, correct physical dysfunction, alter physiological responses, and reduce fears associated with pain-related immobility
32. a. medications – nonopioids and opioids
    b. restorative therapies – physical therapy and occupational therapy
    c. interventional approaches – trigger point injections and neuromodulation
    d. behavioral approaches – for psychological, cognitive, emotional, and social
    e. complementary and integrative health – acupuncture, massage, movement therapies, and spirituality
33. Relaxation is mental and physical freedom from tension or stress that provides individuals with a sense of self-control.
34. Distraction directs a patient's attention to something other than pain and thus reduces the awareness of pain.
35. Music diverts the person's attention away from the pain and creates a relaxation response.
36. Cutaneous stimulation (including massage, warm bath, ice bag, and transcutaneous electrical stimulation [TENS]) reduces pain perception by the release of endorphins, which block the transmission of painful stimuli.
37. Herbals are not sufficiently studied; however, many use herbals such as echinacea, ginseng, gingko biloba, and garlic supplements.

38. One simple way to promote comfort is by removing or preventing painful stimuli; also distraction, prayer, relaxation, guided imagery, music, and biofeedback.
39. a. Nonopioids (acetaminophen and NSAIDs)
    b. Opioids (narcotics)
    c. Adjuvants or coanalgesics
40. Adjuvants or coanalgesics are a variety of medications that enhance analgesics or have analgesic properties that were originally unknown.
41. Refer to Box 44.13.
42. a. Know patient's previous response to analgesics
    b. Select proper medications when more than one is ordered
    c. Know accurate dosage
    d. Assess right time and interval for administration
43. The use of different agents allows for lower than usual doses of each medication, therefore lowering the risk of side effects, while providing pain relief that is good or even better than could be obtained from each of the medications alone.
44. PCA allows patients to self-administer opioids with minimal risk of overdose; the goal is to maintain a constant plasma level of analgesic to avoid the problems of prn dosing.
45. Local anesthesia is intended for local infiltration of an anesthetic medication to induce loss of sensation to a body part.
46. Regional anesthesia is the injection of a local anesthetic to block a group of sensory nerve fibers; perineural local anesthetic infusion.
47. Epidural anesthesia permits control or reduction of severe pain and reduces the patient's overall opioid requirement; can be short or long term.
48. See Table 44.6.
49. a. Incident pain: Pain that is predictable and elicited by specific behaviors such as physical therapy or wound dressing changes
    b. End-of-dose failure pain: Pain that occurs toward the end of the usual dosing interval of a regularly scheduled analgesic
    c. Spontaneous pain: Pain that is unpredictable and not associated with any activity or event
50. a. Patient: Fear of addiction, worry about side effects, fear of tolerance ("won't be there when I need it"), take too many pills already, fear of injections, concern about not being a "good" patient, don't want to worry family and friends, may need more tests, need to suffer to be cured, pain is for past indiscretions, inadequate education, reluctance to discuss pain, pain is inevitable, pain is part of aging, fear of disease progression, primary health care providers and nurses are doing all they can, just forget to take analgesics, fear of distracting primary health care providers from treating illness, primary health care providers have more important or ill patients to see, suffering in silence is noble and expected
    b. Health care provider: Inadequate pain assessment, concern with addiction, opiophobia (fear of opi-

oids), fear of legal repercussions, no visible cause of pain, patients must learn to live with pain, reluctance to deal with side effects of analgesics, fear of giving a dose that will kill the patient, not believing the patient's report of pain, primary health care provider time constraints, inadequate reimbursement, belief that opioids "mask" symptoms, belief that pain is part of aging, overestimation of rates of respiratory depression
    c. Health care system barriers: Concern with creating "addicts," ability to fill prescriptions, absolute dollar restriction on amount reimbursed for prescriptions, mail order pharmacy restrictions, nurse practitioners and physician assistants not used efficiently, extensive documentation requirements, poor pain policies and procedures regarding pain management, lack of money, inadequate access to pain clinics, poor understanding of economic impact of unrelieved pain
51. a. Physical dependence: A state of adaptation that is manifested by a drug class–specific withdrawal syndrome produced by abrupt cessation, rapid dose reduction, decreasing blood level of the drug, or administration of an antagonist
    b. Drug tolerance: A state of adaptation in which exposure to a drug induces changes that result in a diminution of one or more of the drug's effects over time
    c. Addiction: A primary, chronic, neurobiologic disease, with genetic, psychosocial, and environmental factors influencing its development and manifestations. Addictive behaviors include one or more of the following: impaired control over drug use, compulsive use, continued use despite harm, and craving.
52. A placebo is a medication or procedure that produces positive or negative effects in patients that are not related to the placebo's specific physical or chemical properties.
53. Pain clinics treat persons on an inpatient or outpatient basis; multidisciplinary approach to find the most effective pain-relief measures.
54. Palliative care is care provided where the goal is to live life fully with an incurable condition.
55. Hospice care is provided at the end of life; it emphasizes quality of life over quantity.
56. Evaluate the patient for the effectiveness of the pain management after an appropriate period of time; entertain new approaches if no relief; evaluate the patient's perception of pain
57. a,b,d.
58. 2. Only the patient knows whether pain is present and what the experience is like.
59. 1. When the brain perceives pain, there is a release of inhibitory neurotransmitters such as endogenous opioids (e.g., endorphins) that hinder the transmission of pain and help produce an analgesic effect.
60. 2. A patient's self-report of pain is the single most reliable indicator of the existence and intensity of pain.

61. 2. The reticular activating system inhibits painful stimuli if a person receives sufficient or excessive sensory input; with sufficient sensory stimulation, a person is able to ignore or become unaware of pain.

62. a. Determine Mrs. Mays' perspective of pain, including history of pain; its meaning; and its physical, emotional, and social effects. Objectively measure the characteristics of Mrs. Mays' pain. Review potential factors affecting Mrs. Mays' pain.

   b. Physiology of pain. Factors that potentially increase or decrease responses to pain; pathophysiology of conditions causing pain; awareness of biases affecting pain assessment and treatment; cultural variations in how pain is expressed; knowledge of nonverbal communication.

   c. Caring for patients with acute, chronic, and cancer pain; caring for patients who experienced pain as a result of a health care therapy; personal experience with pain

   d. Refer to practice guidelines for acute and chronic pain management. Apply intellectual standards (clarity, specificity, accuracy, and completeness) with gathering assessment. Apply relevance when letting Mrs. Mays explore the pain experience.

   e. Persevere in exploring causes and possible solutions for chronic pain. Display confidence when assessing pain to relieve Mrs. Mays' anxiety. Display integrity and fairness to prevent prejudice from affecting assessment.

63.

Actions to Take	Potential Conditions	Parameters to Monitor
Administer naloxone immediately	Serotonin syndrome	Urinary output
Notify the health care provider	Sepsis	ALT/AST laboratory values
Ensure oxygen is working properly	Opioid toxicity	SpO$_2$
Request order for fluid bolus	Hypoglycemia	Respiratory rate
Administer PRN oral analgesic		Gait stability

Respiratory depression can occur any time a patient is receiving an opioid medication. Even though patient-controlled analgesia (PCA) pumps are programmed, the nurse must still monitor the patient closely, as responses to analgesia are very individualized. When the nurse notices that a patient's blood pressure, pulse, respiratory rate, and oxygen saturation are trending downward, it is important to intervene to ensure the patient does not experience respiratory depression. Due to being placed on a PCA pump following surgery, the most likely explanation for the assessment data is that the patient may be experiencing a degree of opioid toxicity. There is no evidence to suggest that the patient may be experiencing serotonin syndrome which occurs as a result of too much serotonin in the system, or of sepsis (as the temperature would likely be much higher), or hypoglycemia (as blood glucose monitoring over the past 12 hours has been stable).

At this time, the patient's vital signs are not critical; however, there is a definitive downward trend that should be noted in the blood pressure, pulse, respiration rate, temperature, and oxygen saturation. The nurse will need to intervene before problems occur. The first thing the nurse can do is to ensure that the oxygen delivery system is working appropriately; desaturation and respiratory decline could be influenced by lack of oxygen. Mechanisms sometimes malfunction and assuring that everything is working correctly is an appropriate initial intervention. Of the other choices available, the nurse should contact the health care provider to communicate the declining trend that has taken place over the last hour. There is no need to immediately administer naloxone (respiratory depression has not occurred) nor to give a fluid bolus (the patient is already receiving fluids) or PRN oral analgesics (which could increase the risk for respiratory depression if another opioid is given, or induce aspiration if the patient is unable to swallow properly due to being very drowsy).

Once the health care provider has been notified, it is likely there will be a change in opioid dosing. The nurse will need to continue to monitor vital signs including the SpO$_2$ and respiratory rate to watch for any further decline. Monitoring urinary output or ALT/AST laboratory values would be of no significance at this particular time. Asking the patient to ambulate to assess the gait is a safety concern, as the patient is very drowsy and receiving opioid medication.

CHAPTER 45

1. c	19. l
2. h	20. u
3. i	21. t
4. n	22. a
5. o	23. b
6. j	24. f
7. k	25. h
8. v	26. b
9. d	27. g
10. s	28. l
11. p	29. k
12. f	30. j
13. m	31. m
14. e	32. d
15. r	33. e
16. q	34. c
17. w	35. a
18. g	36. i

37. a. The EAR is the recommended amount of nutrition that appears sufficient to maintain a specific body function for 50% of the population based on age and gender.
   b. The RDA is the average needs of 98% of the population, not the individual.
   c. The AI is the suggested intake for individuals based on observed or experimentally determined estimates of nutrient intakes and used when there is not enough evidence to set the RDA.
   d. The UL is the highest level that likely poses no risk of adverse health events.

38. a. Stage of development
   b. Body composition
   c. Activity levels
   d. Pregnancy and lactation
   e. Presence of disease

39. a. Breastfeeding reduces food allergies and intolerances.
   b. Breastfed infants have fewer infections.
   c. Breast milk is easier for an infant to digest.
   d. Breast milk is convenient, available, and fresh.
   e. Breast milk is the correct temperature.
   f. Breastfeeding is economical.
   g. Breastfeeding increases the time for mother and infant interaction.

40. Cow's milk causes GI bleeding, is too concentrated for infants' kidneys to manage, increases the risk of mild product allergies, and is a poor source of iron and vitamins C and E.

41. Honey and corn syrup are potential sources of botulism toxin and should not be used in the infant's diet.

42. a. Nutritional needs
   b. Physical readiness to handle different forms of foods
   c. The need to detect and control allergic reactions

43. a. Diet rich in high-calorie foods
   b. Food advertising targeting children
   c. Inactivity
   d. Genetic predisposition
   e. Use of food for coping mechanism for stress or boredom
   f. Family and social factors

44. a. Body image and appearance
   b. Desire for independence
   c. Eating at fast-food restaurants
   d. Fad diets
   e. Peer pressure

45. a. Anorexia nervosa: Refusal to maintain body weight over a minimal normal weight for age and height such as weight loss leading to maintenance of body weight less than 85% of ideal body weight (IBW) or failure to make expected weight gain during period of growth, leading to body weight less than 85% of that expected; intense fear of gaining weight or becoming fat, although underweight; disturbance in the way in which one's body weight, size, or shape is experienced (e.g., the person claims to "feel fat" even when emaciated, believes that one area of the body is "too fat" even when obviously underweight); in women, absence of at least three consecutive menstrual cycles when otherwise expected to occur (primary or secondary amenorrhea) (A woman is considered to have amenorrhea if her periods occur only after hormone, e.g., estrogen, administration.)
   b. Bulimia nervosa: Recurrent episodes of binge eating (rapid consumption of a large amount of food in a discrete period of time); a feeling of lack of control over eating behavior during the eating binges; the person regularly engages in either self-induced vomiting, use of laxatives or diuretics, strict dieting or fasting, or vigorous exercise to prevent weight gain; a minimum average of two binge eating episodes a week for at least 3 months

46. Folic acid is important for DNA synthesis and the growth of RBCs; inadequate intake will lead to possible neural tube defects, anencephaly, or maternal megaloblastic anemia.

47. a. Age-related gastrointestinal changes that affect digestion of food and maintenance of nutrition include changes in the teeth and gums, reduced saliva production, atrophy of oral mucosal epithelial cells, increased taste threshold, decreased thirst sensation, reduced gag reflex, and decreased esophageal and colonic peristalsis.
   b. The presence of chronic illnesses (e.g., diabetes mellitus, end-stage renal disease, cancer) often affects nutrition intake.
   c. Adequate nutrition in older-adults is affected by multiple causes, such as lifelong eating habits, ethnicity, socialization, income, educational level, physical functional level to meet activities of daily living, loss, dentition, and transportation.

363

d. Adverse effects of medications cause problems such as anorexia, xerostomia, early satiety, and impaired smell and taste perception.

e. Cognitive impairments such as delirium, dementia, and depression affect the ability to obtain, prepare, and eat healthy foods.

48. Ovolactovegetarians avoid meat, fish, and poultry but eat eggs and milk.

49. Lactovegetarians drink milk but avoid eggs, meat, fish, and poultry.

50. Vegans consume only plant foods.

51. a. Screening for malnutrition for risk factors (unintentional weight loss, presence of a modified diet, presence of nutrition impact symptoms)

b. Anthropometry (size and makeup of the body) including IBW and BMI

c. Laboratory and biochemical tests (albumin, transferrin, prealbumin, retinal-binding protein, total iron-binding capacity, and hemoglobin)

d. Dietary history and health history (see Box 45-6)

e. Physical exam: Carefully assessing dysphagia (difficulty swallowing)

52. Dysphagia is difficulty swallowing (neurogenic, myogenic, and obstructive causes).

53. a. General appearance: Listless, apathetic, cachectic

b. Weight: Obesity (usually 10% above IBW) or underweight (special concern for underweight)

c. Posture: Sagging shoulders, sunken chest, humped back

d. Muscles: Flaccid, poor tone, underdeveloped tone; "wasted" appearance; impaired ability to walk properly

e. Nervous system: Inattention, irritability, confusion, burning and tingling of the hands and feet (paresthesia), loss of position and vibratory sense, weakness and tenderness of the muscles (may result in inability to walk), decrease or loss of ankle and knee reflexes, absent vibratory sense

f. Gastrointestinal: Anorexia, indigestion, constipation or diarrhea, liver or spleen enlargement

g. Cardiovascular: Rapid heart rate (> 100 beats/min), enlarged heart, abnormal rhythm, elevated blood pressure

h. General vitality: Easily fatigued, no energy, falls asleep easily, tired and apathetic

i. Hair: Stringy, dull, brittle, dry, thin, sparse, depigmented; easily plucked

j. Skin: Rough, dry, scaly, pale, pigmented, irritated; bruises; petechiae; subcutaneous fat loss

k. Face and neck: Greasy, discolored, scaly, swollen; dark skin over cheeks and under eyes; lumpiness or flakiness of skin around nose and mouth

l. Lips: Dry, scaly, swollen; redness and swelling (cheilosis); angular lesions at corners of mouth; fissures or scars (stomatitis)

m. Mouth, oral membranes: Swollen, boggy oral mucous membranes

n. Gums: Spongy gums that bleed easily; marginal redness, inflammation; receding

o. Tongue: Swelling, scarlet and raw; magenta, beefiness (glossitis); hyperemic and hypertrophic papillae; atrophic papillae

p. Teeth: Unfilled caries; missing teeth; worn surfaces; mottled (fluorosis) or malpositioned

q. Eyes: Eye membranes pale (pale conjunctivas), redness of membrane (conjunctival injection), dryness, signs of infection, Bitot spots, redness and fissuring of eyelid corners (angular palpebritis), dryness of eye membrane (conjunctival xerosis), dull appearance of cornea (corneal xerosis), soft cornea (keratomalacia)

r. Neck (glands): Thyroid or lymph node enlargement

s. Nails: Spoon shape (koilonychia), brittleness, ridges

t. Legs, feet: Edema, tender calf, tingling, weakness

u. Skeleton: Bowlegs, knock-knees, chest deformity at diaphragm, prominent scapulae and ribs

54. a. Impaired low nutrition intake

b. Impaired low nutritional intake

c. Risk for aspiration

d. Overweight

e. Impaired swallowing

55. a. Nutritional intake meets the minimal DRIs.

b. patient will eat well-balanced and healthy snacks every day

c. patient will increase daily protein intake

56. patients who are NPO and receive standard IV fluids for more than 5 to 7 days

57. a. Keep patient's environment free of odors

b. Provide oral hygiene as needed

c. Maintain patient comfort

58. a. Dysphagia puree

b. Dysphagia mechanically altered

c. Dysphagia advanced

d. Regular

59. a. Thin liquids (low viscosity)

b. Nectar-like liquids (medium viscosity)

c. Honey-like liquids

d. Spoon-thick liquids (pudding)

60. a. 1.0 to 2.0 kcal/mL: Milk-based blenderized foods

b. 3.8 to 4.0 kcal/mL: Single macronutrient preparations; not nutritionally complete

c. 1.0 to 3.0 kcal/mL: Predigested nutrients that are easier for a partially dysfunctional GI tract to absorb

d. 1.0 to 2.0 kcal/mL: Designed to meet specific nutritional needs in certain illnesses

61. a. Pulmonary aspiration: Regurgitation of formula, feeding tube displaced, deficient gag reflex, delayed gastric emptying

b. Diarrhea: Hyperosmolar formula or medications, antibiotic therapy, bacterial contamination, malabsorption

c. Constipation: Lack of fiber, lack of free water, inactivity

d. Tube occlusion: Pulverized medications given per tube, sedimentation of formula, reaction of incompatible medications or formula

e. Tube displacement: Coughing, vomiting, not taped securely

f. Abdominal cramping, nausea, or vomiting: High osmolality of formula, rapid increase in rate or volume, lactose intolerance, intestinal obstruction, high-fat formula used, cold formula used

g. Delayed gastric emptying: Diabetic gastroparesis, serious illnesses, inactivity

h. Serum electrolyte imbalance: Excess GI losses, dehydration, presence of disease states such as cirrhosis, renal insufficiency, heart failure, or diabetes mellitus

i. Fluid overload: Refeeding syndrome in malnutrition, excess free water or diluted (hypotonic) formula

j. Hyperosmolar dehydration: Hypertonic formula with insufficient free water

62. a. Appropriate assessment of nutrition needs

b. Meticulous management of the central venous catheter (CVC) line

c. Careful monitoring to prevent or treat metabolic complications

63. Catheter-related problems and metabolic alterations

64. Intravenous fat emulsions provide supplemental kcal, prevent fatty acid deficiencies, and control hyperglycemia.

65. When the patient meets one-third to half of his or her caloric needs per day, PN is usually decreased to half the original volume; increase the EN to meet needs (75%).

66. Medical nutrition therapy is the use of specific nutritional therapies to treat an illness, injury, or condition.

67. *Helicobacter pylori* is a bacteria that causes peptic ulcers and is confirmed by laboratory tests. Infection is treated with antibiotics.

68. Crohn disease and ulcerative colitis are treated with elemental diets or PN, supplemental vitamins, and iron. Manage by increasing fiber, reducing fat, avoiding large meals, and avoiding lactose.

69. Celiac disease is treated with a gluten-free diet.

70. Diverticulitis is treated with moderate- to low-residue and high-fiber diet.

71. Diabetes mellitus is managed with a diet of 45% to 75% carbohydrates; limit fat to less than 7% and cholesterol to less than 200 mg/day.

72. Cardiovascular disease is managed by balancing caloric intake with exercise; a diet high in fruits, vegetables, and whole-grain fiber; fish at least twice per week; limit food high in added sugar and salt.

73. The goal with patients who have cancer is to meet the increased metabolic needs of the patient by maximizing intake of nutrients and fluids.

74. The diets of patients who have HIV should include small, frequent, nutrient-dense meals that limit fatty foods and overly sweet foods.

75. Ongoing comparisons need to be made with baseline measures of weight, serum albumin, and protein and calorie intake and changes in condition.

76. Collaborate with speech-language therapist to identify level of swallowing difficulty

77. 4. Each gram of CHO produces 4 kcal and serves as the main source of fuel (glucose) for the brain, skeletal muscles during exercise, erythrocyte and leukocyte production, and cell function of the renal medulla.

78. 3. When the intake of nitrogen is greater than the output, which is used for building, repairing, and replacing body tissues

79. 4. The growth rate slows during the toddler years (1 to 3 years) and therefore needs fewer kcal but an increased amount of protein in relation to body weight; appetite often decreases at 18 months of age.

80. 1. All of the other patients are at risk for a nutritional imbalance.

81. 2. The measurement of pH of secretions withdrawn from the feeding tubes helps to differentiate the location of the tube.

82. 1. The recommended diet from the AHA to reduce risk factors for the development of hypertension and coronary heart disease

83. a,c,d,f,g

84. a. Select nursing interventions to promote optimal nutrition. Select nursing interventions consistent with therapeutic diets. Consult with other health care professionals (dietitians, nutritionists, physicians, pharmacists, and physical and occupational therapists) to adopt interventions that reflect Mrs. Cooper's needs. Involve the family when designing interventions.

b. Persevere in exploring causes and possible solutions for imbalanced nutrition; display integrity and fairness to prevent prejudice from affecting assessment.

c. Apply intellectual standards (clarity, specificity, accuracy, and completeness) when gathering assessment. Previous patient responses to nursing interventions for altered nutrition; personal experiences with dietary change strategies (what worked and what did not).

d. Integrate knowledge from other disciplines and Healthy People 2020

e. Inquire about her food intake during the last few days; social interaction; weigh patient and assess posture; signs of poor nutrition

85. Correct answers are shown in yellow highlight.

Nurses' Notes:	Patient here for follow-up on weight and general health. Weight today is 92 pounds (41.7 kg). Parent and patient report an increase in daily green vegetable consumption. At school, patient takes part in required physical education classes twice weekly and has joined an after-school marching band program. Breakfast and lunch are provided by the patient's school. Patient reports getting a vending machine snack and soda before each marching band practice. Dinner is usually consumed in the car watching a video between evening appointments while the patient's parent carpools older siblings for sports. No changes in bowel or bladder habits; no chest pain or respiratory difficulties; no headaches reported.

Childhood obesity rates continue to rise. Nurses can intervene early as soon as a weight concern identified to help the patient and family develop better nutrition habits that will enhance wellness over the lifespan. Areas where the nurse will need to provide further education include teaching about vending machine foods and eating in car.

Vending machines are often supplied with snack foods that are high in fat, sugar, and sale, and that have little nutrition density. Although having a snack can be helpful to maintain energy expended during physical activity (such as marching band), the nurse will encourage the patient and parent to pack a nutrition snack from home that can be easily accessed and consumed. Examples include snack foods from the dairy, fruit and vegetable groups. String cheese, apples, and carrots are easily packed and provide much more nutrition density than vending machine snacks.

The nurse will also address eating in the car while watching a video. Although families' lives are often very busy, eating on the go is discouraged as much as possible. This creates a scenario in which people often choose unhealthy fast food because of convenience. Watching videos or television, and video gaming, are also actions that decrease awareness of the types and volumes of food being consumed. The nurse can again suggest packing a healthy dinner when possible, and discouraging the use of videos while eating.

The demonstrated weight loss is a favorable finding, as is increasing daily green vegetables and engaging in physical activity like marching band. It is also favorable that the patient has not experienced changes in elimination, nor reports any other findings such as chest pain, respiratory difficulty, or headaches.

CHAPTER 46

1. d
2. c
3. g
4. f
5. b
6. e
7. a
8. a. Growth and development – voluntary control, readiness, older-adults (decease in bladder capacity and risk of urinary incontinence)
   b. Sociocultural factors – privacy issues, religious norms, social expectations
   c. Psychological factors – anxiety and stress, depression
   d. Personal habits – need for privacy and adequate time to void
   e. Fluid intake – balances, alcohol decreases the release of ADH thus increasing urine production, caffeine and bladder irritants
   f. Pathological conditions – diabetes, multiple sclerosis, stroke (alter bladder contractility); arthritis, Parkinson's dementia (interfere with timely access to a toilet); spinal cord injury or intervertebral disk disease (loss of urine control); prostatic enlargement (obstruction)
   g. Surgical procedures – local trauma; mechanical obstruction or altered neural control of bladder
   h. Medications – diuretics (increase output), drugs change color of urine, anticholinergics (retention), hypnotics and sedatives (reduce ability to recognize and act on the urge to void)
   i. Diagnostic exams – cystoscopy (localized trauma), catheterizations
9. Caused by medical conditions that in many cases are reversible
10. Causes outside the urinary tract, usually related to functional deficits (altered mobility and manual dexterity, cognitive impairment, poor motivation or environmental barriers)
11. Involuntary loss of urine caused by an overdistended bladder often related to bladder outlet obstruction or poor bladder emptying because of weak contractions
12. Leakage of small volumes of urine usually related to urethral hypermobility of incompetent sphincter
13. Involuntary passage of urine associated with a strong sense of urgency usually related to neurological or infectious processes
14. Involuntary loss usually at predictable intervals with specific bladder volumes
15. Hospital-acquired UTIs result from catheterization; *Escherichia coli* is the most common pathogen.
16. Created from a distal portion of the ileum and proximal portion of the colon; a catheter needs to be inserted through the stoma to empty the urine 4 to 6 times a day.

17. Ileal pouch to replace the bladder; able to void using a Valsalva technique
18. Permanent diversion created by transplanting the ureters into closed-off position of the ileum and then creating a stoma with continuous flow of urine collected in a pouch
19. Small tubes into the renal pelvis to relieve obstruction
20. An immediate and strong desire to void that is not easily deferred
21. Pain or discomfort associated with voiding
22. Voiding more than eight times during waking hours
23. Delay in start of urinary stream when voiding
24. Voiding excessive amounts
25. Diminished urinary output in relation to fluid intake
26. Awakened from sleep because of the urge to void
27. Leakage of small amounts of urine despite voluntary control of micturition
28. Presence of blood in urine
29. Unable to void when bladder is adequately full or overfull
30. a. Self-care ability
    b. Cultural considerations
    c. Health literacy
31. Pale, straw-colored to amber-colored depending on its concentration
32. Appears transparent at voiding; becomes more cloudy on standing in a container
33. Has a characteristic ammonia odor; the more concentrated the urine, the stronger the odor
34. a. Random: Collect during normal voiding from an indwelling catheter or urinary diversion collection bag. Use a clean specimen cup.
    b. Clean-voided or midstream: Use a sterile specimen cup. For girls and women: After donning sterile gloves, spread the labia with thumb and forefinger of the nondominant hand. Cleanse the area with a cotton ball or gauze, moving from front (above urethral orifice) to back (toward anus). Using a fresh swab each time, repeat the front-to-back motion three times (begin with the center, then left side, then right side). If agency policy indicates, rinse the area with sterile water and dry with dry cotton ball or gauze. While continuing to hold the labia apart, have the patient initiate the urine stream. After the patient achieves a stream, pass the container into the stream and collect 30 to 60 mL. Remove the specimen container before the flow of urine stops and before releasing the labia. The patient finishes voiding in a bedpan or toilet. For boys and men: After donning sterile gloves, hold the penis with one hand, and using circular motion and antiseptic swab, cleanse the end of the penis, moving from the center to the outside. In uncircumcised men, retract the foreskin before cleansing. If agency procedure indicates, rinse the area with sterile water and dry with cotton or gauze. After the patient has initiated the urine stream, pass the specimen collec-

tion container into the stream and collect 30 to 60 mL. Remove the specimen container before the flow of urine stops and before releasing the penis. The patient finishes voiding in a bedpan or toilet.
    c. Sterile: If the patient has an indwelling catheter, collect a sterile specimen by using aseptic technique through the special sampling port (Fig. 46-12) found on the side of the catheter. Clamp the tubing below the port, allowing fresh, uncontaminated urine to collect in the tube. After the nurse wipes the port with an antimicrobial swab, insert a sterile syringe hub and withdraw at least 3 to 5 mL of urine (check agency policy). Using sterile aseptic technique, transfer the urine to a sterile container.
    d. Timed urine: Time required may be 2-, 12-, or 24-hour collections. The timed period begins after the patient urinates and ends with a final voiding at the end of the time period. The patient voids into a clean receptacle, and the urine is transferred to the special collection container, which often contains special preservatives. Each specimen must be free of feces and toilet tissue. Missed specimens make the whole collection inaccurate. Check with agency policy and the laboratory for specific instructions.
35. A urinalysis will analyze values of pH (4.6 to 8.0), protein (none or ≤ 8 mg/100 mL), glucose (none), ketones (none), specific gravity (1.0053 to 1.030), and microscopic values for RBCs (up to 2), WBCs (0 to 4 per low-power field), bacteria (none), casts (none), and crystals (none).
36. Specific gravity measures concentration particles in the urine. High specific gravity in the urine reflects concentrated and low reflects diluted urine.
37. A urine culture is performed on a sterile or clean voided sample of urine and can report bacterial growth in 24 to 48 hours.
38. a. Abdominal radiography: Determines the size, shape, symmetry, and location of the kidneys.
    b. IVP: Views the collecting ducts and renal pelvis and outlines the ureters, bladder, and urethra. A special intravenous injection (iodine based) that converts to a dye in urine is injected intravenously.
    c. Direct visualization, specimen collection, and treatment
    d. CT scan: Obtains detailed images of structures within a selected plane of the body. The computer reconstructs cross-sectional images and thus allows the health care provider to view pathologic conditions such as tumors and obstructions.
    e. Ultrasonography: Renal ultrasonography identifies gross renal structures and structural abnormalities in the kidney using high-frequency, inaudible sound waves. Bladder ultrasonography identifies structural abnormalities of bladder or lower urinary tract. It can also be used to estimate the volume of urine in the bladder.

367

Answer Key

39. a. Urinary Incontinence (Functional, Reflex, Stress, Urge)
   b. Infection
   c. Impaired Self-Toileting
   d. Impaired Skin Integrity
   e. Urinary Retention
40. a. Normal elimination
   b. Patient will be able to independently use the toilet
   c. Decrease the number of pads by one to two within 8 weeks
41. a. Maintain adequate fluid intake
   b. Keep good voiding habits
   c. Keep the bowels regular
   d. Prevent urinary tract infection
   e. Stop smoking
   f. Report to your health care provider any changes in bladder habits
42. a. Intermittent: Used to measure post void residual (PVR) when a bladder scanner is not available or as a way to manage chronic urinary retention
   b. Short- or long-term indwelling: Used for accurate monitoring of urinary output, perioperative or postoperative after urologic or GYN procedures, and when the bladder inadequately empties due to obstruction or neurological condition
43. The nurse should perform personal hygiene at least three times a day for a patient with an indwelling catheter with soap and water.
44. Catheter care requires special care three times a day and after defecation.
45. Fluid intake should be 2000 to 2500 mL if permitted.
46. To maintain the patency of indwelling catheters, it may be necessary to irrigate or flush with sterile normal saline (NS). Blood, pus, or sediment can collect within the tubing, resulting in the need to change the catheter.
47. For a suprapubic catheter, a catheter is surgically placed through the abdominal wall above the symphysis pubis and into the urinary bladder.
48. An external catheter is suitable for incontinent or comatose men who still have complete and spontaneous bladder emptying.
49. Improve the strength of pelvic muscles and consist of repetitive contractions of muscle groups. They are effective in treating stress incontinence, overactive bladders, and mixed causes of urinary incontinence.

50. Bladder retraining is used to reduce the voiding frequency and to increase the bladder capacity, specifically for patients with urge incontinence related to overactive bladder.
51. Benefits patients with functional incontinence by improving voluntary control over urination
52. A nurse would evaluate for change in the patient's voiding pattern and continued presence of urinary tract alterations.
53. Identify if the patient is at risk for a latex allergy. Identify if patient has an allergy to povidone-iodine (Betadine). Follow asepsis techniques when performing catheter insertion.
54. 2. Involuntary leakage of urine during increased abdominal pressure in the absence of bladder muscle contraction
55. 1. Pain or burning (dysuria), 5. fever, chills, 6. nausea or vomiting, and 7. malaise
56. 3. Symptoms of an allergic response
57. 4. Antibiotics help the situation; the other choices are interventions to teach the patient to prevent UTIs.
58. a. Gather nursing history of the urination pattern, symptoms, and factors affecting urination. Conduct a physical assessment of body systems potentially affected by urinary change. Assess the characteristics of urine. Assess perceptions of urinary problems as they affect self-concept and sexuality.
   b. Physiology of fluid balance; anatomy and physiology of normal urine production and urination; pathophysiology of selected urinary alterations; factors affecting urination; principles of communication used to address issues related to self-concept and sexuality
   c. Caring for patients with alterations in urinary elimination; caring for patients at risk for UTI; personal experience with changes in urinary elimination
   d. Maintain privacy and dignity. Apply intellectual standards to ensure history and assessment are complete and in depth. Apply professional standards of care from professional organizations such as ANA and AHCPR.
   e. Display humility in recognizing limitations in knowledge.

59.

Laboratory Results	Parameter	Result	Reference Range
	Color	Yellow	Clear or yellow
	Clarity	Cloudy	Clear
	Specific gravity	1.020	1.005 – 1.030
	pH	7.0	4.5 – 8.0
	Protein	120 mg/dL	Negative
	Glucose	Negative	Negative
	Ketone	Negative	Negative
	Bilirubin	Negative	Negative
	Blood	Negative	Negative
	Urobilinogen	< 2 mg/dL	0 – 2 mg/dL
	White blood cells (microscope)	6 – 10 HPF	0 – 5 HPF
	Red blood cells (microscope)	0 – 5 HPF	0 – 5 HPF
	Bacteria	Present	Absent

Urinalysis findings consistent with a urinary tract infection include variation in clarity, as well as the presence of white blood cells and bacteria. Thick and/or cloudy appearance can indicate the present of infection and/or white blood cells. White blood cells in the urine indicate infection (or inflammation). Bacteria in the urine indicates infection (or colonization, in the absence of other clinical findings).

Although the patient also has protein in the urine, this is not indicative of infection. Protein is an indicator of kidney function; this finding could indicate glomerular membrane damage.

All other findings within this urinalysis are within normal and expected parameters, and do not indicate presence of a urinary tract infection.

CHAPTER 47

1. The teeth masticate food, breaking it down to swallow, and saliva is produced to dilute and soften the food for easier swallowing.
2. The bolus of food travels down and is pushed along by peristalsis, which propels the food through the length of the GI tract.
3. The stomach stores swallowed food and liquid; mixing of food, liquid, and digestive juices and empties its contents into the small intestine; produces HCl, mucus, pepsin, and intrinsic factor, which is essential for the absorption of vitamin B12.
4. Segmentation and peristaltic movement facilitate both digestion and absorption; chyme mixes with digestive juices.
5. The lower GI tract (colon) is divided into the cecum, colon, and rectum. It is the primary organ of elimination.
6. Contraction and relaxation of the internal and external sphincters, innervated by sympathetic and parasympathetic stimuli, aid in control of defecation.
7. a. Normal GI tract function
   b. Sensory awareness of rectal distention and rectal contents
   c. Voluntary sphincter control
   d. Adequate rectal capacity and compliance
8. a. Age
   b. Diet – fiber provides bulk in fecal material; good sources include whole grains, fresh fruits, and vegetables.
   c. Fluid intake – recommended 2.7 L/day; fluid liquefies the intestinal contents, easing its passage through the colon; reduced fluid intake slows the passage of food through the intestine and results in hardening of stool contents.
   d. Physical activity – promote peristalsis, immobilization depresses it; weakened abdominal and pelvic floor muscles impair the ability to increase intraabdominal pressure and to control the external sphincter.
   e. Psychological factors – during emotional stress the digestive process is accelerated, and peristalsis is increased; stress is associated with ulcerative colitis, irritable bowel syndrome, certain gastric and duodenal ulcers, and Crohn disease.
   f. Personal habits – work habits and best time for elimination
   g. Position during defecation – squatting is the normal position
   h. Pain – hemorrhoids, rectal surgery, anal fissures
   i. Pregnancy – temporary obstruction created by fetus impairs passage of feces

j. Surgery and anesthesia – action of the anesthetic slows or stops peristaltic waves; direct manipulation of the bowel temporarily stops peristalsis (paralytic ileus).

k. Medications – slow peristalsis and contractions (constipation)

l. Diagnostic tests – increased gas or loose stool

9. a. Hemorrhoids
   b. Rectal surgery
   c. Rectal fistulas
   d. Abdominal surgery

10. a. Improper diet
    b. Reduced fluid intake
    c. Lack of exercise
    d. Certain medications

11. a. Infrequent bowel movements <3 per week
    b. Hard, dry stools that are difficult to pass

12. Fecal impaction occurs when a collection of hardened feces that a person cannot expel (as a result of unrelieved constipation) becomes wedged in the rectum.

13. a. Oozing of diarrhea
    b. Loss of appetite (anorexia)
    c. Nausea or vomiting
    d. Abdominal distention and cramping
    e. Rectal pain

14. Diarrhea is an increased number of stools and the passage of liquid, unformed feces associated with disorders affecting digestion, absorption, and secretion.

15. a. Contamination and risk of skin ulceration
    b. Fluid and electrolyte or acid–base imbalances

16. *C. difficile* is a causative agent of mild diarrhea to severe colitis acquired by the use of antibiotics, chemotherapy, invasive bowel procedures, or a health care worker's hands or direct contact with environmental surfaces.

17. a. Fecal incontinence is the inability to control passage of feces and gas from the anus caused by physical conditions that impair anal sphincter function or control.
    b. Flatulence is a gas accumulation in the lumen of the intestine; stretches and distends (a common cause of abdominal fullness, pain, and cramping).

18. Dilated, engorged veins in the lining of the rectum; either internal or external

19. A stoma is an artificial opening in the abdominal wall.

20. An ileostomy is a surgical opening in the ileum.

21. A colostomy is a surgical opening in the colon.

22. a. Determination of the usual elimination pattern
    b. Patient's description of usual stool characteristics
    c. Identification of routines followed to promote normal elimination
    d. Presence and status of bowel diversions
    e. Changes in appetite
    f. Diet history
    g. Description of daily fluid intake
    h. History of surgery or illness affecting the GI tract

i. Medication history
j. Emotional state
k. History of exercise
l. History of pain or discomfort
m. Social history
n. Mobility and dexterity

23. Inspect all four quadrants for contour, shape, symmetry, and skin color. Note masses, peristaltic waves, scars, venous patterns, stomas, and lesions.

24. Assess bowel sounds in all four quadrants

25. Palpate for masses or areas of tenderness

26. Use percussion to detect lesions, fluid, or gas

27. Fecal occult blood testing, measures microscopic amounts of blood in feces; useful as a screening tool for colon cancer

28. a. Endoscopy
    b. Anorectal manometry
    c. Plain film of abdomen/kidneys, ureter, and bladder (KUB)
    d. Barium enema
    e. Ultrasonography
    f. Computed tomography
    g. Colonic transit study
    h. Magnetic resonance imaging

29. a. Bowel Incontinence
    b. Constipation
    c. fecal impaction
    d. impaired defecation
    e. Lack of Knowledge of Dietary Regime

30. a. Patient establishes a regular defecation schedule.
    b. Patient is able to list proper fluid and food intake needed to achieve elimination.
    c. Patient implements a regular exercise program.
    d. Patient reports daily passage of soft, formed brown stool.
    e. Patient does not report any discomfort associated with defecation.

31. a. Establishes a regular defecation schedule
    b. Lists proper fluid and food intake needed to soften stool and promote regular bowel elimination
    c. Implements a regular exercise program
    d. Reports daily passage of soft, formed brown stool
    e. Does not report straining or discomfort associated with defecation

32. Cathartics and laxatives (bulk forming, emollient or wetting, saline, stimulant, lubricant) have the short-term action of emptying the bowel.

33. Antidiarrheal opiate agents decrease intestinal muscle tone to slow passage of feces.

34. Enemas provide temporary relief of constipation, emptying the bowel before diagnostic tests, and bowel training.

35. Cleansing enemas include tap water, normal saline, soapsuds solution, and low-volume hypertonic saline. Cleansing enemas promote the complete evacuation of feces from the colon.

36. A tap water enema is hypotonic and exerts a lower osmotic pressure than fluid in interstitial spaces.

37. Normal saline enema is the safest enema solution; it exerts the same osmotic pressure as fluids in interstitial spaces surrounding the bowel.

38. Hypertonic solutions exert osmotic pressure that pulls out of interstitial spaces; they are contraindicated in patients who are dehydrated and in young infants.

39. Soapsuds create the effect of interstitial irritation to stimulate peristalsis.

40. Oil retention enemas lubricate the rectum and the colon and make the feces softer and easier to pass.

41. A carminative enema provides relief from gaseous distention; it improves the ability to pass flatus.

42. a. Can cause irritation to the mucosa
    b. Can cause bleeding
    c. Can cause stimulation of the vagus nerve, which results in a reflex slowing of the heart rate

43. a. Decompression – removal of secretions and gaseous substances from GI tract
    b. Enteral feeding – nutritional supplements for patients with impaired swallowing
    c. Compression – internal application of pressure by inflated balloon to prevent GI hemorrhage
    d. Lavage – irrigation of the stomach

44. The nurse should assess the condition of the nares and mucosa for inflammation and excoriation, frequent changing of the tape and lubrication of the nares, and frequent mouth care.

45. a. Assessing the normal elimination pattern and recording times when the patient is incontinent
    b. Incorporating principles of gerontologic nursing when providing bowel training programs for older-adults
    c. Choosing a time in the patient's pattern to initiate defecation-control measures
    d. Offering a hot drink or fruit juice before the defecation time
    e. Assisting the patient to the toilet at the designated time
    f. Providing privacy
    g. Instructing the patient to lean forward at the hips when on the toilet, apply manual pressure with the hands over the abdomen, and bear down but not strain to stimulate colon emptying
    h. Unhurried environment and a nonjudgmental caregiver
    i. Maintaining normal exercise within the patient's physical ability

46. Patient is able to have regular, pain-free defecation of soft, formed stool.

47. a,c,e

48. 4. Reabsorption in the small intestine is very efficient.

49. 1. See Box 47.5.

50. 1. An infant's stool is yellow, and an adult's stool is brown.

51. 2. In a supine position, it is impossible to contract the muscles used during defecation; raising the HOB assists the patient to a more normal sitting position, enhancing the ability to defecate.

52. 3. Correct volume for a school-aged child

53. a. Javier needs to select nursing interventions to promote normal bowel elimination. Consult with nutritionists and enteral stoma therapists. Involve Mr. Johnson and his family in designing nursing interventions.
    b. Role of the other health care professionals in returning the patient's bowel elimination pattern to normal; impact of specific therapeutic diets and medication on bowel elimination patterns; expected results of cathartics, laxatives, and enemas on bowel elimination
    c. Previous patient response to planned nursing therapies for improving bowel elimination (what worked and what did not)
    d. Individualize therapies to Mr. Johnson's bowel elimination needs. Select therapies consistent within wound and ostomy professional practice standards.
    e. Javier needs to be creative when planning interventions for Mr. Johnson to achieve normal elimination patterns. Display independence when integrating interventions from other disciplines in Mr. Johnson's plan of care. Act responsibly by ensuring that interventions are consistent within standards.

54. The patient is at risk for developing <u>ileus</u>, <u>constipation</u>, and <u>decreased peristalsis</u>.

Patients who have had surgery involving the abdominal cavity and direct manipulation of the bowel are at risk for developing an ileus. This condition, in which peristalsis is temporarily stopped, usually lasts 24-48 hours. Opioid medication also slows peristalsis and contractions, often culminating in constipation. The patient is not at risk for developing diarrhea, due to use of opioid medication. The patient is not at risk for fecal incontinence, as stool is not passing loosely during the postsurgical period and while using opioids. There is no evidence to indicate the patient is at any risk of developing *C. difficile*.

CHAPTER 48

1. e
2. f
3. a
4. b
5. d
6. c
7. a. Pressure intensity
   b. Pressure duration
   c. Tissue tolerance
8. a. Impaired sensory perception – unable to feel when a part of their body undergoes increased, prolonged pressure or pain
   b. Impaired mobility – unable to change their positions independently
   c. Alteration in level of consciousness – unable to protect themselves

d. Shear – occurs when the head of the bed is elevated and the sliding of the skeleton starts but the skin is fixed because of friction with the bed

e. Friction – skin is dragged across a coarse surface affecting the epidermis layer

f. Moisture – reduces the resistance of the skin to other physical factors (pressure, friction, or shearing)

9. I. Intact skin with nonblanchable redness of a localized area over a bony prominence

II. Partial-thickness skin loss involving epidermis, dermis, or both

III. Full-thickness with tissue loss

IV. Full-thickness tissue loss with exposed bone, tendon, or muscle

10. Intact or nonintact skin with localized area of persistent nonblanchable deep red, maroon, purple discoloration or epidermal separation revealing a dark wound bed or blood-filled blister. This injury results from intense and/or prolonged pressure and shear forces at the bone–muscle interface.

11. Red, moist tissue composed of new blood vessels, which indicates wound healing

12. Stringy substance attached to wound bed that is soft, yellow, or white tissue

13. Black or brown necrotic tissue

14. Describes the amount, color, consistency, and odor of wound drainage; excessive drainage indicates an infection

15. Wound that is closed by epithelialization with minimal scar formation as long as infection and secondary breakdown are prevented

16. Wound is left open until it becomes filled by scar tissue; chance of infection is greater; healing takes longer.

17. a. Inflammatory response – causing redness and swelling to the area with moderate amount of serous exudate

b. Epithelial proliferation (reproduction) – cells begin to regenerate, providing new cells to replace the lost cells

c. Migration with reestablishment of the epidermal layers

18. a. Injured blood vessels constrict, and platelets gather to stop bleeding; clots form a fibrin matrix for cellular repair.

b. Damaged tissues and mast cells secrete histamine (vasodilates) with exudation of serum and WBC into damaged tissues.

c. With the appearance of new blood vessels as reconstruction progresses, the proliferative phase begins and lasts from 3 to 24 days. The main activities during this phase are the filling of the wound with granulation tissue, contraction of the wound, and resurfacing of the wound by epithelialization.

d. Maturation, the final stage, may take up to 1 year; the collagen scar continues to reorganize and gain strength for several months.

19. a. Bleeding from a wound site that occurs after hemostasis indicates a slipped surgical suture, a dislodged clot, infection, or erosion of a blood vessel by a foreign object (internal or external).

b. Localized collection of blood underneath the tissue

c. Second most common health care–associated infection; purulent material drains from the wound (yellow, green, or brown, depending on the organism)

d. A partial or total separation of wound layers; risks are poor nutritional status, infection, or obesity

e. Total separation of wound layers with protrusion of visceral organs through a wound opening requiring surgical repair

20. a. Sensory perception – ability to respond appropriately to pressure-related discomfort

b. Moisture – degree to which the skin is exposed to moisture

c. Activity – degree of physical activity

d. Mobility – ability to change and control body position

e. Nutrition – usual food intake pattern

f. Friction or shear

21. a. Nutrition – deficiencies in any of the nutrients result in impaired or delayed healing

b. Tissue perfusion – the ability to perfuse the tissues with adequate amounts of oxygenated blood is critical to wound healing

c. Infection – prolongs the inflammatory phase, delays collagen synthesis, prevents epithelialization, and increases the production of proinflammatory cytokines

d. Age – increased age causes a decrease in the functioning of the macrophages, which leads to a delayed inflammatory response, delayed collagen synthesis, and slower epithelialization

e. Psychosocial impact of wounds – stress on a patient's adaptive mechanisms

22. a. Potential effects of impaired mobility; muscle tone and strength

b. Malnutrition is a major risk factor; a loss of 5% of usual weight, weight less than 90% of ideal body weight, or a decrease of 10 lb in a brief period.

c. Continuous exposure of the skin to body fluids, especially gastric and pancreatic drainage, increases the risk for breakdown.

d. Adequate pain control and patient comfort will increase mobility, which in turn reduces risk.

23. a. Is superficial with little bleeding and is considered a partial-thickness wound

b. Sometimes bleeds more profusely depending on depth and location (> 5 cm or 2.5 cm in depth)

c. Bleeds in relation to the depth and size, with a high risk of internal bleeding and infection

24. Whether the wound edges are closed, the condition of tissue at the wound base; look for complications and skin coloration

25. Amount, color, odor, and consistency of drainage, which depend on the location and the extent of the wound
26. See Table 48.3.
27. Observe the security of the drain and its location with respect to the wound and the character of the drainage; measure the amount
28. Surgical wounds are closed with staples, sutures, or wound closures. Look for irritation around staple or suture sites and note whether the closures are intact.
29. Lightly press the wound edges, detecting localized areas of tenderness or drainage collection
30. a. Risk for Infection
    b. Acute or Chronic Pain
    c. Impaired Mobility
    d. Impaired Peripheral Tissue Perfusion
31. a. Increase in the percentage of granulation tissue in the wound base
    b. no wound erythema or renderness to palpation
    c. No further skin breakdown
    d. An increase in the caloric intake by 10%
32. a. Skin care and management of incontinence
    b. Mechanical loading and support devices
    c. Education
33. a. Prevent and manage infection
    b. Cleanse the wound
    c. Remove nonviable tissue
    d. Maintain the wound in moist environment
    e. Eliminate dead space
    f. Control odor
    g. Eliminate or minimize pain
    h. Protect the wound
34. Remove nonviable necrotic tissue to rid the ulcer of a source of infection, enable visualization of the wound bed, and provide a clean base necessary for healing
35. a. Mechanical
    b. Autolytic – removal of dead tissue via lysis of necrotic tissue by the WBCs and natural enzymes of the body
    c. Chemical – topical enzyme preparation (Dakin's solution or sterile maggots)
    d. Sharp or surgical
36. Control bleeding by applying direct pressure in the wound site with a sterile or clean dressing, usually after trauma, for 24 to 48 hours
37. Appropriate cleaning solution and using a mechanical means of delivering the solution without causing injury to healing wound tissue. Normal saline is the preferred solution.
38. Applying sterile or clean dressings and immobilizing the body part
39. a. Protects a wound from microorganism contamination
    b. Aids in hemostasis
    c. Promotes healing by absorbing drainage and debriding a wound
    d. Supports or splints the wound site

e. Promotes thermal insulation of the wound surface
f. Provides a moist environment
40. See Box 48.8.
41. a. Promotes a moist environment
    b. Ideal for small wounds
    c. Serves as a barrier to external fluids and bacteria
    d. Adheres to undamaged skin, does not need a secondary dressing
    e. Permits viewing
42. a. Absorbs drainage through the use of exudate absorbers
    b. Maintains wound moisture
    c. Slowly liquefies necrotic debris
    d. Impermeable to bacteria
    e. Self-adhesive and occlusive
    f. Acts as a preventive dressing for high-risk friction areas
    g. May be left in place for 3 to 5 days, minimizing skin trauma and disruption of healing
43. a. Soothing and reduces pain
    b. Provides a moist environment
    c. Debrides the wound
    d. Does not adhere to the wound base and is easy to remove
44. a. Know the type of dressing, the presence of underlying drains or tubing and type of supplies needed
    b. Use of medical aseptic technique
    c. Teach the patient how to change dressings in preparation for home care
45. Assess the size, depth, and shape of the wound; dressing (moist) needs to be flexible and in contact with all of the wound surface; do not pack tightly (overpacking causes pressure); do not overlap the wound edges (maceration of the tissue).
46. Applies localized negative pressure to draw the edges of a wound together by evacuating wound fluids and stimulating granulation tissue formation, reduces the bacterial burden of a wound, and maintains a moist environment
47. a. Cleanse in a direction from the least contaminated area to the surrounding skin
    b. Use gentle friction when applying solutions locally to the skin
    c. When irrigating, allow the solution to flow from the least to the most contaminated area
48. Use of an irrigating syringe to flush the area with a constant low-pressure flow of solution of exudates and debris. Never occlude a wound opening with a syringe.
49. Portable units that connect tubular drains lying within a wound bed and exert a safe, constant low-pressure vacuum to remove and collect drainage
50. a. Creating pressure over a body part
    b. Immobilizing a body part
    c. Supporting a wound
    d. Reducing or preventing edema
    e. Securing a splint
    f. Securing dressings

373

51. a. Inspecting the skin for abrasions, edema, discoloration, or exposed wound edges
    b. Covering exposed wounds or open abrasions with a sterile dressing
    c. Assessing the condition of underlying dressings and changing if soiled
    d. Assessing the skin for underlying areas that will be distal to the bandage for signs of circulatory impairment
52. a. Improves blood flow to an injured part; if applied for more than 1 hour, the body reduces blood flow by reflex vasoconstriction to control heat loss from the area
    b. Diminishes swelling and pain, prolonged results in reflex vasodilation
53. a. A person is better able to tolerate short exposure to temperature extremes.
    b. More sensitive to temperature variations: neck, inner aspect of the wrist and forearm, and perineal region
    c. The body responds best to minor temperature adjustments.
    d. A person has less tolerance to temperature changes to which a large area of the body is exposed.
    e. Tolerance to temperature variations changes with age.
    f. Physical conditions that reduce the reception or perception of sensory stimuli
    g. Uneven temperature distribution suggests that the equipment is functioning improperly.
54. Improve circulation, relieve edema, and promote consolidation of pus and drainage
55. Promotes circulation, lessens edema, increases muscle relaxation, and provides a means to debride wounds and apply medicated solutions
56. The pelvic area is immersed in warm fluid, causing wide vasodilation.
57. Disposable hot packs that apply warm, dry heat to an area
58. Relieves inflammation and swelling
59. Immersing a body part for 20 minutes
60. Used for muscle sprain, localized hemorrhage, or hematoma
61. a. Was the etiology of the skin impairment addressed?
    b. Was wound healing supported by providing the wound base with a moist, protected environment?
    c. Were issues such as nutrition assessed and a plan of care developed?
62. Frequent perineal and sacral skin assessments; use an incontinence cleanser, followed by application of a moisture-barrier ointment; offering frequent ambulation and help to the toilet
63. 3. The force exerted parallel to the skin resulting from both gravity pushing down on the body and resistance between the patient and the surface

64. 1. Age is not a subscale. Perception, moisture, activity, mobility, nutrition, friction, and shear are the subscales.
65. 3. The recommended protein intake for adults is 0.8 g/kg; a higher intake of up to 1.8 g/kg/day is necessary for healing.
66. 2. See Table 48.8 for choice and rationale for dressings for injury stages.
67. 4,3,2,5,1
68. a. Identify the risk for developing impaired skin integrity. Identify signs and symptoms associated with impaired skin integrity or poor wound healing. Examine Mrs. Stein's skin for actual impairment in skin integrity.
    b. Pathogenesis of pressure injuries; factors contributing to pressure injury formation or poor wound healing; factors contributing to wound healing; impact of underlying disease process on skin integrity; impact of medication on skin integrity and wound healing
    c. Caring for patients with impaired skin integrity or wounds; observation of normal wound healing
    d. Apply intellectual standards of accuracy, relevance, completeness, and precision when obtaining health history regarding skin integrity and wound management; knowledge of AHCPR standards for prevention of pressure injuries
    e. Use discipline to obtain complete and correct assessment data regarding Mrs. Stein's skin and wound integrity. Demonstrate responsibility for collecting appropriate specimens for diagnostic and laboratory tests related to wound management.
69. Mr. Montoya is a 70-year-old Hispanic male with a history of type II diabetes mellitus (DM). He has been admitted to the medical-surgical unit for stabilization of his blood sugar. Mr. Montoya has lived in the US for 40 years, and shares in a two-story house with his wife. His son, daughter, and son in law and their three children also live in the home. Mr. Montoya had a below the knee amputation (BKA) of the right leg 2 years ago, after he developed gangrene in his right foot. Mr. Montoya states for 3 weeks, he had frequent urination and blurry vision. In addition, he has lost 12 lbs in the last month. Since his surgery has been less physically active. He has seen a dietician, self-monitors his BS occasionally. He takes Glucophage 500 mg BID. He drinks 8 ounces of beer with dinner each evening and smokes ½ pack of cigarettes per day. His peripheral pulses are 2+ radial, left dorsalis pedis 1+. His left foot is cool, with capillary refill of 5 seconds. BP 158/98, HR 84 and respirations 20.

70.

Assessment Finding	Evisceration	Dehiscence	Both evisceration and dehiscence
Wound layers separated			X
Opening noted after light coughing		X	
Reports a sensation of "something giving way"			X
Portion of incision line minimally open		X	
Blood pressure 70/30 mm Hg	X		
Visceral organs visible	X		
Partial opening in surgical wound		X	
Pulse 150 beats per minute	X		

Patients who have had surgery are at risk for dehiscence, the partial or total separation of wound layers, and evisceration, the total separation of wound layers with protrusion of visceral organs. Although these risks are minimal, either can happen and nurses must recognize critical assessment findings to intervene appropriately.

Both conditions are characterized by a separation in wound layers; the degree of separation, and presence or absence of visceral organ protrusion differentiates evisceration from dehiscence. Both conditions can cause the sensation of something "giving way" under a dressing.

Assessment findings associated with evisceration include signs of shock (e.g., low blood pressure like 70/30 mm Hg and rapid pulse such as 150 beats/minute), and visualization of visceral organs protruding through the wound opening.

Assessment findings associated with dehiscence include occurrence after coughing or straining to have a bowel movement, and a portion of the incision line partially open (often small in size).

CHAPTER 49

1. c
2. f
3. d
4. b
5. a
6. e
7. c
8. f
9. h
10. j
11. l
12. d
13. i
14. k
15. b
16. g
17. a
18. e

19. The patient receives multiple sensory stimuli and cannot perceptually disregard or selectively ignore some stimuli. Overload prevents meaningful response by the brain, the patient's thoughts race, attention scatters in many directions, and anxiety and restlessness occur.

20. a. Age – proprioceptive changes occur after the age of 60, including increased difficulty with balance, spatial orientation, and coordination
    b. Meaningful stimuli – reduce the incidence of sensory deprivation
    c. Amount of stimuli – excessive can cause overload
    d. Social interaction – absence of visitors influences the degree of isolate a patient feels
    e. Environmental factors – occupational
    f. Cultural factors – some sensory alterations occur more commonly in select cultural groups
21. Older-adults because of normal physiological changes involving sensory organs, individuals who live in confined environments, acutely ill patients
22. a. Has your family member shown any recent mood swings (outbursts of anger, nervousness, fear, or irritability)?
    b. Have you noticed the family member avoiding social activities?

23.

Sense	Assessment Technique	Child Behavior	Adult Behavior
Vision	Ask patient to read newspaper, magazine, or lettering on menu. Ask patient to identify colors on color chart or crayons. Observe patient performing ADLs.	Self-stimulation, including eye rubbing, body rocking, sniffing or smelling, arm twirling; hitching (using legs to propel while in sitting position) instead of crawling	Poor coordination, squinting, underreaching or overreaching for objects, persistent reposition- ing of objects, impaired night vision, accidental falls
Hearing	Assess patient's hearing acuity and history of tinnitus. Observe patient conversing with others. Inspect ear canal for hardened cerumen. Observe patient behaviors in a group.	Frightened when unfamiliar people approach, no reflex or purposeful response to sounds, failure to be awakened by loud noise, slow or absent development of speech, greater response to movement than to sound, avoidance of social interaction with other children	Blank looks, decreased attention span, lack of reaction to loud noises, increased volume of speech, positioning of head toward sound, smiling and nodding of head in approval when someone speaks, use of other means of communication such as lip-reading or writing, complaints of ringing in ears
Touch	Check patient's ability to discriminate between sharp and dull stimuli. Assess whether patient is able to distinguish objects (coin or safety pin) in the hand with eyes closed. Ask whether patient feels unusual sensations.	Inability to perform developmental tasks related to grasping objects or drawing, repeated injury from handling of harmful objects (e.g., hot stove, sharp knife)	Clumsiness, overreaction or underreaction to painful stimulus, failure to respond when touched, avoidance of touch, sensation of pins and needles, numbness Unable to identify object placed in hand
Smell	Have patient close eyes and identify several nonirritating odors (e.g., coffee, vanilla).	Difficult to assess until child is 6 or 7 years old, difficulty discriminating noxious odors	Failure to react to noxious or strong odor, increased body odor, increased sensitivity to odors
Taste	Ask patient to sample and distinguish different tastes (e.g., lemon, sugar, salt). (Have patient drink or sip water and wait 1 minute between each taste.)	Inability to tell whether food is salty or sweet, possible ingestion of strange-tasting things	Inability to tell whether food is salty or sweet, possible ingestion of strange-tasting things

24. a. Uneven, cracked walkways leading to front and back doors
    b. Extension and phone cords in main route of walking traffic
    c. Loose area rugs and runners over carpeting
    d. Bathrooms without shower or tub grab bars
    e. Unmarked water faucets designating hot or cold
    f. Unlit stairways, lack of handrails
    g. Poor lighting in stairways, halls, and entrance doors
25. a. Expressive aphasia, a motor type, is the inability to name common objects or to express simple ideas in words or writing.
    b. Receptive aphasia, a sensory type, is the inability to understand written or spoken language.
26. a. Antibiotics can be ototoxic and permanently damage the auditory nerve
    b. Opioids, sedatives, and antidepressants alter the perception of stimuli
27. a. Impaired Verbal Communication
    b. Risk for Injury
    c. Impaired Mobility
    d. Impaired Socialization
    e. Risk for Falls

28. a. Use communication techniques to send and receive messages
    b. Demonstrate technique for cleansing hearing aid within 1 week
    c. Self-report improved hearing acuity
29. a. Screening for rubella, syphilis, chlamydia, and gonorrhea in women who are considering pregnancy
    b. Advocate adequate prenatal care to prevent premature birth (danger of exposure of the infant to excessive oxygen)
    c. Administer eye prophylaxis in the form of erythromycin ointment approximately 1 hour after an infant's birth
    d. Periodic screening of children, especially newborns through preschoolers, for congenital blindness and visual impairment caused by refractive error and strabismus
30. Refractive error such as nearsightedness
31. a. Family history of childhood hearing impairment
    b. Prenatal infection (rubella, herpes, or CMV)
    c. Low-birth-weight
    d. Chronic ear infection
    e. Down syndrome

32.

Senses	Common Sensory Deficits	Interventions to Minimize Loss
Vision	Presbyopia: A gradual decline in the ability of the lens to accommodate or to focus on close objects. Individual is unable to see near objects clearly. Cataract: Cloudy or opaque areas in part of the lens or the entire lens that interfere with passage of light through the lens, causing problems with glare and blurred vision. Cataracts usually develop gradually without pain, redness, or tearing in the eye. Dry eyes: Result when tear glands produce too few tears, resulting in itching, burning, or even reduced vision. Glaucoma: A slowly progressive increase in intraocular pressure that causes progressive pressure against the optic nerve, resulting in peripheral visual loss, decreased visual acuity with difficulty adapting to darkness, and a halo effect around lights if left untreated. Diabetic retinopathy: Pathological changes occur in the blood vessels of the retina, resulting in decreased vision or vision loss caused by hemorrhage and macular edema.	Wearing sunglasses Use of yellow or amber lenses and shades or blinds on windows to minimize the glare Warm incandescent lighting Use glasses A pocket magnifier
	Macular degeneration: Condition in which the macula (specialized portion of the retina responsible for central vision) loses its ability to function efficiently. First signs include blurring of reading matter, distortion or loss of central vision, and distortion of vertical lines.	Larger print in books
Hearing	Presbycusis: A common progressive hearing disorder in older-adults.	Amplify the sound of telephones and TVs
	Cerumen accumulation: Buildup of earwax in the external auditory canal. Cerumen becomes hard, collects in the canal, and causes a conduction deafness.	Ensure that the problem is not cerumen
Taste and Smell	Xerostomia: Decrease in salivary production that leads to thicker mucus and a dry mouth. Often interferes with the ability to eat and leads to appetite and nutritional problems.	Good oral hygiene keeps the taste buds well hydrated. Well-seasoned, differently textured food eaten separately heightens taste perception. Flavored vinegar or lemon juice adds tartness to food. Always ask the patient what foods are most appealing. Improvement in taste perception improves food intake and appetite as well.
		Stimulation of the sense of smell with aromas such as brewed coffee, cooked garlic, and baked bread heightens taste sensation. The patient needs to avoid blending or mixing foods because these actions make it difficult to identify tastes. Older persons need to chew food thoroughly to allow more food to contact remaining taste buds.
		You improve smell by strengthening pleasant olfactory stimulation. Make the patient's environment more pleasant with smells such as cologne, mild room deodorizers, fragrant flowers, and sachets. The removal of unpleasant odors (e.g., bedpans, soiled dressings) will also improve the quality of a patient's environment.

Answer Key

Senses	Common Sensory Deficits	Interventions to Minimize Loss
Touch		Providing touch therapy stimulates existing function. If the patient is willing to be touched, hair brushing and combing, a back rub, and touching of the arms or shoulders are ways of increasing tactile contact. When sensation is reduced, firm pressure is often necessary for the patient to feel the nurse's hand. Turning and repositioning will also improve the quality of tactile sensation. When performing invasive procedures, it is important to use touch by holding the patient's hands and keeping them warm and dry.
		If a patient is overly sensitive to tactile stimuli (hyperesthesia), minimize irritating stimuli. Keeping bed linens loose to minimize direct contact with the patient and protecting the skin from exposure to irritants are helpful measures.

33. a. Listen to the patient and wait for the patient to communicate. Do not shout or speak loudly (hearing loss is not the problem). If the patient has problems with comprehension, use simple, short questions and facial gestures to give additional clues. Speak of things familiar and of interest to the patient. If the patient has problems speaking, ask questions that require simple yes or no answers or blinking of the eyes. Offer pictures or a communication board so the patient can point. Give the patient time to understand; be calm and patient; do not pressure or tire the patient. Avoid patronizing and childish phrases.

   b. Use pictures, objects, or word cards so that the patient can point. Offer a pad and pencil or Magic Slate for the patient to write messages. Do not shout or speak loudly. Give the patient time to write messages because these patients become easily fatigued. Provide an artificial voice box (vibrator) for the patient with a laryngectomy to use to speak.

   c. Get the patient's attention. Do not startle the patient when entering the room. Do not approach a patient from behind. Be sure the patient knows that you wish to speak. Face the patient and stand or sit on the same level. Be sure your face and lips are illuminated to promote lip-reading. Keep your hands away from your mouth. Be sure that patients keep eyeglasses clean so they are able to see your gestures and face. If the patient wears a hearing aid, make sure it is in place and working. Speak slowly and articulate clearly. Older-adults often take longer to process verbal messages. Use a normal tone of voice and inflections of speech. Do not speak with something in your mouth. When you are not understood, rephrase rather than repeat the conversation. Use visible expressions. Speak with your hands, your face, and your eyes. Do not shout. Loud sounds are usually higher pitched and often impede hearing by accentuating vowel sounds and concealing consonants. If you need to raise your voice, speak in lower tones. Talk toward the patient's best or normal ear. Use written information to enhance the spoken word. Do not restrict a deaf patient's hands. Never have IV lines in both of the patient's hands if the preferred method of communication is sign language. Avoid eating, chewing, or smoking while speaking. Avoid speaking from another room or while walking away.

34. a. Orientation to the environment: name tags are visible, address the patient by name, explain to the patient any transfers, note physical boundaries

   b. Communication: Depends on the type of aphasia (See Box 49-7)

   c. Control sensory stimuli: Prevent overload by organizing patient's care with periods of rest; control extraneous noise

   d. Safety measures: Help with ambulation, sighted guide, frequent repositioning

35. a. Spend time with a person in silence or conversation

   b. When culturally supportive, use physical contact (holding a hand, embracing a shoulder) to convey caring

   c. Help recommend alterations in living arrangements if physical isolation is a factor

   d. Assist older-adults in keeping in contact with people important to them

   e. Help obtain information about support groups

   f. Arrange for security escort services as needed

   g. Bring a pet that is easy to care for into the home

   h. Link a person with organizations attuned to the social needs of older-adults

36. The nature of a patient's alterations influences how the nurse would evaluate the outcome of care. If the expected outcomes have not been achieved, there needs to be a change in the interventions or an alteration in the patient's environment. The nurse also needs to evaluate the integrity of the sensory organs and the patient's ability to perceive stimuli.

37. Introduce yourself and use face-to-face communication. Ask the patient about how he or she would like to be assisted. Orient the patient to the room and keep pathways clear of obstacles.

38. 1. Caused by sensory deprivation related to restrictive environment of the hospital

39. 1,3,5,6

40. 3. Priorities need to be set in regard to the type and extent of the sensory alteration, and safety is always a top priority.

41. 4. Motor type of aphasia

42. 1,4,5

43. a. Understanding of how a sensory deficit can affect the patient's functional status; knowledge of therapies that promote or restore sensory function; the role of other health care professionals that might provide sensory function management; services of community resources; adult learning principles to apply when educating the patient and the family

b. Previous patient responses to planned nursing interventions to promote sensory function

c. Individualized therapies that allow the patient to adapt to sensory loss in any setting; standards of safety

d. Using creativity to find interventions that help the patient adapt to the home environment

e. Ms. Long will maintain independence in a safe home environment by selecting strategies to assist the patient in remaining functional at home, adapting therapies for any sensory deficit, involving the family in helping the patient; refer to appropriate health care professional agencies

44.

Sense	Potential Nursing Interventions
Sight (visual)	Remove all throw rugs in the living area Remind to use eyeglasses to overcome clouded vision Ensure adequate lighting in rooms and hallways Decrease clutter in the living environment
Hearing (auditory)	Face the patient when speaking Encourage regular use of hearing aids Write all directions for patient to read Assess for presence of cerumen in the ear canal
Taste (gustatory)	Ask which foods are favorites Increase seasonings in foods to enhance flavor Remove environmental distractors before meals Provide foods that are separated and not mixed together

Patients with sensory deficits can benefit from interventions that enhance the degree of sense present. To provide care to the patient with a visual deficit due to cataracts, the nurse will enhance safety by removing throw rugs (which may not be seen, causing the patient to slip and fall), ensure adequate lighting in rooms and hallways (so the patient can see objects to the best of their ability), and decrease clutter in the living environment (which can again cause the patient to fall if they do not see something).

To ensure communication when a patient is hard of hearing, the nurse will face the patient when speaking. Regular use of hearing aids can be helpful, so a reminder about using them consistently can provide the patient with more opportunities to hear noise and conversation around them. Assessing for the presence of cerumen in the ear canal is important, as this may be the cause of hearing difficulties. Cerumen can cause conductive hearing loss by blocking stimuli; when removed, hearing can increase.

A decrease in taste is common in older-adults, as taste buds are not as sensitive. The nurse can enhance appetite and enjoyment of eating by asking about the patient's favorite foods and then ensuring they are served. Seasoning of foods with spices, herbs, flavored vinegar, or lemon juice can add flavor to foods. Creating a pleasant environment in which to eat can also enhance appetite and taste; therefore the nurse will remove any environmental distractors (e.g., unpleasant sights or odors) prior to meals. Foods should be served without being blended or touching whenever possible, as these processes can make it difficult to identify tastes.

The nurse will not remind the patient with cataracts to use eyeglasses to overcome clouded vision, as the only treatment for cataracts is surgical removal. Writing directions for a patient to read may be helpful to a patient who only has a hearing deficit; however, this patient also has cataracts so reading the written directions will not be effective.

CHAPTER 50

1. a. Preoperative (before)
   b. Intraoperative (during)
   c. Postoperative (after surgery)
2. d
3. h
4. j
5. c
6. g
7. i
8. b
9. l
10. f
11. k
12. a
13. e
14. See Table 50.2.
15. a. Smoking/vaping: risk for pneumonia, atelectasis, and delayed wound healing
    b. Age: Very young and older-adult as a result of an immature or a declining physiological status
    c. Nutrition: tissue repair and resistance to infection. Poor tolerance to anesthesia, negative nitrogen balance.
    d. Obesity: Atelectasis, pneumonia, and death
    e. Obstructive sleep apnea: Oxygen desaturation
    f. Immunosuppression: Infection
    g. Fluid and electrolyte imbalance – stress response
    h. Postop nausea and vomiting – younger age, woman, volatile anesthetics, types of surgery
    i. postoperative urinary retention – specific to patient, procedure, and anesthesia
    j. Venous thromboembolism – preventable
16. See Table 50.3.
17. Identify a patient's normal preoperative function and the presence of any risks to recognize, prevent, and minimize possible postoperative complications
18. a. Patient's tolerance to a pressure injury insult (altered nutrition, deceased mobility, older age, decreased mental status, infection, incontinence, impaired sensory perception, and comorbidities)
    b. Variables that increase tissue susceptibility to sustain external pressure (temperature, friction and shearing forces, and moisture)
    c. Length of surgery, position on OR table, devices, anesthetic agents, length of time
19. See Table 50.4.
20. See Table 50.5.
21. a. Smoking places the patient at greater risk for pulmonary complication because of an increased amount and thickness of mucous secretions in the lungs.
    b. Alcohol and substance use predisposes the patient to adverse reactions to anesthetic agents and cross-tolerance to anesthetic agents; malnourishment also leads to delayed wound healing.
22. a. The patient and family's expectations for pain management after surgery
    b. The patient's perceived tolerance to pain

c. Exploring past experiences and prior successful interventions used
23. Have the patient identify personal strengths and weaknesses; poor self-concept hinders the ability to adapt to the stress of surgery and aggravates feelings of guilt or inadequacy.
24. Assess for body image alterations that patients perceive will result, taking into consideration culture, age, self-concept, and self-esteem; removal of body parts often leaves permanent disfigurement, alteration in body function, or concern over mutilation, loss of body function.
25. Discussion of feelings and self-concept reveals whether the patient is able to cope with the stress of surgery, past stress management and behaviors used, and coping resources.
26. a. General survey
    b. Head and neck
    c. Integument
    d. Thorax and lungs
    e. Heart and vascular system
    f. Abdomen
    g. Neurologic status
27. See Table 50.6.
28. a. Ineffective Airway Clearance
    b. Anxiety
    c. Impaired Skin Integrity
    d. Risk for Infection
    e. Acute Pain
29. a. remains free of pressure injury 24 hours after surgery
    b. Performs deep breathing and coughing exercises upon awakening from anesthesia
    c. Performs postoperative leg exercises and early ambulation 12 hours after surgery
    d. Performs incentive spirometry upon return to patient care after surgery
    e. Patient verbalizes rationale for early ambulation 24 hours postoperatively.
30. Informed consent for surgery (surgeon's responsibility) involves the patient's understanding of the need for a procedure, steps involved, risks, expected results, and alternative treatments.
31. a. Improves the ability and willingness to deep breathe and cough effectively
    b. Improves understanding and willingness to ambulate and resume activities of ADL
    c. Have less anxiety
    d. Reduces stay by preventing or minimizing complications
    e. Less anxious about pain; ask what they need and require less after surgery
32. a. Patient understands reasons for preoperative instructions and exercises.
    b. Preoperative routines
    c. Surgical procedure
    d. Time of surgery
    e. Postoperative unit and location of family during surgery and recovery
    f. Anticipated postoperative monitoring and therapies
    g. Sensory preparation

h. Postoperative activity resumption
i. Pain-relief measures
j. Rest
k. Feelings regarding surgery

33. a. Reduction of risk of surgical wound infection – skin asepsis, hair removal (limit)
   b. Maintain normal fluid and electrolyte balance – NPO 2 to 6 hours
   c. Prevention of bowel incontinence and contamination

34. a. Hygiene
   b. Preparation of hair and removal of cosmetics
   c. Removal of prostheses (artificial limbs, partial or complete dentures, artificial eyes, and hearing aids)
   d. Safeguarding valuables – remove all
   e. Preparing the bowel and bladder
   f. Vital signs
   g. Prevention of deep vein thrombosis (DVT) – antiembolism devices
   h. Administering preoperative medications – to reduce anxiety, the amount of anesthesia required, respiratory tract secretions and the risk of nausea, vomiting and possible aspiration
   i. Documentation and handoff
   j. Eliminating the wrong site and wrong procedure surgery – all relevant documents and results are available, mark the operative site, a "time out"

35. a. The circulating nurse (does not scrub) reviews the preoperative assessment, establishes and implements the intraoperative plan of care, evaluates the care, and provides for continuity of care postoperatively.
   b. The scrub nurse maintains a sterile field during the surgical procedure and assists with supplies.

36. a. Ineffective Airway Clearance
   b. Risk for Deep Vein Thrombosis
   c. Risk for Perioperative Positioning Injury
   d. Risk for Impaired Skin Integrity
   e. Risk for Latex Injury

37. General anesthesia is given by IV and inhalation routes through three phases (induction, maintenance, and emergence), resulting in an immobile, quiet patient who does not recall the surgical procedure.

38. Regional anesthesia results in loss of sensation in an area of the body via spinal, epidural, or a peripheral nerve block with no loss of consciousness.

39. Local anesthesia involves the loss of sensation at the desired site; common for minor procedures.

40. Conscious sedation is routinely used for procedures that do not require complete anesthesia but rather a depressed level of consciousness.

41. a. Immediate postoperative recovery (phase I) begins when the patient leaves the OR to the time he is stabilized in the recovery area, discharged or transferred.
   b. Progression to home (phase II)
   c. Convalescence (phase III) ongoing care

42. Responsibilities include maintaining the patient's airway, respiratory, circulatory, and neurologic status and managing pain.

43. The patient will show vital sign stability, temperature control, good ventilatory function and oxygenation status, orientation to surroundings, absence of complications, minimal pain and nausea, controlled wound drainage, adequate output, and fluid and electrolyte balance.

44. Every 15 minutes twice, every 30 minutes twice, and then hourly for 2 hours and then every 4 hours or per orders

45. a. snoring
   b. little or no air movement on auscultation
   c. retraction of intercostal muscles
   d. decreased oxygen saturation

46. Careful assessment of heart rate and rhythm, along with blood pressure, reveals the patient's cardiovascular status; capillary perfusion—note refill, pulses, and the color and temperature of the nail beds.

47. Hypercarbia, tachypnea, tachycardia, premature ventricular contractions (PVC), unstable blood pressure, cyanosis, skin mottling, and muscular rigidity

48. a. Assess the hydration status and monitor cardiac and neurological function
   b. Monitor and compare laboratory values
   c. Maintain patency of IV lines
   d. Record accurately the I & O, daily weights
   e. Assess daily weight for the first several days after surgery and compare with the preoperative weight

49. a. Orientation to self and the hospital
   b. Pupil and gag reflexes, hand grips, and movement of all extremities
   c. Neurologic assessment
   d. Extremity strength

50. a. A rash can indicate a drug sensitivity or allergy.
   b. Abrasions or petechiae result from inappropriate positioning or restraining that injures skin layers or from a clotting disorder.
   c. Burns may indicate that an electrical cautery grounding pad was incorrectly placed.

51. a. Accumulation of gas
   b. Development of a paralytic ileus

52. a. Impaired Airway Clearance
   b. Risk for Infection
   c. Impaired Mobility
   d. Impaired Skin Integrity
   e. Acute Pain

53. a. Frequency of VS monitoring and special assessments
   b. Types of IV fluids and rates of infusions
   c. Postoperative medications
   d. Resumption of preoperative medications
   e. Fluid and food allowed by mouth
   f. Level of activity
   g. Measures to prevent DVT
   h. Positions while in bed
   i. Intake and output and daily weights
   j. Laboratory tests and radiography studies
   k. Special directions related to drains, irrigations, and dressings

54. a. Patient's incision remains closed and intact by discharge

b. Patient's incision remains free of infectious drainage by discharge.

c. Patient remains afebrile.

55. a. Encourage diaphragmatic breathing exercises every hour

b. Administer CPAP or NIPPV to patients who use this modality at home

c. Instruct patients to use incentive spirometer for maximum inspiration

d. Encourage early ambulation

e. Turn the patient on his or her sides every 1 to 2 hours and have the patient sit when possible

f. Keep the patient comfortable

g. Encourage coughing exercises every 1 to 2 hours and maintain pain control

h. Provide oral hygiene

i. Initiate orotracheal or nasotracheal suction for inability to cough

j. Administer oxygen and monitor saturation

56. See Table 50.8.

57. a. Provide pain medications to ensure early ambulation

b. Encourage the patient to perform leg exercises at least every hour while awake

c. Apply graded compression stockings or pneumatic compression stockings

d. Encourage early ambulation

e. Before ambulation, assess vital signs at rest

f. Avoid positioning the patient in a manner that interrupts blood flow to the extremities

g. Administer anticoagulant drugs as ordered

h. Provide adequate fluid intake orally or IV

58. Incision area, drainage tubes, tight dressing or casts, muscular strains caused by positioning

59. a. Maintain a gradual progression in dietary intake

b. Promote ambulation and exercise

c. Maintain an adequate fluid intake

d. Promote adequate food intake by stimulating the patient's appetite (remove noxious odors)

e. Avoid moving a patient suddenly to minimize nausea

f. Comfortable position for mealtime

g. Frequent oral hygiene

h. Fiber supplements, stool softeners

i. Provide meals when patient is rested and free from pain

60. a. Assume their normal position

b. Check frequently for the need to void

c. Assess for bladder distention (void 8–12 hours after surgery)

d. Monitor I & O

61. a. Provide privacy with dressing changes or inspection of the wound

b. Maintain patient's hygiene

c. Prevent drainage devices from overflowing

d. Provide a pleasant environment

e. Offer opportunities for the patient to discuss fears or concerns

f. Provide the families with opportunities to discuss ways to promote self-concept

62. Delayed ambulation, reduced ventilation, retained pulmonary secretions, and reduced appetite

63. 1. Increases susceptibility to infection and impairs wound healing from altered glucose metabolism and associated circulatory impairment

64. 1. That is a medical decision and the responsibility of the provider.

65. 1,2,4. These patients are at risk for developing serious fluid and electrolyte imbalances.

66. 2,4. Promoting venous return and joint mobility.

67. 2. Not always a sign of hypothermia but rather a side effect of certain anesthetic agents

68. 2,3,5

69. a. Evaluate Mrs. Campana's knowledge of surgical procedure and planned postoperative care. Have Mrs. Campana demonstrate postoperative exercises. Observe behaviors or nonverbal expressions of anxiety or fear. Ask if patient's expectations are being met.

b. Behaviors that demonstrate learning; characteristics of anxiety or fear; signs and symptoms or conditions that contraindicate surgery

c. Previous patient responses to planned preoperative care; any personal experience with surgery

d. Use established expected outcomes to evaluate Mrs. Campana's plan of care (ability to perform postoperative exercises).

e. Demonstrate perseverance when Mrs. Campana has difficulty performing postoperative exercises

70. Temperature 104.2°F (40°C)

Heart rate 140 beats/minute

Respirations 28/minute

Ventricular fibrillation

Skin mottling

Malignant hyperthermia (MH) is a life-threatening complication associated with anesthesia. In this hypermetabolic state that occurs within skeletal muscle cells, in increase in intracellular calcium ion concentration occurs. The condition manifests with high carbon dioxide levels, metabolic and respiratory acidosis, increased oxygen consumption, heat production, sympathetic nervous system activation, high serum potassium levels, and multiple organ dysfunction and failure.

Early signs of MH include tachycardia (heart rate 140 beats/minute), tachypnea (respirations 28/minute), heart arrhythmias (ventricular fibrillation), hyperkalemia, hypercarbia, and muscular rigidity. The skin becomes mottled due to changes in oxygenation. Later signs include elevated temperature (104.2°F [40°C]), myoglobinuria, and multiple organ failure.

MH involves muscular rigidity (not muscular flaccidity), a high pulse rate (instead of a low pulse rate like 50 beats/minute), and increasing blood pressure (instead of hypotension).